# EXERCISE PSYCHOLOGY

WILEY SERIES ON
HEALTH PSYCHOLOGY/BEHAVIORAL MEDICINE

Thomas J. Boll, Series Editor

# Exercise Psychology: The Influence of Physical Exercise on Psychological Processes

Edited by

**Peter Seraganian**
Concordia University

**A Wiley-Interscience Publication**

**JOHN WILEY & SONS, INC.**

New York / Chichester / Brisbane / Toronto / Singapore

98010024
27|10|98

*Library of Congress Cataloging-in-Publication Data:*

Exercise psychology : the influence of physical exercise on
    psychological processes / edited by Peter Seraganian.
        p. ca.—(Wiley series on health psychology/behavioral
    medicine)
    Includes index.
    ISBN 0-471-52701-7 (cloth)
    1. Exercise—Psychological aspects. I. Seraganian, Peter, 1946–
    II. Series.
    [DNLM: 1. Exercise. 2. Physical Fitness—psychology. 3. Stress.
    Psychological—therapy. QT 255 E9558]
    QP301.E975    1993
    616.89'13—dc20
    DNLM/DLC
    for Library of Congress                                    92-5498

Coventry University

# Contributors

James A. Blumenthal, Ph.D., Associate Professor of Medical Psychology, Department of Psychiatry, Duke University Medical Center, Durham, North Carolina

Stephen H. Boutcher, Ph.D., Senior Lecturer, Department of Human Movement Science, University of Wollongong, New South Wales, Australia

Lawrence R. Brawley, Ph.D., Associate Professor, Department of Kinesiology, University of Waterloo, Waterloo, Ontario, Canada

Randal P. Claytor, Ph.D., Associate Professor, Department of Physical Education, Health, and Sport Studies, Miami University, Oxford, Ohio

Jennifer L. Etnier, Ph.D. Exercise & Sport Research Institute, Arizona State University, Tempe, Arizona

Roger B. Fillingim, Ph.D., Clinical Director, Treasure Coast Rehabilitation Hospital, Vero Beach, Florida

Karen R. Flood, M.A., Psychology Department, Lakehead University, Thunder Bay, Ontario, Canada

Lise Gauvin, Ph.D., Associate Professor, Department of Exercise Science, Concordia University, Montreal, Quebec, Canada

David S. Holmes, Ph.D., Professor, Department of Psychology, The University of Kansas, Lawrence, Kansas

Thelma S. Horn, Ph.D., Associate Professor, Department of Physical Education, Health, and Sport Studies, Miami University, Oxford, Ohio

John L. Jamieson, Ph.D., Professor, Psychology Department, Lakehead University, Thunder Bay, Ontario, Canada

Karla A. Kubitz, Ph.D., Department of Physical Education and Leisure Studies, Kansas State University, Manhattan, Kansas

Daniel M. Landers, Ph.D., Professor, Exercise & Sport Research Institute, Arizona State University, Tempe, Arizona

Bonita C. Long, Ph.D., Associate Professor, Department of Counselling Psychology, University of British Columbia, Vancouver, British Columbia, Canada

François Péronnet, Ph.D., Professor, Department of Physical Education, University of Montreal, Montreal, Quebec, Canada

Steven J. Petruzzello, Ph.D. Exercise & Sport Research Institute, Arizona State University, Tempe, Arizona

Thomas G. Plante, Ph.D., Clinical Instructor, Department of Psychiatry and Behavioral Sciences, Stanford University Medical School, Stanford, California

W. Jack Rejeski, Ph.D., Professor, Department of Health and Sport Science, Wake Forest University, Winston-Salem, North Carolina

Wendy M. Rodgers, Ph.D., Department of Kinesiology, University of Windsor, Windsor, Ontario, Canada

Walter Salazar, Ph.D. Exercise & Sport Research Institute, Arizona State University, Tempe, Arizona

Peter Seraganian, Ph.D., Associate Professor, Psychology Department, Concordia University, Montreal, Quebec, Canada

David Sinyor, Ph.D., Psychologist, Royal Victoria Hospital, Allan Memorial Institute, Montreal, Quebec, Canada

Attila Szabo, M.Sc., Department of Physical Education, University of Montreal, Montreal, Quebec, Canada

Amy Thompson, M.A., Department of Health and Sport Science, Wake Forest University, Winston-Salem, North Carolina

Kim M. Tuson, B.A., School of Psychology, University of Ottawa, Ottawa, Ontario, Canada

# Series Preface

This series is addressed to clinicians and scientists who are interested in human behavior relevant to the promotion and maintenance of health and the prevention and treatment of illness. *Health psychology* and *behavioral medicine* are terms that refer to both the scientific investigation and interdisciplinary integration of behavioral and biomedical knowledge and technology to prevention, diagnosis, treatment, and rehabilitation.

The major and purposely somewhat general areas of both health psychology and behavioral medicine that will receive greatest emphasis in this series are theoretical issues of biopsychosocial function, diagnosis, treatment, and maintenance; issues of organizational impact on human performance and an individual's impact on organizational functioning; development and implementation of technology for understanding, enhancing, or remediating human behavior and its impact on health and function; and clinical considerations with children and adults, alone, in groups, or in families that contribute to the scientific and practical/clinical knowledge of those charged with the care of patients.

The series encompasses considerations as intellectually broad as psychology and as numerous as the multitude of areas of evaluation, treatment, prevention, and maintenance that make up the field of medicine. It is the aim of the series to provide a vehicle that will focus attention on both the breadth and the interrelated nature of the sciences and practices making up health psychology and behavioral medicine.

THOMAS J. BOLL

*The University of Alabama at Birmingham*
*Birmingham, Alabama*

# Preface

The emergence of this multidisciplinary volume in the domain of exercise psychology can be linked to a number of academic, political, and historical factors. By providing some indication of these undercurrents, a clearer picture of the overall endeavor may emerge.

First, from an academic perspective, the book's orientation reflects what has been characterized as a "behavioral," as opposed to a "medical," model. Accordingly, greater emphasis is placed on overt behavior patterns rather than on more molecular substrates of behavior. These opposing models contrast with each other along a number of dimensions. From both preventive and rehabilitative perspectives, a behavioral model seeks to establish linkage between patterns of physical activity and psychological states. Thus, instead of focusing on drugs as an agent of change, emphasis shifts to the analysis of patterns of physical activity. Drugs may bring about more immediate changes but can yield longer-term detrimental consequences. The more gradual changes typically observed with behavioral interventions are less likely to elicit undesirable side effects.

With behavioral interventions, the individual often assumes increased responsibility for health maintenance. Regular participation in vigorous physical pursuits can place scheduling demands on the busy contemporary life-style, but this sustained personal commitment is part of the cost that is incurred when the individual assumes greater personal involvement for health promotion. A pharmacological outlook associated with the medical model gives much less emphasis to such individual responsibility and instead relies heavily on strict compliance with drug prescription to combat symptomatology.

Within the academic tradition, the research methodology employed by medical and behavioral researchers can differ. The vast majority of medical research falls within a reductionistic framework, in which one searches for simpler elements that are presumed to lie at the source of complex problems. Indeed, the focus on pharmacological interventions can be seen as a natural extension of the exploration of the chemical substrates of behavior. Although some behavioral research works within a reductionistic framework, a prominent and growing segment of behavioral researchers use a more holistic or gestalt outlook. With this more holistic approach, it is felt that one loses some of the richness of the phenomenon as a whole if one seeks endlessly to break down behavior into constituent elements. Rather, it is argued that the whole is greater than the sum of its parts. Thus, within the behavioral model, research paradigms can be more eclectic.

From a political perspective, a different set of forces seem to be at play. In both Canada and the United States, health-care costs have become major legislative concerns. Although Canada has enjoyed universal publicly funded health care for almost three decades, its spiraling expense has accelerated the search for preventive interventions that might decrease demands on the overtaxed health delivery system. Physical exercise, along with weight control, stress management, and smoking cessation, are viewed as major behavioral strategies that might contribute to health promotion and thereby reduce future demands on an overextended health-delivery system. In the United States, the absence of publicly funded health care has deprived a growing segment of the population of necessary health services. As the federal government is increasingly pressured to introduce universal health care, the means to pay for such services looms as a major deterrent. Programs such as the President's Council on Physical Fitness and Sports, which seek to enhance regular participation in physical activities, particularly in America's children, may serve as cost-containment strategies for future health-care programs. By encouraging greater individual responsibility for health maintenance, particularly in early formative stages, less subsequent utilization of costly rehabilitative services may result.

From a historical perspective, exercise psychology can be seen as a facet of one of the oldest issues in both psychology and physical education curriculums—namely, the mind–body problem. The aspect of this problem that comes to the fore in exercise psychology is exploration of the impact of vigorous physical activity on mental states. For Western culture, the roots of this issue can be traced back 24 centuries to the time known as the "Golden Age of Greece," as can so much of our political, philosophical, and educational heritage. During this period, in stark contrast to current practice, regular physical activity played a prominent role in many citizens' lives. A substantial portion of the daily schedule (for children, adults, and the elderly alike) was committed to vigorous physical activity. Such practice was promoted not just for its own sake but also for the contribution that exercise was felt to make toward mental well-being. This volume seeks to bring this historical position back into contemporary prominence.

Acknowledgments to several sources are in order, for their contribution to this volume. If, some 15 years ago, Sandra Keller had not kindled my interest in the experimental analysis of the influence of aerobic fitness on psychophysiological reactivity, I might still be conducting studies on discrimination learning in pigeons. Nancy K. Innis and R. W. J. Neufeld of the University of Western Ontario provided needed encouragement at early formative stages of this undertaking. Brad Hatfield cosponsored a conference at the University of Maryland in the spring of 1989, at which several of the contributors of the present volume first met to discuss their views. Over the past two years, Naomi Rappaport has taken on a variety of administrative responsibilities that have contributed immeasurably to keeping the project moving forward. Thomas G. Brown assisted in the adaptation of a software package that streamlined creation of the author index. Herb Reich, senior editor at John Wiley & Sons, has provided invaluable counsel, which helped to steer the project through some rough spots. Finally, Concordia University has willingly followed my shift in research focus, even though my current pursuits differ markedly from those for which I was originally hired.

Peter Seraganian

*September 1992*
*Montreal, Canada*

# Contents

## Part III:  Applications

PART **I**

# HISTORICAL AND CONCEPTUAL UNDERPINNINGS

# 1

# Historical and Conceptual Roots of Exercise Psychology

## W. JACK REJESKI AND AMY THOMPSON

## BACKGROUND

### Introduction

The purpose of this chapter is to provide an overview of the historical and conceptual roots of exercise psychology and the highly visible interface that has developed between exercise and health psychology. As the introductory chapter to the text, the information presented is based on two key beliefs shared by the editor and the authors. First, it is important that the reader appreciate the relationship of the research presented in this text to the field of study known as "exercise psychology." Such a perspective reveals limitations in our current knowledge base and provides direction for future study. Second, there are historical events, conceptual directions, and technological developments that either have served as or continue to constitute either barriers or facilitating forces in the development of exercise psychology and related fields of study. Awareness of these can elevate the quality of research, creating a more systematic, productive science.

Before we can begin examining historical and conceptual issues, however, we need a clear definition for the field of exercise psychology. As Rejeski and Brawley (1988) have noted, definitional ambiguity inherent in this subspecialty has contributed to a number of problems. For example, many legitimate and important areas of study have gone unrecognized, whereas, from a pragmatic viewpoint, there has been little agreement regarding the appropriate academic training of professionals. With respect to the present chapter, a historical caricature of exercise psychology and health outcomes that may be associated with exercise is impossible without specifying what the term *exercise* denotes.

## Defining Exercise Psychology

If you asked 50 different individuals what *exercise* means, chances are that no two responses would be the same. To some, *exercise* includes just about any form of physical exertion, from walking to work to planting the garden. Others, however, believe that the term *exercise* is reserved for vigorous aerobic activity or vigorous resistance training. Indeed, even in the scientific literature, the word *exercise* is used freely without qualification. For example, one conclusion we often hear quoted from the literature is that exercise is a tenable treatment for depression. Are we to assume that this refers to aerobic training conducted according to standards published by the American College of Sports Medicine? Would a circuit training program in a local health spa serve the same purpose?

To understand what the word *exercise* entails, and thus the breadth and boundaries of the subspecialty of exercise psychology, it behooves us to reflect momentarily on the field of exercise physiology. Typically, exercise physiologists define the content of their field around the parameters of physical fitness. These include muscular strength, muscular endurance, cardiopulmonary endurance, flexibility, and body composition. Also, exercise physiologists have a role in science, education, and clinical programs, such as cardiac rehabilitation and corporate fitness. Parallel to the insightful work of Matarazzo (1980) in health psychology, it is also important to note that exercise physiologists contribute knowledge that is important to the explanation, promotion, and maintenance of strength, flexibility, aerobic power, and body composition. What then are the implications of the historical basis of exercise physiology for the developing field of exercise psychology?

First of all, it is important to have consistency across fields of study. For example, if exercise psychology was defined in a manner that placed restrictions on the content already established by exercise physiology, it would create problems in the design of curricula. Moreover, professionals would be inadequately trained, and important areas of study would remain underdeveloped. Second, exercise psychology is not limited to the study of aerobic fitness, which was the craze of the 1980s. It also involves exercise forms that enhance strength and range of motion. Moreover, consideration needs to be given to psychological factors that influence perceptions related to physique, as well as actual changes in body composition. In 1988, Rejeski and Brawley, following the lead of Matarazzo (1980) in health psychology, suggested that exercise psychology represented "the application of the educational, scientific, and professional contributions of psychology to the promotion, explanation, maintenance, and enhancement of behaviors related to physical work capacity" (p. 239). The only modification we are suggesting is to replace the words "behaviors related to physical work capacity" with the phrase "the parameters of physical fitness." Thus, *exercise psychology* is the "application of the educational, scientific, and professional contributions of psychology to promoting, explaining, maintaining, and enhancing the parameters of physical fitness." It is concerned with cognitions, emotions, and behaviors that are related to the perception of and/or objective changes in muscular strength and endurance, range of motion, cardiopulmonary endurance, and body composition.

## How Exercise and Health Psychology Differ

At this point, a logical question is how to distinguish exercise psychology from health psychology. After all, a major area of research for the past decade has been the role of exercise in enhancing various aspects of psychological well-being. Does this type of research rightfully fall under the umbrella of exercise or of health psychology? Rejeski and Brawley (1988) proposed that a very simple yet effective means of resolving this problem is to further define boundaries through the identification of the primary dependent variables. Hence, if one examined the role of self-efficacy in exertional responses during exercise, it is clearly a study within the field of exercise psychology because the dependent measure in question is exercise based. On the other hand, if the experimental hypothesis was that exercise training enhanced physical self-efficacy, then the study would be more appropriately labeled as health psychology.

In a general exercise psychology course, content would probably include investigations in which exercise is considered as both an independent and a dependent variable. This arrangement is similar to that found in health psychology. For example, health psychologists would want to understand compliance to exercise in order to maximize the efficacy of this health behavior. Additionally, properly trained exercise psychologists can make important contributions to the study of how exercise influences psychological well-being. In particular, most health psychologists do not have formal training in exercise physiology and lack the measurement expertise that is critical to understanding and interpreting exercise manipulations. The interface of exercise and health psychology is essential to the future development of both fields. This is precisely the belief that motivated Seraganian to invite both exercise and health scientists as contributing authors to this text. The outcome should be rewarding for everyone involved.

## THE HISTORICAL ROOTS OF EXERCISE PSYCHOLOGY

According to our reconstruction, the case study of a female subject in 1884 represents the first published work in exercise psychology. The investigator, C. Rieger, suggested that hypnotic catalepsy greatly facilitated muscular endurance (see Morgan, 1972). Several years later, Norman Triplett (1897), in the *American Journal of Psychology*, published the first experimental study in exercise. In an intriguing paper, Triplett recounted trends that were observed from bicycle records obtained from the Racing Board of the League of American Wheelman. Triplett was fascinated by the apparent facilitative effects of interpersonal competition, and the second part of his paper described an experimental study in which he developed the first hand ergometer to evaluate the performance effects of working alone versus working in competition with another. In his concluding remarks, Triplett noted, "we infer that the bodily presence of another individual contestant participating simultaneously in the race serves to liberate latent energy not ordinarily available" (p. 533). Although not mentioned in the summary, Triplett partitioned his data on the basis of difference scores computed between the alone and the dyadic conditions. He noted that not all individuals experienced a facilitative effect with competition; for some, the competitive environment was debilitating. He described these individuals as overstimulated, exhibiting a feature described as "rigidity of the arms" (p. 523). It would appear that Triplett was the first investigator to observe the adverse effects of competitive anxiety.

Despite this auspicious beginning, between the years 1897 and the late 1970s, the growth of exercise psychology—and of research in which exercise had been treated as an independent variable—was relatively slow. We believe the explanation for this secular trend is the fact that the early part of the twentieth century was a period of history in which attitudes toward sport and exercise were, at best, mixed. For certain, the enhancement of physical skills and physiological potentials were viewed as secondary to intellectual activity. This *competition* between mind and body was also evident in the field of medicine, a perspective that can be traced to the concept of dualism fostered by Plato, Galen, and Descartes, among others (Sarafino, 1990). This split between mind and body in medicine is painfully evident in the biomedical model—the view that all diseases and physical disorders are linked to disturbances in physiological processes. Interestingly, as late as 1986, Taylor argued that the biomedical model continued to be the dominant force in medicine, despite significant challenges to the contrary from contemporary study within the fields of psychosomatic medicine, behavioral medicine, and health psychology.

Despite Taylor's (1986) position, she readily admits that since the late 1970s, there has been a growing awareness on the part of the medical community, and within the general population at large, that dualism is neither a correct nor a constructive philosophical position. Additionally, escalating health-care costs have spawned considerable interest in life-style modification as a means of primary intervention. Coupled with increased leisure time in our society, the past 15 years or so have resulted in new meaning being attributed to exercise and other forms of physical activity. Indeed, exercise is not only linked to physical well-being. As can be seen in this text, there is ample evidence that physical abilities and physical conceptions of the self play an integral role in mental health. The mind–body distinction has slowly, but noticeably yielded to the concept of biopsychosocial interactions—the position that the body, the mind, and the social context of human existence are reciprocally interdependent on one another.

It should not come as a surprise then to find that the 1980s gave rise to a surge of scientific interest in exercise, particularly work in which exercise was studied for its potential therapeutic value in the arena of mental health. Historically, exercise-related investigations fall into 1 of 10 categories: (1) fitness and mental health, (2) body image/esteem, (3) stress reactivity, (4) fatigue/exertion, (5) motivation, (6) exercise performance and metabolic responses, (7) sleep, (8) cognition, (9) the corporate/industrial environment, or (10) exercise addiction.

In the following pages, we provide a selective historical overview of this literature. We have attempted to be particularly sensitive to early investigations, yet provide a contemporary perspective on the field (1983–1990) through the use of a PsychINFO computer search. Although it was impossible to be comprehensive in a single chapter, we have attempted to include key developments and weaknesses that have characterized various lines of research. Additionally, due to restrictions in the length of individual chapters and the focus of the present text, we elected to concentrate on the areas of research that have clear implications for the interface between exercise and mental health. We have omitted research from the final four of the preceding categories: sleep, cognition, the corporate/industrial environment, and exercise addiction. Deleting these areas of study did not hinder the historical sketch we sought to provide.

## Fitness and Mental Health

One of the earliest reports in the psychological literature to discuss a connection between exercise and mental health appeared in the 1926 issue of *Occupational Therapy and Rehabilitation*. In this journal, Vaux proposed that exercise helps to relieve cases of depression by promoting nervous-system stimulation and improving glandular secretion. In 1934, Linton, Hamelink, and Hoskins compared the cardiovascular fitness of a group of schizophrenics to a control group drawn from the hospital staff. The mean score of the psychiatric group (Schneider test) was 19% lower than the control group, a finding that was attributed to inactivity of the mental patients. A review paper by Morgan (1969) critiqued six other preexperimental investigations conducted between the years 1936 and 1962. Collectively, these empirical studies suggested that individuals with personality dysfunction also have weakness in their physical-fitness profile. Furthermore, in his review, Morgan (1969) reported on data that were initially quite striking. He found a moderate negative correlation (–0.50) between physical work capacity and depth of depression. We should remember, however, that physical inactivity may be a *consequence* rather than an *antecedent* of poor mental health. Also, the research cited by Morgan involved a very small sample of depressed patients ($n = 7$).

The most comprehensive and informative review of the pre-1980 literature dealing with exercise and mental health appeared in the *American Psychologist* (Folkins & Sime, 1981). Based on an analysis of study designs, these authors concluded that physical fitness training leads to improved mood, self-concept, and work behavior (i.e., reduced absenteeism, reduced errors, and improved output). There was no evidence that exercise interventions altered personality or psychotic symptomatology. Folkins and Sime also noted that the interpretation of published data was complicated by variation across studies in both the intensity and the duration of activity. Moreover, subjects employed in most exercise interventions were volunteers. If individual differences such as preferred coping styles or beliefs in the efficacy of exercise as a therapeutic tool mediate mental health outcomes, then there may well be a positive bias in this literature.

Finally, Folkins and Sime (1981) were highly critical of the theoretical positions evoked to explain the effects of fitness on depression; in fact, as they pointed out, a significant segment of this research literature has been atheoretical. When theoretical explanations were present, it was criticized as being too mechanistic or simplistic. Examples of these include (a) the endorphin hypothesis, (b) the position that exercise exerts a positive effect on mental health through reductions in resting muscle-action potential, (c) the fact that exercise may compete with anxiety-provoking stimuli for limited channel capacity, (d) the impact of exercise on an improved sense of control or mastery, and (e) the meditative experience provided by exercise through altered states of consciousness (see Morgan, 1985a, for a review of the literature pertinent to most of these hypotheses). One alternative offered by Folkins and Sime was to conceptualize exercise as a self-regulatory (coping) process similar to Lazarus's (1975) interpretation of biofeedback. Such a model places cognitive appraisal in a central position for understanding why and how exercise has positive affective consequences. For example, for an executive who is having to deal with occupational stress, acute exercise may have the immediate effect of increasing vigor and decreasing negative affect. However, in such a context, it is likely that exercise serves two purposes: (1) An immediate effect is enhanced affect, and (2) awareness of being able to curb stress responses (secondary appraisal) effectively then strengthens self-efficacy toward coping with job strain.

Through a psychINFO computer search covering 1983 to 1990, we located 23 investigations dealing with the antidepressive effects of exercise and 42 related to anxiety, mood, and various other self-reported symptoms. It is to the credit of those investigating exercise and depression that we have seen increased attention given to groups with documented depressive disorders ($\approx 40\%$). Across the general area of mental health there has been an interest in women (25%), gender comparisons (57%), and groups with diverse subject characteristics. In addition, significant additions to the mental health literature have been meta-analyses in the areas of depression (North, McCullagh, & Vu Tran (1990), anxiety (Petruzzello, Landers, Hatfield, Kubitz, & Salazar, 1991), and self-concept (McDonald & Hodgdon, 1991).

The quantitative review on depression by North and his colleagues (1990) led to the conclusion that both chronic and acute exercise significantly reduce both state and trait depression, but that the combined effect of exercise and psychotherapy is greater than exercise alone. While the efficacy of exercise as a treatment for depression appears robust across various populations, the largest decreases are seen in medical and psychological rehabilitation settings and in studies that demonstrate sound internal validity. To the surprise of some, anaerobic work (weight training) was found to be an effective form of therapy, and there was evidence that changes in depression occurred early in several programs of research, at a time before physiological training effects had occurred. At the same time, however, it does appear that length of time spent in exercise therapy correlates positively with the decreases seen in depression.

The meta-analysis by Petruzzello et al. (1991) revealed a general anxiolyic effect for aerobic exercise on state anxiety, trait anxiety, and the psychophysiological correlates of anxiety (blood pressure, heart rate, muscle tension, skin responses, brain-wave activity, and the Hoffman reflex). There was some support for the proposition that at least 20 minutes of activity is required to reduce state and trait anxiety; however, this effect was confounded by the fact that a significant number of the investigations that employed 20 minutes of exercise or less compared exercise to other treatments, as opposed to no-treatment controls, possibly creating a negative bias. When the authors restricted their analyses to exercise versus no-treatment control comparisons, there was no support for the proposed 20-minute cut point. Also of interest was an analysis of how duration of activity influenced psychophysiological correlates of anxiety. The largest effect sizes were found for exercise of 30 minutes or less. In other words, it appears that the psychophysiological correlates of anxiety are adversely affected by duration of each training session.

Finally, McDonald and Hodgdon's (1991) review of the self-concept literature found that exercise leads to improved conceptions of the self across diverse psychometric measures that differ both in the construct being assessed and in the measure's level of specificity (e.g., body cathexis vs. global self-esteem). There was no evidence for gender differences; however, the largest effect size was obtained for senior citizens. It is also interesting to note that aerobic dance was found to be as effective in improving self-concept as standard aerobic exercise (i.e., jogging or running). It is also important to emphasize that recent theoretical developments in this area call for a hierarchical structure of concepts, based on level of specificity. For example, Sonstroem and Morgan (1989) have hypothesized that changes in physical self-efficacy enhance more general levels of physical competence and physical acceptance, which jointly contribute to global self-esteem. Indeed, research in cardiac rehabilitation has shown that resistance training can substantially improve patients' confidence in strength-related abilities, consequences that have ramifications for both mental health and physical recovery (Ewart, 1989). Also, Fox and Corbin (1989), in developing the Physical Self-perception Profile, have provided preliminary data to support the position that conceptions of the physical self are related in a hierarchical fashion to more global aspects of self-esteem. It is surprising, however, that these new developments have failed to incorporate important conceptual distinctions into their models. For example, self-esteem and body image do not simply differ in their degree of specificity. This problem is addressed in greater detail in the following section on body image and related constructs.

In summary, it is unfortunate that 50% of the empirical studies on exercise and mental health issues identified in our search employed preexperimental designs. There is very restricted information on how depressive symptoms are influenced by acute bouts of physical work, and most studies involving chronic exercise continue to provide insufficient information concerning the intensity of the exercise stimulus. Interestingly, one study in the literature on the chronic effects of physical work manipulated the intensity of exercise (Blumenthal, Emery, & Rejeski, 1988). In that study, cardiac patients exercised for 3 months at either 65–75% of heart rate reserve (HRR) or below 45% HRR. Contrary to expectations, both groups made significant improvements in cardiovascular function; however, there was no main effect of time in relation to psychosocial status. It is worth noting that individuals who were clinically depressed at the onset of the study did appear to derive some therapeutic value from exercise; however, due to the absence of a no-treatment control, the possibility of regression to the mean cannot be ignored. Parenthetically, not all literature reviews have placed the same degree of confidence in the antidepressive effects of exercise as the North et al. (1990) meta-analysis. For example, Dunn and Dishman (1991) have argued that the existing research is too weak and varied for any firm consensus statement.

An additional concern we have with the mental-health literature pertains to the assessment of mood in acute exercise settings. In our own laboratory (Rejeski, Hardy, & Shaw, 1991), we have shown that traditional psychometric measures, when they are used either during or in close proximity to exercise, may be confounded by somatic changes induced by the accompanying physical stress. Quite frankly, in this area of exercise psychology, research is needed to verify the construct validity of measures such as the State–Trait Anxiety Inventory (STAI) and the Profile of Mood States (POMS). A simple example of interpretational problems that can exist is found in an abstract published by Morgan and Horstman (1976). Using the STAI, these investigators described an increase in anxiety with exercise. When we attempted to replicate these data using the short form of the STAI (Rejeski et al., 1991), we found that increased anxiety during exercise was due to elevation in two STAI items. Other measures taken permitted us to verify that these changes were due to elevated biological responses that had nothing whatsoever to do with cognitive or somatic anxiety. In fact, the internal consistency of the STAI during exercise was totally unacceptable (0.33). Another study conducted by Steptoe and Cox (1988) is subject to similar problems. These investigators reported that high-intensity exercise has negative effects on mood when assessments are taken immediately following exercise. The concern here is that it is incorrect to assume that all changes in arousal denote negative psychological states. For example, is it any surprise that subjects report feeling more tense or shaky after they just exercised at 100 watts for 8 minutes? Is this the same tension that people feel when they are under job strain? Along these same lines, the meta-analysis by Petruzzello et al. (1991) is characterized as a review of the anxiety literature. However, their work does not acknowledge differences between tension and anxiety. Furthermore, they found that the psychophysiological correlates of anxiety were adversely affected by duration of activity. It is important to underscore the fact that physiological measures alone cannot be taken as evidence that anxiety is present or absent, a point that was made earlier in our discussion of the STAI.

Finally, a major challenge that remains in the literature on exercise and mental health is teasing out the conceptual basis for observed effects. Although, it is beyond the scope of this chapter to explore this point in any detail, from a historical perspective, several comments seem relevant. First, there is considerable evidence that psychological outcomes of exercise therapy need not be contingent on changes in physiological parameters. As one example, Rodin (1988) found that consistent high-efficacy feedback to exercisers (e.g., "You are doing something you should be proud of") greatly facilitated a variety of positive mental-health outcomes when contrasted with a group of exercisers who received no such feedback. Second, both human and lower-animal research leave open the possibility that enhanced aminergic synaptic transmission plays a role in at least some cases where exercise has antidepressant effects (Dunn & Dishman, 1991; Ransford, 1982). It seems judicious to encourage the study of both biological and social cognitive variables simultaneously. Third, in chronic programs of exercise, it may well be the repeated acute bouts of exercise that explain positive mental-health outcomes. Training effects may or may not be necessary. Rather than simply using a pretest/posttest design, previous research suggests that psychological outcomes should be monitored using continuous assessments. Along these lines, the comments of Lise Gauvin and Lawrence Brawley's (see Chapter 6) concerning experiential sampling are particularly relevant.

### Body Image, Physical Self-Concept, Body Esteem, and Physique Anxiety

In 1935, Schilder first defined the concept of *body image* as "the picture of our body which we form in own mind" (p. 11). Another related concept, *body affect* (also called "body esteem"), refers to how satisfied or dissatisfied individuals are with various aspects of their body (Secord & Jourard, 1953). In fact Secord and Jourard (1953) originally used the term *body cathexis* to separate feelings that people had about their body from perceptions concerning its objective size and shape.

Early research on body image and affect focused on body-image disturbances that were evident in clinical populations, such as individuals with neurological impairment (Kolb, 1959) or physical deformities (Schonfeld, 1962). However, it was soon realized that perceptual distortions of body image were more ubiquitous and were present in normal populations as well (Cappon & Banks, 1968). For instance, Miller, Linke, and Linke (1980) reported that 54% of college undergraduates were dissatisfied with their weight, a trend that has been found to be gender dependent. In particular, women tend to consistently overestimate their body size when compared to men (e.g., Clifford, 1971) and to express a desired weight that is 14 pounds lighter than their actual weight (Miller et al. (1980). An intriguing fact about the work of Miller and his colleagues (1980) is that only 39% of the women could be classified as overweight by objective standards, yet 70% reported that they were at least slightly overweight. It should be noted, however, that a significant portion of the variance in dysfunctions of body image/esteem frequently has an objective basis. That is to say, individuals with a higher percentage of body fat are particularly prone to disturbances in body image (Young & Reeve, 1980) and body-esteem (Mendelson & White, 1985).

An important finding is that disturbances in body image/esteem are related to general conceptions and feelings about the self (Rosen & Ross, 1968; Rohrbacker, 1973). For both males and females, dissatisfaction with body image has been found to correlate with low self-esteem, (Hawkins, Turrell, & Jackson, 1983), insecurity (Hurlock, 1967), and depression (Marsella, Shizuru, Brennan, & Kameoka, 1981). Tucker (1983a) studied the relationships between muscular strength and mental health in college men. After covarying body weight, he found that strength was positively related to body esteem, emotional stability, facets of extroversion, and confidence. In a related training study, Tucker (1983b) evaluated the impact of weight training on the self-concept of college males. Although there are limitations in the design due to static group comparisons, he did find that individuals enrolled in weight-training classes experienced significant improvements in self-concept when contrasted with subjects taking coursework in personal health. Also of interest was the finding that improvements in self-concept were related to changes in neuroticism, body cathexis, and muscular-strength scores.

Since 1984, several studies have examined the relationship between various physical activities and changes in women's body image/esteem. For example, Skrinar, Bullen, Cheek, and McArthur (1986), using a single-group preexperimental design, reported that aerobic exercise improves middle-aged women's perception of internal body consciousness and en-hances feelings of body competence. Riddick and Freitag (1984) suggested that exercise has a positive influence on the body image of elderly women; however, the design of this study was also preexperimental. The best study to date was conducted by Ben-Shlomo and Short (1985–1986). They ran-domized middle-aged women into one of three conditions: 6 weeks of arm training, 6 weeks of leg training, or no-treatment control. Those who ex-ercised had improved physical self-concepts and showed marginally sig-nificant improvement in body cathexis.

An important development in the body-image/esteem literature has been the gradual realization that critical gender differences exist. Specifi-cally, Franzoi and Shields (1984) found that dimensions of body esteem for male college students consist of physical attractiveness, upper-body strength, and physical condition. Conversely, for college women, the di-mensions of esteem were sexual attractiveness, weight concern, and physical condition. An independent report by Silberstein, Striegel-Moore, Timko, and Rodin (1988) found that men were as likely to want to be heavier as thinner, whereas virtually no women wished to be heavier. These two studies suggest that men and women have different motives for and will seek different outcomes from physical training. Based on these data, it is odd to discover that the recent development of a physical self-perception profile (Fox & Corbin, 1989) appears not to have considered gender differences in the development of the subscales. Moreover, investigators in exercise science have not been careful in their use of constructs such as "self-efficacy," "body image," "body-concept," "body esteem," and so forth. For example, Sonstroem and Morgan (1989) have offered a hierarchical model of self-perceptions that are influenced by exercise. The model's hierarchy ascends from the specific to the general and proposes that "self-efficacy statements relative to particular physical tasks represent the lowest generality level of the competence dimension" (p. 333). Moreover, self-efficacy is proposed to feed a higher level of physical competence (the general evaluation of physical fitness), which combines with physical acceptance (i.e., body cathexis) to determine global self-esteem. One problem with this model is the lack of congruence among the levels of construction. For example, self-efficacy toward specific physical tasks need not translate into more general feelings of competence about *one's level of physical fitness*. A single bout of exercise via a treadmill exam can bring cardiac patients to the realization that they were not as disabled as they once thought. While this may increase their physical competence, there need not be (and probably is not) a change in the evaluation of their physical fitness per se. Similarly, increasing coordination through aerobic dance has important ramifications for physical competence and more global conceptions of the self, yet these increases are unrelated to fitness.

There is an enormous amount of literature on body-image/esteem. Several hundred entries were located across a 7-year period. Unfortunately, many studies published during the past decade continue to be correlational, and there has been limited interest in the interface between these topics and exercise behavior. Hart, Leary, and Rejeski (1989) have suggested that an interesting and neglected area of study is the socially based anxiety that people have regarding their physiques. They constructed a social-physique anxiety measure and argued that self-presentational motives related to this form of anxiety have implications for (a) the physical activities in which people engage, (b) where and with whom they do so, and (c) the enjoyment they derive from such involvement. "Research should begin to explore the impact of physique anxiety on recreational activities, particularly on the degree to which concerns with others' evaluations inhibit people from participating in physical activities that would be beneficial to them. Ironically, individuals who have the greatest need for aerobic exercise may be the most reluctant to engage in it because of their concerns with others' impressions of them" (p. 102).

## Exercise as a Buffer to Stress Reactivity

In the past decade, there has been substantial interest in the potential effects that exercise may have on reducing the biological consequences of stress. Although most of the attention has been directed toward the effects of fitness training on reactivity, there has been some work on the effects that acute bouts of exercise have on subsequent responses to psychological stress. Even though most of the research activity is recent, there are traces of work in this area as early as the 1950s. For example, in 1957, Michael published a review on "Stress Adaption Through Exercise." He cited Van Liere as one of the first investigators to study the effects of exercise and the autonomic nervous system. Van Liere had found that exercising rats manifested increased propulsive motility of the small intestine, as compared to a group of nonexercising rats. This was attributed to the positive influence of exercise on the parasympathetic nervous system. Michael (1957) also reviewed work on stress and the adrenal glands, concluding— largely from indirect evidence—that "the increased adrenal activity resulting from repeated exercise seems to cause an increase in the reserve of steroids available to counter stress" (p. 53).

In 1987, Crews and Landers conducted "A Meta-analytic Review of Aerobic Fitness and Reactivity to Psychosocial Stressors." From examining their data and the research published over the past 3 years, a fairly clear historical picture emerged. First, despite the early efforts of Michael (1957), research on this topic really did not blossom until the late 1970s (Cantor, Zillman, & Day, 1978; Cox, Evans, & Jamieson, 1979; Sime, 1977). Up until 1987, 74% of the studies conducted dealt with chronic exercise, and the majority were correlational (77%). For the most part, dependent measures have focused on cardiovascular function via blood pressure and heart rate; however, recent publications suggest that this trend may be changing. In their conclusion, Crews and Landers (1987) stated that "the mean ES was 0.48 which was significantly different from zero (P<.01). Thus, the effect of aerobic exercise on psychosocial stress response amounts to approximately one-half of a standard deviation above that of the control group or baseline value" (p. S118). We should add, however, that recent longitudinal studies have challenged the conclusions reached by Crews and Landers (1987). For example, a carefully executed investigation by de Geus, Lorenz, vanDoornen, de Visser, and Orlebeke (1990) has compared cross-sectional and training data in the same study. Interestingly, they found support for the proposition that exercise buffers stress reactivity using a cross-sectional approach; however, they failed to support this hypothesis using a 7-week training program. It is possible, of course, that there is a dose–response relationship involved. In other words, subjects may have to train for 3 months or more before exercise has a noticeable effect on stress reactivity. Perhaps this explains why the stress-buffering hypothesis of exercise is supported by cross-sectional data. On the other hand, de Geus and his colleagues (1990) point out that the "concurrent effects of constitution on both aerobic exercise and diastolic or vagal reactivity cannot be excluded by correlational analyses" p. 473.

There are three points that we would like to consider from a historical perspective. First, until recently, much of the research addressed the therapeutic value of chronic as opposed to acute exercise. More important, in Crews and Landers's review, the mean effect size for investigations involving acute bouts of activity (0.11) was considerably lower than that reported for chronic training effects (0.59). Regrettably, however, previous studies involving acute exercise and stress reactivity have been poorly designed (see Rejeski, Gregg, Thompson, & Berry, 1991). For example, one shortcoming in early work was the heavy emphasis placed on the use of heart rate (HR) as an index of stress reactivity. The dilemma facing investigators is that HR remains elevated for an extended period following exercise, a condition that confounds its use as an index of change in subsequent stress manipulations. Moreover, there has been some indication that researchers would benefit from focusing on peripheral, as opposed to central, factors. In particular, vanDoornen, de Geus, and Orlebeke (1988) argue that "the effect of fitness on adrenoceptor sensitivity suggests that the most important effect of fitness might be found in the vascular part of the stress response" p. 303). A second problem is that many of the early studies on acute exercise elected to use very low doses of work. It is not uncommon to find intensities lower than 60% of maximum aerobic capacity and durations less than 15 minutes. Interestingly, we (Rejeski et al., 1991) produced evidence in support of a positive dose–response relationship between acute exercise and subsequent blood-pressure reactivity to stress.

Second, the recent availability of reliable ambulatory blood pressure devices now makes it possible to examine how long the effects of acute exercise persist. In fact, data from a paper delivered by Ebbesen, Prkachin, and Mills (1989) suggest that exercise may buffer blood-pressure responses to some stressors for as long as 3 hours postexercise. This same technology can be used to track the effects of fitness training on responses to daily stress or to examine the influence of acute and chronic physical activity on average responses across different phases of daily living. It is also worth noting that the data reported by Ebbesen et al. revealed a potential confound in studies involving chronic exercise and stress reactivity. That is, if investigators do not ensure that subjects have refrained from acute exercise for as long as 3 or 4 hours prior to psychophysiological studies, it is possible that significant findings are inappropriately attributed to training.

Third, we question the suitability of the conceptual model that has dominated this line of empirical inquiry. Typically, investigators rely exclusively on physiological mechanisms to explain the positive effects that exercise—either acute or chronic—has on various biological stress responses. In our view, this historical trend has created a number of methodological shortcomings and ignores the possibility that a broader social-psychobiological framework is required to understand the problem at hand. For example, far too many experiments now in the literature have failed to provide documentation that their stress manipulations were successful. It is well recognized in the psychological literature that stress is an interactive process between individuals and their environments. It is inappropriate to *assume* that an objective demand selected by the experimenter places subjects in a position of threat or challenge. Furthermore, we might ask whether the effects of exercise on stress reactivity are similar for perceptions of threat versus challenge and how other features of the stressor (e.g., whether an active coping response is elicited) influence various outcomes. A broader conceptual model integrating social, psychological, and biological variables is also essential to teasing out potential cognitive and/or emotive-based causal networks. For example, as mentioned earlier in this chapter, work by Lazarus (1975) places exercise in the realm of *secondary appraisal*; that is, once the threat of challenge or harm is realized, a major determinant of physiological reactivity is subjects' cognitive evaluation of skills and resources that they have to combat the demand. The perception that exercise is beneficial or that it has enhanced an individual's hardiness in some way could constitute critical mediating variables.

## The Study of Fatigue/Exertion and In-Task Emotional Responses

It is beyond the scope of this chapter to provide a detailed historical treatise on fatigue. Its importance as a psychological construct can be traced to the work of Thorndike at the beginning of the twentieth century (e.g., Thorndike, 1912), but the term has been used to describe various forms of incapacitation, including such diverse topics as (a) cellular activity, (b) x-ray irradiation, (c) changes in the visual and auditory systems, (d) deterioration in intellectual functioning, and (e) studies of exertion in various work situations (Bartley, 1976). It is this lack of specificity that made the work of Gunnar Borg particularly appealing. In 1962, he published a monograph on "Physical Performance and Perceived Exertion." Although Borg had conducted research as early as 1960, it was his publications from 1962 through 1968 that appear to have served as the impetus for the large volume of exercise research that followed in the 1970s and 1980s. Indeed, a significant feature of Borg's work is that in addition to presenting a clearly defined construct, he offered a simple and psychometrically sound approach to reliably assess ratings of perceived exertion (RPE).

From a conceptual viewpoint, it is instructive to track the history of this construct. Borg is a psychophysicist whose assumptions place RPE within a unidirectional sensory model. What this means is that, much like motor reflexes, subjective estimates of exertion are believed to be automatic, the function of direct sensory input (Borg, 1985, personal communication). Thus, for the first decade or so, RPE existed as a construct independent of emotion and conscious thought processes. Most of the attention was directed toward investigating the physiological correlates of RPE and documenting the manner in which individual differences such as disease or level of fitness moderated such responses. Much like B. F. Skinner's (1990) position, there was no need for theory.

There were, however, three important exceptions to this exclusive physiological orientation. Specifically, in the early 1970s, Morgan (1973) published a paper on the role of personality in perceived exertion. He demonstrated that anxious neurotics and depressives at moderate workloads and extroverts at heavy workloads tend to underestimate RPE. These conclusions, however, were based on data from very small sample sizes and had to be viewed cautiously. In a second line of research, Morgan and his colleagues (e.g., Morgan, Raven, Drinkwater, & Horvath, 1973) studied the effect of hypnotic suggestion on ratings of perceived exertion. Their data provided the first indication that a cognitive manipulation (i.e., suggestion) could alter perceptual responses.

In that same year, Weiser and his colleagues (Weiser, Kinsman, & Stamper, 1973), working with bicycle ergometry, demonstrated that subjective responses during exercise could be differentiated into local, central, and general fatigue. More important, they offered a conceptual model, which introduced the proposition that subjective factors such as motivation contributed to the fatigue experience. It is important to note that the work of these researchers represented a departure from Borg's conception of perceived exertion. Unfortunately, their model was reductionistic; that is, the origin of all subjective experience was proposed to be rooted in physiological substrata. Furthermore, despite two chapters dedicated to the "Introspective Aspects of Work and Fatigue," which appeared in a 1976 text (Simonson & Weiser), the main influence of this work on RPE research was that it led to the measurement of specific, as well as generalized, responses. For example, in a typical experiment, subjects might be asked to provide local (e.g., ratings of the legs) as well as general RPEs. As one might suspect, research in the late 1970s was designed to evaluate the physiological basis of these differentiated ratings (cf. Pandolf, 1977).

A paper in the early 1980s (Rejeski, 1981) was designed to integrate the RPE research that had been conducted during the 1960s and 1970s. The major objective of this review was to underscore the fact that exertional responses are *not* analogous to muscle reflexes or amenable to a strict psychophysical paradigm. Rather, psychological dispositions and social-cognitive variables constitute potent mediating mechanisms in the perceived sense of effort. Morgan's work (Morgan 1973, Morgan et al., 1983) certainly offered support for this supposition, as did research in our own laboratory (Rejeski & Ribisl, 1980), which had demonstrated that RPEs given at a particular point in exercise are affected by the expected duration of a task. In the 1981 review, I also proposed (Rejeski, 1981) that the relative contribution of subjective and objective input to perceptions of exertion will depend on the intensity and duration of the exercise stimulus. For example, when a physical demand is excessive, powerful metabolic changes may preclude cognitive manipulations from enabling someone to continue an activity.

In the mid-1980s, a conceptual paper appeared (Rejeski, 1985), which reinforced the idea that self-reported exertion involves an "active" rather than a "passive" subject. In this report, discussion and empirical support was provided for Leventhal and Everhart's (1979) parallel process model of pain. For example, we have published data indicating that preconscious cognitive and emotional schemas influence the extent to which subjects rate the difficulty of physical work (e.g., Hochstetler, Rejeski, & Best, 1985). Moreover, in an experimental context (Rejeski & Sanford, 1984), we have shown that emotional schemas concerning exercise can be primed and altered using social models. That is, RPEs are influenced by how negatively subjects view physical activity. In 1986, in an independent laboratory, Hardy, Hall, and Presholdt demonstrated that RPEs can be influenced by self-presentational motives. This position was corroborated by the work of Boutcher, Fleischer-Curtian, and Gines (1988), who found that males gave lower RPEs with female than with male experimenters.

When we examined the trends in the RPE research since 1985, 20 entries were found, 10 of which involved college students. There was a fairly even split on gender and a propensity toward the study of social cognitive variables (35%). Moreover, 50% of the study designs were experimental or quasi-experimental. Overall, these data are quite encouraging. In contrast to earlier work, more of the contemporary research is theory driven, with a balance of attention now being given to the study of both men and women. For the future, it is important to build on the social-psychobiological framework that was precipitated by the psychometric contributions of Borg and the early research on cognition by Morgan (see Rejeski, 1985). We would encourage more experimental work on the possible social basis of schemata that are pertinent to the processing of exercise-induced changes in various biological systems. Based on recent data from our own laboratory, we suspect that aversion to exercise symptoms profoundly influence responses both to acute episodes of work and to chronic patterns of physical activity.

The concern that we have for subjects' both preconscious and conscious affective responses toward exercise symptoms (see Rejeski, 1985) motivated us to study a central in-task dimensional feature of affect—that is, how good or bad a person feels when involved in exercise (Hardy & Rejeski, 1989; Rejeski, Best, Griffith, & Kenney, 1987). It has become quite clear that the measurement of RPE and positive or negative "feelings" are distinct enough from a measurement perspective to warrant individual instruments (Hardy & Rejeski, 1989). For example, Boutcher and Trenske (1990) found that the introduction of music to controlled bouts of exercise did not alter RPE; however, subjects reported a better feeling about working under these conditions. Similarly, Kenney, Rejeski, and Messier (1988) reported that distress-management training provided for novice women runners resulted in improved feelings but no change in the RPEs of fixed workloads. Because data also indicate that feminine-typed men (e.g., submissive, emotional, dependent) are, in general, less positive toward exercise symptoms (Rejeski et al., 1987), it appears that both dispositional and situational variables can influence the feelings that subjects experience during exercise. We think that an interesting area of study for the future is the manner in which in-task feelings contribute to motivational states, as well as to the acute and chronic effects of exercise on various mental-health outcomes. Finally, we would encourage investigators to further explore the subjective realm of exercise behavior because we readily admit to the limitations inherent in a single-item affect measure.

## Exercise Motivation

An issue that is interconnected with nearly every topic discussed in this opening chapter is the problem of motivating people to exercise. What is the key to keeping depressed patients involved in exercise therapy? How are subjective responses to exercise-related symptoms related to participant motivation? Do concerns regarding peer evaluation of physique or feelings of low self-efficacy serve as deterrents to physically active life-styles? These and related questions suggest that the topic of exercise motivation may be the most important of all. However, other than Kenyon's (1968) work in the mid-1960s, interest in this facet of exercise psychology did not blossom until the late 1970s and early 1980s.

Rod Dishman and his colleagues (Dishman, 1982, 1986, 1988; Dishman, Sallis, & Orenstein, 1985) have provided extensive reviews of research on factors that correlate with the initiation of and compliance with programs of exercise. In his 1986 review, Dishman concluded the following:

It is clear that (1) blue-collar workers, smokers, and the obese appear less likely to adopt or maintain a supervised or spontaneous fitness program; (2) high self-motivation reliably predicts compliance but not dropout, suggesting that self-motivated individuals are likely to continue an exercise routine without supervision; (3) perceived inconvenience and lack of time correlate with dropout, but some exercisers keep participating despite the same barriers; (4) reinforcements from health or exercise professionals, peers, and family and from feelings of well-being or goal attainment appear more important to continued participation than beliefs about health benefits, though such beliefs can influence adoption; (5) intentions and perceived ability to exercise are related to adoption of a program but do not predict dropout; and (6) exercise prescriptions that are tailored to the exerciser's initial fitness level often fail to satisfy the exertion preferences of dropouts. (p. 143)

What we wish to emphasize in this chapter is how various conceptual/ theoretical models may have limited what we know and why some of the conclusions reached may be misdirected.

It is our impression that the growth of interest in exercise motivation during the late 1970s was precipitated, in part, by the increased popularity of applied programs in behavioral medicine (e.g., cardiac rehabilitation), which relied on exercise therapy as its principal mode of intervention. As one would expect, the early research was characterized by descriptive investigations that were largely atheoretical (e.g., Andrew & Parker, 1979; Oldridge & Jones, 1983). Despite this limitation, these data brought to our attention the potential importance of both individual differences and situational/environmental barriers as determinants of exercise behavior. The following decade gave rise to several different lines of research that were designed to increase the systematic study of compliance. For example, Dishman, Ickes, and Morgan (1980) introduced the self-motivation inventory as an individual difference measure of behavioral persistence. There were investigations based on the health-belief model (e.g., Lindsey-Reid & Osborn, 1980), social-learning theory (e.g., Long & Haney, 1986), and self-efficacy theory (e.g., Dzewaltowski, 1989). Fishbein and Ajzen's theory of reasoned action was touted as an improved conceptual model for studying the combined effects of attitudes, beliefs, and intentions (e.g., Riddle, 1980), while a number of investigators examined various facets of cognitive-behavioral modification (see Martin & Dubbert, 1984).

On the bright side, researchers employing different conceptual models have consistently found that compliance to organized exercise programs is significantly related to perceived barriers such as the physical demands of exercise and the time required for training (Dzewaltowski, 1989; Godin, Shephard, & Colantonio, 1986; Sonstroem, 1982). There is evidence that various forms of social support play a significant part in exercise motivation (King, Taylor, Haskell, & Debusk, 1988; Wankel, 1984), and a number of different studies have reinforced the value of various cognitive-behavioral interventions (Martin & Dubbert, 1984). Furthermore, McAuley (1992) recently reviewed research on self-efficacy and was very optimistic about research from both primary and secondary preventive perspectives. By implication, he argued that self-efficacy is a common mechanism that can be employed to explain the effects of seemingly diverse processes such as goal setting and social support. The movement toward parsimonious theoretical explanations ought to be viewed as a step in the right direction; however, according to Rejeski (1992), there are several characteristics of the historical record that create confusion and will continue to cause problems if left uncorrected.

Take for example, the conclusion that "attitudes toward physical activity have not predicted who will eventually adhere or drop-out" (Dishman, 1982, p. 240). Dishman is correct about the studies reviewed; yet, if you examined these investigations, you would find several different operational definitions of *attitudes*, none of which reflected contemporary theory or established measurement protocols. In short, in 1982, it was premature to suggest that attitudes were unrelated to either initiation of or continued involvement in physical activity. Another more complex problem surfaces in the conclusion that "high self-motivation reliably predicts compliance" (Dishman, 1986, p. 143). First of all, not all published results on the self-motivation inventory (SMI) have been positive (see Wankel, 1984). More important, however, are current limitations in the SMI, created by the fact that it was developed independent of any systematic theory. Our point here is simple. Self-motivation may be an important psychological construct; however, the history of psychology tells us that general levels of construction (e.g., "I seldom work to my full capacity") and reliance on single constructs will yield disappointing levels of behavioral prediction (Rotter, 1954). This would suggest that even research on self-efficacy—a situation-specific theory—must be reexamined. For example, freedom from barriers may yield high levels of self-efficacy, yet this cognitive set is unlikely to lead to persistence if the individual involved does not value the outcomes associated with exercise. To reiterate, single constructs are ineffective in providing stable behavioral predictions. We believe that investigators—ourselves included—need to step back and closely reexamine the integrity of conceptual models and theories that serve as the basis for hypothesis testing (see Rejeski, 1992).

## Psychological Influences on Exercise Performance and Metabolic Parameters

**Exercise Performance.**   As indicated in the opening paragraph of this section, the earliest recorded investigations in exercise psychology can be traced to the performance research of Reiger and Triplett in the late 1880s. Unfortunately, Triplett's pioneering work did not stimulate systematic study of how social factors influence exercise behavior. In fact, other than studies by Ayres (1911) and Voor, Lloyd, and Cole (1969), there was practically no interest in the social psychology of exercise prior to the late 1970s.

The earlier of the two studies (i.e., Ayres, 1911), utilized an annual bicycle race in Madison Square Garden to test the hypothesis that music enhances performance. It so happened that part of the competition involved routine play by a military band; they would play a musical selection, rest, and repeat this cycle throughout 46 miles of competition. Although there were no statistical comparisons of the two experimental conditions (music vs. no music), Ayres reported that the average speed of the group while the band played was 19.6 mph, whereas when the band stopped, the speed decreased to 17.9 mph! Voor and his colleagues (1969) brought the study of social facilitation to the laboratory. In their study, male college students who participated on intramural teams were tested in one of two conditions: individually or in a group ostensibly involving team competition ($25 was given to the winning team). All subjects were required to hold a submaximal isometric contraction for as long as possible. In the group condition, three individuals performed one at a time, with the average score taken as the team score. During each subject's performance, the two remaining team members were present, to provide whatever encouragement they desired. Contrary to expectations, social facilitation did not improve performance. However, the team atmosphere did lead to higher electromyographic (EMG) responses, which was interpreted as an index of increased stress.

Throughout the early twentieth century and into the 1970s, the principal focus of performance-based research in psychology centered around the *ergogenic* (performance-enhancing) properties of hypnosis (Barber, 1966; Hull, 1933; Morgan, 1972); however, in recent years there have been several lines of research emphasizing the active role that subjects may play in performance enhancement. Shelton and Mahoney (1978), for example, have been able to show that emotional "psych-up" prior to a weightlifting task dramatically increases performance, a finding that has been replicated since in several laboratories (see Weinberg, Gould, Yukelson, & Jackson, 1981). Nelson and Furst (1972) manipulated perceived superiority in a muscular strength/endurance competition and found that objectively weaker opponents who thought they were stronger won 83% of their bouts. Along similar lines, Weinberg et al. (1981) have shown that preexisting and manipulated self-efficacy significantly influence muscular endurance. Yet another direction of empirical inquiry has been the role of active coping in managing exercise distress. Several investigators have reported that distracting attention from the distress of exercise can result in enhanced performance (e.g., Gill & Strom, 1985; Morgan, Horstman, Cymerman, & Stokes, 1983; Weinberg, Smith, Jackson, & Gould, 1984); however, the term *distraction* has been used to describe several different methods that are not conceptually equivalent. Also, no systematic attention has been given to individual differences. This may well be an important consideration, given Rejeski and Kenney's (1987) data, which suggest that cognitive complexity is an important determining factor in the effectiveness of cognitively involved dissociative strategies.

Like other areas of research in exercise psychology, there are general lessons to be learned from the historical footprints left by research on cognition and performance. Morgan (1972) mentioned several methodological problems in his review on hypnosis, which have implications for other programs of research. Most significant, we believe, are the concerns that he expressed regarding confounds between hypnosis and suggestion. Frequently, independent variables in the exercise-psychology literature are too broad and combine variance from multiple sources. For example, in a paper on dissociative cognitive strategies by Morgan and his colleagues (1983), the manipulation of dissociation involved suggestions of "psych-up" and reduced distress in conjunction with some aspects of noncultic relaxation. In reflecting on these data, one is compelled to ask, "Just what was responsible for the observed effect?" This criticism could also be lodged against chronic exercise interventions because they typically involve more than exercise alone. For example, subjects in rehabilitation programs are frequently praised for their performance and typically gain social support from other group members. How then can one be confident that it is the exercise that buffers stress or reduces depression?

A second point related to the first, which was made less explicit by Morgan (1972), is that across investigations, there is substantial variation in the operational definition of *suggestion*, a problem that increases the difficulty of synthesizing information from different laboratories. This concern reminds us of a study in the cognitive-behavioral literature, which examined the relative efficacy of association versus dissociation in improving the attendance rates of males and females in a 12-week exercise program (Martin et al., 1984). The authors reported that dissociation yielded better compliance than association.

> Close inspection of the cognitive strategies, however, suggests that their operational definitions of association and dissociation were inconsistent with contemporary theory (cf. Rejeski, 1985). Normally, association is used to refer to a focus on physical sensations, the attempt is to tune subjects into physiological input so that less cognitive capacity is available for negative affective processing of sensory cues. In contrast, dissociation refers to attentional strategies designed to cover-up or distract subjects from the fatigue-producing effects of exercise. In the Martin et al. study, subjects who associated did focus on physiologic cues, but they were encouraged to "be their own coach," to set high personal standards, and to reemphasize in their own minds that they could do better than they had in the past. By contrast, those in the dissociation condition were told to attend to the environment and pleasant stimuli, to set realistic goals, and to replace self-defeating thoughts with positive coping statements. Thus, at best, their results imply that positive realistic cognitive restructuring is superior to cognitive sets in which performance is the focal point and continued improvement is the mark of success. (Rejeski, 1992, p. 154)

A third point made by Morgan concerns the importance of establishing stable baseline data. As he noted, stable baselines are crucial to drawing inferences about the effects of hypnosis or cognitive manipulations on performance. This is another problem with broad implications. For example, an investigator may employ a field test of cardiovascular fitness as a manipulation check of aerobic conditioning. Let us suppose that an experimental group trained for 15 minutes, twice weekly for 12 weeks, whereas a control group remained sedentary. Improvement in pacing alone would create group differences on the posttest. Parenthetically, such a confound may even exist on submaximal tests, where HR is employed as the criterion, or in measuring baseline blood pressure when one is attempting to study the influence of exercise on resting hemodynamics. As reported in a subsequent section, metabolism can be altered by mental processes.

As a final lesson from history, research in cognition and performance reaffirms the importance of emphasizing theory-based research. In light of this, it is unfortunate that work on dissociative strategies has proceeded largely independent of formal theory. Trial and error has yielded some important lessons; however, conceptual models from the pain literature provide the starting point for a much more systematic plan of inquiry (cf. Rejeski, 1985). Additionally, after reading the research in hypnosis, one cannot help but wonder why this technique should enhance performance. Actually, there are several possible hypotheses, yet no agreed-upon theoretical structure to guide research. If this does not change, our sense is that a decade from now, another review on hypnosis will conclude similar to Morgan's (1972): "Hull stated in 1933 that the literature in this area was contradictory, and unfortunately the present review suggests that 40 years of research have failed to provide any clarification" (p. 216).

**Psychological Factors and Exercise Metabolism.**    An interesting area of study, with a 60-year history is the influence that cognition, affect, and the perceived intensity of physical work have on metabolic responses. This body of literature offers strong support to the position that anticipatory reactions to an exercise stimulus and the manner in which subjects process information during exercise significantly alter metabolism. As early as 1939, two Russian scientists, Nemtzova and Shatenstein, reported that hypnotic suggestions of heavy work increased ventilation 14.5 L/min$^{-1}$ and elevated oxygen uptake by 409 mL/min$^{-1}$ (reported in Morgan 1985b). In a clever comparison, Dudlye and his colleagues (Dudlye, Holmes, Martin, & Ripley, 1964), using hypnotic suggestion, contrasted the metabolic effects of thinking about active and passive behavior/emotions. When subjects were given suggestions of exercise, anxiety, or anger (active responses), their ventilation and oxygen consumption increased, whereas carbon dioxide decreased. The opposite was true for relaxation and depression (passive responses): Ventilation and oxygen consumption decreased while carbon dioxide increased. As Morgan (1985b) stated in a recent review of psychogenic factors in metabolism, data support the position that the mere image of exercise—like other action-oriented responses (e.g., anxiety)—can elevate HR, cardiac output, ventilation, and oxygen uptake.

As noted previously, research also indicates that metabolic responses *during exercise* can be influenced by the way in which exercise stimuli are processed. A demonstration of this effect was published by Morgan (see 1985b review). Subjects in this investigation were required to exercise on a bicycle ergometer in a control waking state and in several hypnotic states. During the control condition, subjects were given the suggestion that the work was of moderate intensity, whereas in the hypnotic states, subjects exercised under the suggestion of light, moderate, or heavy exercise. The principal finding, according to Morgan, was the pattern in the ventilatory data. The suggestion of heavy exercise resulted in a ventilatory response that was 15 L/min higher than the suggestion of moderate work in the waking state. Also, the observed effect for suggestions of heavy work in a hypnotic state was accompanied by increases in both carbon dioxide and the respiratory exchange ratio. Incidentally, an interesting pattern in Morgan's data was the similarity in responses between the suggestion of moderate work, which was given in either a waking or a hypnotic state. In other words, it seems highly probable that suggestion rather than hypnosis is responsible for many effects attributed to the hypnotic trance (Barber, 1966).

The position that conscious cognitive processes can alter metabolic responses has garnered some interesting, yet limited support (Morgan, 1985b). In particular, research suggests that relaxation training (Benson, Dryer, & Hartley, 1978) and stress-management training (Ziegler, Klinzing, & Williamson, 1982) can increase the efficiency with which oxygen is utilized during exercise. Benson and his colleagues studied subjects who had had a minimum of 6 months training in noncultic relaxation. Compared to a control run, the use of relaxation improved oxygen consumption by 4%. Ziegler and her associates (1982) found similar effects with stress-management training; however, these investigators used collegiate cross-country runners. This latter finding has particular significance, in that it is believed to be more difficult to find support for cognitive manipulations in trained, as compared to untrained populations (Morgan, 1972). Finally, there is some indication that the physiological effects of physical warm-up are, in part, psychologically based (see Franks, 1972). Unfortunately, to our knowledge, no additional attention has been given to the study of this important topic.

## GENERAL SUMMARY

This chapter was designed to provide a historical critique of exercise psychology and related investigations where exercise has been employed as an independent variable. With few exceptions, this field of inquiry has had a relatively brief history of about 25 years. In commenting on various research directions in the literature, our principal goal was to track methodological and conceptual idiosyncrasies. These footprints assist us in understanding limitations of knowledge and provide important lessons for the future. The following sections underscore the major issues raised.

## Modifying the Scope of Empirical Inquiry and Professional Involvement

In the very beginning of this chapter, we defined *exercise psychology* as "the application of the educational, scientific, and professional contributions of psychology to promoting, explaining, maintaining, and enhancing the parameters of physical fitness." We also argued that exercise psychologists should concern themselves with research questions where exercise is treated as an independent variable. For example, properly trained exercise psychologists can make significant contributions to the study of exercise therapy in enhancing mental health. Moreover, mental-health outcomes are closely connected with exercise topics such as compliance and subjective responses to exercise symptoms. From a historical viewpoint, a major consequence of not having a formally defined field of study is that the scope of empirical inquiry has been restricted. There are only a handful of studies on strength, not a single investigation involving range of motion, most exercise psychologists do not even consider body image to be a part of the field, and investigators have chosen to essentially ignore topics such as the psychology of warm-up. Moreover, psychologists have not been extensively involved in national educational programs such as the committee for Preventive and Rehabilitative Exercise Programs within the American College of Sports Medicine. There are national certifications for fitness instructors and program directors, yet little input from the profession of psychology. If, as a field of study, we are to experience significant change in the future, then it is critical to define what we are about and to promote a broad-based educational, scientific, and professional growth.

### Historical Lessons in Experimental Methods

The historical sketch of exercise psychology presented in this chapter has provided some valuable lessons in the realm of experimental methods. First, much of the chronic-exercise research in mental health suffers from a common problem: There are multiple sources of variance in experimental manipulations. Truthfully, when we say that exercise programs can provide an effective means of combating depression, the word *program* should probably be taken to mean exercise, social support, performance feedback, and so on. Unfortunately, in many published investigations it is not even possible to discern what the term *exercise therapy* meant. Along these same lines, a second limiting factor has been the failure both to quantify treatment effects (i.e., ensure that subjects' physiology has been modified as a function of training) and to verify that subjects complied with therapeutic protocols. Third, across several areas of study, it has become apparent that investigators should consider both alternative endpoints and novel approaches to assessment. For example, experiential sampling (discussed by Lise Gauvin and Lawrence Brawley in Chapter 6) and ambulatory blood pressure monitoring (see Chapter 8 by John Jamieson and Karen R. Flood) enable researchers to increase the ecological validity of research. Fourth, we are quick to look toward tightly designed experiments for verification of theory yet largely ignore external validity. How can we rule particular constructs or entire theoretical approaches as invalid in the absence of random samples? Attitudes may be unimportant when you deal with volunteer populations; however, they might well have a lot to do with explaining the behavior of individuals who normally would not choose to exercise. Fifth, construct validity is an ongoing process that is extremely critical to the study of acute exercise. Exercise symptoms can be easily misinterpreted by investigators. Whereas changes in HR and muscle activity may imply the onset of anxiety or feelings of fatigue—the presence of depression—these same sensations can signify energetic arousal and, as one power lifter has described, "the positive cathartic effects of a good pump."

## Issues Related to Theory

The final comments in the chapter, those related to theory, may be the most significant historical lessons of all. Our initial challenge in the future is to define research problems concisely and unambiguously, to seek theoretical frameworks that combine input from social, psychological, and biological perspectives. We will have to fight to resist recurring historical setbacks created by reductionism and dualism. As we have seen in the physical-exertion literature and in the study of exercise with stress reactivity, it is easy to be lured by the concrete nature of objective measures; it has been tempting for investigators who work with RPE to attempt to discover the single critical physiological cue that determines perceived sense of effort (cf. Mihevic, 1981). However, in doing so, the fact is ignored that social cognition and human biological responses are reciprocal systems that cannot be studied in isolation—not if we are to reject dualistic thinking as we attempt to understand phenomena such as aversion to physical work or the role of exercise in mediating responses to threat and challenge.

The study of explanatory concepts/processes in exercise psychology underscores the importance of considering theoretical models that cut across multiple disciplines and diverse measurement strategies. For example, research in depression (North et al., 1990) has shown that some of the therapeutic benefits of exercise programs occur before training effects are realized; yet, among these same data, there is evidence that changes in depression covary with length of time in training. Rodin (1988) has shown that efficacy feedback in conjunction with exercise yields more favorable psychological outcomes than exercise alone; however, there are some indications that the ability of exercise to buffer subsequent physiological responses to stress are dose dependent (Rejeski et al., 1991). In reality, positive psychological outcomes attributed to exercise are probably determined by multiple causes, the specific factors varying with the nature of the disorder and the needs of the individual. A nomothetic approach treats this source of variance as error.

Finally, our choice of theories and conceptual frameworks has been as much of a problem to exercise psychology as was the atheoretical stance found in early research. Put differently, there are ample instances where constructs, theories, and conceptual models have been inappropriately applied; moreover, some theories and models offer very poorly articulated blueprints for the construction of knowledge. As a gold standard, theories that guide our research programs ought to (a) involve multiple levels of construction, (b) include content-related as well as process-oriented constructs, and (c) offer clear, systematic operational definitions of constructs (cf. Rejeski, 1992). The problem of not having multiple levels of construction is that historically single constructs used in isolation have offered very poor behavioral prediction (Rotter, 1954). The distinction between content-related and process-oriented constructs implies that theories must recognize individual differences (i.e., content-related constructs), yet include constructs that assist in explaining why behavior occurs and how it is changed. The recent success of self-efficacy theory is a testimony to the value inherent in this level of construction. Finally, we have mentioned several times how vague operational definitions have confused rather than assisted research in exercise psychology. Ideally, constructs within a theory, via their operational definitions, should be systematically tied to one another (see Rotter, 1954).

If those who work in the field of exercise psychology reflect on its relatively brief history, we believe that significant advancements will be made during the 1990s. Unfortunately, ignoring the past will mean that we repeat our failures.

## REFERENCES

Andrew, G. M., & Parker, J. O. (1979). Factors related to dropout of postmyocardial infarction patients from exercise programs. *Medicine and Science in Sports, 11,* 376–378.

Ayres, L. P. (1911). *American Physical Education Review, 16,* 321.

Barber, T. X. (1966). *British Journal of Social and Clinical Psychology, 5,* 42.

Bartley, S. H. (1976). Visual fatigue. In E. Simonso & P. C. Weiser (Eds.), *Psychological aspects and physiological correlates of work and fatigue.* Springfield, IL: Charles C. Thomas.

Ben-Shlomo, L. S., & Short, M. A. (1985–1986). The effects of physical conditioning on selected dimensions of self-concept in sedentary females. *Occupational Therapy in Mental Health, 5,* 27–46.

Benson, H., Dryer, B. A., & Hartley, H. H. (1978). Decreased $\dot{V}O_2$ consumption exercise with elicitation of the relaxation response. *Journal of Human Stress, 4*(2), 38–42.

Blumenthal, J. A., Emery, C. F., & Rejeski, W. J. (1988). The effects of exercise training on psychosocial functioning after myocardial infarction. *Journal of Cardiopulmonary Rehabilitation, 8*, 183–193.

Borg, G. (1962). *Physical performance and perceived exertion.* Lund: Gleerup, 1962.

Boutcher, S. H., & Trenske, M. (1990). The effects of sensory deprivation and music on perceived exertion and affect during exercise. *Journal of Sport & Exercise Psychology, 12*, 442–447.

Boutcher, S. H., Fleischer-Curtian, L. A., & Gines, S. D. (1988). The effects of self-presentation on perceived exertion. *Journal of Sport and Exercise Psychology, 10*, 270–280.

Cantor, J. R., Zillman, D., & Day, K. D. (1978). Relationship between cardiovascular fitness and physiological responses to films. *Perceptual Motor Skills, 46*, 1123–1130.

Cappon, D., & Banks, R. (1968). Distorted body perception in obesity. *Journal of Nervous and Mental Disorders, 46*, 465–467.

Clifford, E. (1971). Body satisfaction in adolescence. *Perceptual and Motor Skills, 33*, 119–125.

Cox, J. P., Evans, J. F., & Jamieson, J. L. (1979). Aerobic power and tonic heart rate responses to psychosocial stressors. *Personality and Social Psychology Bulletin, 5*, 160–163.

Crews, D. J., & Landers, D. M. (1987). A meta-analytic review of aerobic fitness and reactivity to psychosocial stressors. *Medicine and Science in Sports and Exercise, 19*, 114–120.

de Geus, E. C. J., Lorenz, J. P., van Doornen, L. J. P., de Visser, D. C., & Orlebeke, J. F. (1990). Existing and training induced differences in aerobic fitness: Their relationship to physiological response patterns during different types of stress. *Psychophysiology, 27*, 457–478.

Dishman, R. K. (1982). Compliance/adherence in health related exercise. *Health Psychology, 1*, 237–267.

Dishman, R. K. (1986). Exercise compliance: A new view for public health. *The Physician and Sports Medicine, 14*, 127–145.

Dishman, R. K. (1988). *Exercise adherence: Its impact on public health.* Champaign, IL: Human Kinetics.

Dishman, R. K., Ickes, W., & Morgan, W. P. (1980). Self-motivation and adherence to habitual physical activity. *Journal of Applied Social Psychology, 2*, 115–132.

Dishman, R. K., Sallis, J. F., & Orenstein, D. R. (1985). The determinants of physical activity and exercise. *Public Health Report, 100*, 158–171.

Dudlye, D. L., Holmes, T. H., Martin, C. J., & Ripley, H. S. (1964). Changes in respiration associated with hypnotically induced emotion, pain, and exercise. *Psychosomatic Medicine, 26*, 46–57.

Dunn, A. L., & Dishman, R. K. (1991). Exercise and the neurobiology of depression. In J. O. Holloszy (Ed.), *Exercise and sport science reviews* (pp. 41–98). Baltimore, MD: Williams & Wilkins.

Dzewaltowski, D. A. (1989). Toward a model of exercise motivation. *Journal of Sport and Exercise Psychology, 11*, 251–269.

Ebbesen, B. L., Prkachin, K. M., & Mills, D. E. (1989). *Effects of acute exercise on car-*

*diovascular reactivity.* Paper presented at the tenth annual meeting of the Society of Behavioral Medicine, San Francisco.

Ewart, C. K. (1989). Psychological effects of resistive weight training: Implications for cardiac patients. *Medicine and Science in Sports and Exercise, 21,* 683–688.

Folkins, C. H., & Sime, W. E. (1981). Physical fitness training and mental health. *American Psychologist, 36,* 373–389.

Fox, K. R., & Corbin, C. B. (1989). The physical self-perception profile: Development and preliminary validation. *Journal of Sport and Exercise Psychology, 11,* 408–430.

Franks, D. (1972). Physical warm-up. In W. P. Morgan (Ed.), *Ergogenic aids and muscular performance* (pp. 159–191). New York: Academic Press.

Franzoi, S. L., & Shields, S. A. (1984). The Body Esteem Scale: Multidimensional structure and sex differences on a college population. *Journal of Personality Assessment, 48,* 173–178.

Gill, D., & Strom, E. H. (1985). The effect of attentional focus on performance of an endurance task. *International Journal of Sport Psychology, 16,* 217–223.

Godin, G., Shephard, R. J., & Colantonio, A. (1986). The cognitive profile of those who intend to exercise but do not. *Public Health Reports, 101,* 521–526.

Hardy, C. J., Hall, E. G., & Presholdt, P. H. (1986). The mediational role of social influence in the perception of exertion. *Journal of Sport and Exercise Psychology, 8,* 88–104.

Hardy, C. J., & Rejeski, W. J. (1989). Not what, but how one feels: The measurement of affect during exercise. *Journal of Sport and Exercise Psychology, 11,* 304–317.

Hart, E. A., Leary, M. R., & Rejeski, W. J. (1989). The measurement of social physique anxiety. *Journal of Sport and Exercise Psychology, 11,* 94–104.

Hawkins, R. C., Turell, S., & Jackson, L. J. (1983). Desirable and undesirable masculine and feminine traits in relation to students' dieting tendencies and body image dissatisfaction. *Sex Roles, 9,* 6.

Hochstetler, S. A., Rejeski, W. J., & Best, D. L. (1985). The influence of sex-role orientation on ratings of perceived exertion. *Sex Roles, 12,* 825–835.

Hull, C. L. (1933). *Hypnosis and suggestibility.* New York: Appleton.

Hurlock, E. B. (1967). *Adolescent development.* New York: McGraw-Hill.

Kenney, E. A., Rejeski, W. J., & Messier, S. P. (1988). Managing exercise distress: The effect of broad spectrum intervention on affect, RPE, and running efficiency. *Canadian Journal of Sport Sciences, 12,* 97–105.

Kenyon, G. S. (1968). A conceptual model for characterizing physical activity. *Research Quarterly, 39,* 96–105.

King, A. C., Taylor, C. B., Haskell, W. L., & Debusk, R. F. (1988). Strategies for increasing early adherence to and long-term maintenance of home-based exercise training in healthy middle-aged men and women. *American Journal of Cardiology, 61,* 628–632.

Kolb, L. C. (1959). Disturbances of body image. In S. Arieti (Ed.), *American handbook of psychiatry* (Vol. 1, pp. 749–769). New York: Basic Books.

Lazarus, R. S. (1975). A cognitively oriented psychologist looks at biofeedback. *American Psychologist, 30,* 553–561.

Leventhal, H., & Everhart, D. (1979). Emotion, pain, and physical illness. In C. E.

Izard (Ed.), *Emotions in personality and psychopathology* (pp. 263–298). New York: Plenum.

Lindsey-Reid, E., & Osborn, R. W. (1980). Readiness for exercise adoption. *Social Science Medicine, 14,* 139–146.

Linton, J. M., Hamelink, M. H., & Hoskins, R. G. (1934). Cardiovascular system in schizophrenia studied by the Schneider method. *Archives of Neurological Psychiatry, 32,* 712–722.

Long, B. C., & Haney, C. J. (1986). Enhancing physical activity in sedentary women: Information, locus of control, and attitudes. *Journal of Sport Psychology, 8,* 8–24.

Marsella, A. J., Schizuru, L., Brennan, J., & Kameoka, J. (1981). Depression and body image satisfaction. *Journal of Cross-Cultural Psychology, 12,* 360–371.

Martin, J. E., & Dubbert, P. M. (1984). Behavioral management strategies for improving health and fitness. *Journal of Cardiac Rehabilitation, 4,* 200–208.

Martin, J. E., Dubbert, P. M., Kattell, A. D., Thompson, J. K., Raczynski, J. R., Lake, M., Smith, P. O., Webster, J. S., Sisora, T., & Cohen, R. A. (1984). Behavioral control of exercise in sedentary adults: Studies 1 through 6. *Journal of Consulting and Clinical Psychology, 52,* 795–811.

Matarazzo, J. D. (1980). Behavioral health medicine: Frontiers for a new health psychology. *American Psychologist, 42,* 893–903.

McAuley, E. (1992). Understanding exercise behavior: A self-efficacy perspective. In G. C. Roberts (Ed.), *Motivation in sport and exercise* (pp. 107–128). Chicago, IL: Human Kinetics.

McDonald, D. G., & Hodgdon, J. A. (1991). *Psychological effects of aerobic fitness training.* New York: Springer-Verlag.

Mendelson, B. K., & White, D. R. (1985). Development of self- body-esteem in overweight youngsters. *Developmental Psychology, 21* (1), 90–96.

Michael, E. D. (1957). Stress adaptation through exercise. *Research Quarterly, 28,* 50–54.

Mihevic, P. M. (1981). Sensory cues for perceived exertion: A review. *Medicine and Science in Sports and Exercise, 13,* 150–163.

Miller, T. M., Linke, J. G., & Linke, R. A. (1980). Survey on body image, weight, and diet of college students. *Journal of the American Dietetic Association, 77,* 561–566.

Morgan, W. P. (1969). Physical fitness and emotional health: A review. *American Correctional Therapy Journal, 23,* 124–127.

Morgan, W. P. (1972). Hypnosis and muscular performance. In W. P. Morgan (Ed.), *Ergogenic aids and muscular performance* (pp. 193–231). New York: Academic Press.

Morgan, W. P. (1973). Psychological factors influencing perceived exertion. *Medicine and Science in Sports, 5,* 97–103.

Morgan, W. P. (1985a). Affective beneficence of vigorous physical activity. American College of Sports Medicine Symposium: Exercise and endorphins (1983, Montreal, Canada). *Medicine and Science in Sports and Exercise, 17,* 94–100.

Morgan, W. P. (1985b). Psychogenic factors and exercise metabolism: A review. *Medicine and Science in Sports and Exercise, 17,* 309–316.

Morgan, W. P., & Horstman, D. H. (1976). Anxiety reduction following acute physical activity. *Medicine and Science in Sports, 8,* 62.

Morgan, W. P., Horstman, D. H., Cymerman, A., & Stokes, J. (1983). Facilitation of physical performance by means of a cognitive strategy. *Cognitive Therapy and Research, 7*, 251–264.

Morgan, W. P., Raven, P. B., Drinkwater, B. L., & Horvath (1973). Perceptual and metabolic responsivity to standard bicycle ergometry following various hypnotic suggestions. *International Journal of Clinical and Experimental Hypnosis, 21*, 86–101.

Nelson, L. R., & Furst, M. L. (1972). An objective study of the effects of expectation on competitive performance. *Journal of Psychology, 81*, 69–72.

Nemtzova, O. L., & Shatenstein, D. I. (1939). The effect of the central nervous system upon some physiological processes during work. (From *Psychological Abstracts*, p. 422.)

North, C. T., McCullagh, P., & Vu Tran, W. (1990). Effect of exercise on depression. In R. Terjung (Ed.), *Exercise and Sport Science Reviews, 19*, 379–415.

Oldridge, N. B., & Jones, N. L. (1983). Improving patient compliance in cardiac exercise rehabilitation: Effects of written agreement and self-monitoring. *Journal of Cardiac Rehabilitation, 3*, 257–262.

Pandolf, K. B. (1977). Psychological and physiological factors influencing perceived exertion. In G. Borg (Ed.), *Physical work and effort*. New York: Pergamon.

Petruzzello, S. J., Landers, D. M., Hatfield, B. D., Kubitz, K. A., & Salazar, W. (1991). A meta-analysis on the anxiety reducing effects of acute and chronic exercise: outcomes and mechanisms. *Sports Medicine, 11*, 143–180.

Ransford, C. P. (1982). A role for amines in the antidepressant effect of exercise: A review. *Medicine and Science in Sports and Exercise, 14*, 1–10.

Rejeski, W. J. (1981). The perception of exertion: A social psychophysiological integration. *Journal of Sport Psychology, 4*, 305–320.

Rejeski, W. J. (1985). Perceived exertion: An active or passive process? *Journal of Sport Psychology, 7*, 371–378.

Rejeski, W. J. (1992). Motivation for exercise behavior: A critique of theoretical directions. In G. C. Roberts (Ed.), *Motivation in sport and exercise* (pp. 129–158). Chicago, IL: Human Kinetics.

Rejeski, W. J., Best, D. L., Griffith, P., & Kenney, E. (1987). Sex-role orientation and the responses of men to exercise stress. *Research Quarterly for Exercise and Sport, 58*, 260–264.

Rejeski, W. J., & Brawley, L. R. (1988). Defining the boundaries of sport psychology. *The Sport Psychologist, 2*, 231–242.

Rejeski, W. J., Gregg, E., Thompson, A., & Berry, M. (1991). The effects of varying doses of aerobic exercise on psychophysiological stress responses in highly trained cyclists. *Journal of Sport and Exercise Psychology, 13*, 188–199.

Rejeski, W. J., Hardy, C. J., & Shaw, J. (1991). Psychometric confounds of assessing state anxiety in conjunction with bouts of vigorous exercise. *Journal of Sport and Exercise Psychology, 13*, 65–74.

Rejeski, W. J., & Kenney, E. (1987). Distracting attentional focus from fatigue: Does task complexity make a difference? *Journal of Sport Psychology, 9*, 66–73.

Rejeski, W. J., & Ribisl, P. M. (1980). Expected task duration and perceived effort: An attributional analysis. *Journal of Sport Psychology, 2*, 227–236.

Rejeski, W. J., & Sanford, B. (1984). Feminine-typed females: The role of affective schema in the perception of exercise intensity. *Journal of Sport Psychology, 6,* 197–207.

Riddick, C. C., & Freitag, R. S. (1984). The impact of aerobic fitness programs on the body image of older women. *Activities, Adaptation, and Aging, 6,* 59–70.

Riddle, P. K. (1980). Attitudes, beliefs, behavioral intentions, and behaviors of women and men toward regular jogging. *Research Quarterly for Exercise and Sport, 51,* 663–674.

Rodin, J. (1988). *The psychological effects of exercise.* Unpublished manuscript, Yale University.

Rohrbacker, R. (1973). Influence of special camp program for obese boys on weight loss, self-concept, and body image. *Research Quarterly, 44,* 150–157.

Rosen, G. M., & Ross, A. D. (1968). Relationship of body image to self-concept. *Journal of Consulting and Clinical Psychology, 32,* 100.

Rotter, J. B. (1954). *Social learning and clinical psychology.* Englewood Cliffs, NJ: Prentice-Hall.

Sarafino, E. P. (1990). *Health psychology: Biopsychosocial interactions.* New York: Wiley.

Schilder, P. (1935). *The image and appearance of the human body.* New York: International Universities Press.

Schonfield, W. A. (1962). Gynecomastia in adolescence: Effect on body image and personality adaptation. *Psychosomatic Medicine, 24,* 379–389.

Secord, P. F., & Jourard, S. M. (1953). The appraisal of body cathexis: Body cathexis and the self. *Journal of Consulting Psychology, 17*(5), 343–347.

Shelton, T. O., & Mahoney, M. J. (1978). The content and effect of "psyching-up" strategies in weight lifters. *Cognitive Therapy and Research, 2,* 275–284.

Silberstein, L. R., Striegel-Moore, R. H., Timko, C., & Rodin, J. (1988). Behavioral and psychological implications of body dissatisfaction: Do men and women differ? *Sex-Roles, 19,* 291–232.

Sime, W. E. (1977). A comparison of exercise and meditation in reducing physiological responses to stress. *Medicine and Science in Sports and Exercise, 9,* 55.

Simonson, E., & Weiser, P. C. (1976). Psychological and physiological correlation of work and fatigue. Springfield, IL: Charles C. Thomas.

Skinner, B. F. (1990). Can psychology be a science of mind? *American Psychologist, 45,* 1206–1209.

Skrinar, G. S., Bullen, B. A., Creek, J. M., McArthur J. W., et al. (1986). Effects of endurance training on body-consciousness in women. *Perceptual and Motor Skills, 62,* 485–490.

Sonstroem, R. J. (1982). Attitudes and beliefs in the prediction of exercise participation. In R. C. Cantu & W. J. Gillespie (Eds.), *Sports medicine, sports sciences: Bridging the gap.* Lexington, MA: Collamore Press.

Sonstroem, R. J., & Morgan, W. P. (1989). Exercise and self-esteem: Rationale and model. *Medicine and Science in Sports and Exercise, 21,* 329–337.

Steptoe, A., & Cox, S. (1988). Acute effects of aerobic exercise on mood. *Health Psychology, 7,* 329–340.

Taylor, S. E. (1986). *Health psychology.* New York: Random House.

Thorndike, E. (1912). The curve of work. *Psychological Reviews, 19,* 165–194.

Triplett, N. (1897). The dynamogenic factors in pacemaking and competition. *American Journal of Psychology, 9,* 507–553.

Tucker, L. A. (1983a). Effect of weight training on self-concept: A profile of those influenced most. *Research Quarterly for Exercise and Sport, 54,* 389–397.

Tucker, L. A. (1983b). Muscular strength and mental health. *Journal of Personality and Social Psychology, 45,* 1355–1360.

van Doornen, L. J. P., de Geus, E. J. C., & Orlebeke, J. F. (1988). Aerobic fitness and the physiological stress response: A critical evaluation. *Science and Medicine, 26,* 303–307.

Vaux, C. L. (1926). A discussion of physical exercise and recreation. *Occupational Therapy and Rehabilitation, 5,* 329–333.

Voor, V. H., Lloyd, A. J., & Cole, R. J. (1969). *Journal of Motivational Behavior, 1,* 210.

Wankel, L. M. (1984). Decision-making and social support strategies for increasing exercise involvement. *Journal of Cardiac Rehabilitation, 4,* 124–135.

Weinberg, R. S., Gould, D., Yukelson, D., & Jackson, A. (1981). The effect of pre-existing and manipulated self-efficacy on a competitive muscular endurance task. *Journal of Sport Psychology, 4,* 345–354.

Weinberg, R. S., Smith, J., Jackson, A., & Gould, D. (1984). Effect of association, dissociation and positive self-talk strategies on endurance performance. *Canadian Journal of Applied Sport Sciences, 9,* 25–32.

Weiser, P. C., Kinsman, R. A., & Stamper, D. A. (1973). Task specific symptomatology changes resulting from prolonged submaximal bicycle riding. *Medicine and Science in Sports, 5,* 79–85.

Young, M., & Reeve, G. (1980). Discrimination analysis of personality and body image factors of females differing in percent body fat. *Perceptual and Motor Skills, 50,* 547–552.

Ziegler, S. G., Klinzing, J., & Williamson, K. (1982). The effects of two stress management training programs on cardiorespiratory efficiency. *Journal of Sport Psychology, 4,* 280–289.

# PART II

## THE STATUS OF
## RELEVANT RESEARCH

# 2

# Aerobic Fitness and the Response to Psychological Stress

**DAVID S. HOLMES**

## INTRODUCTION AND BACKGROUND

Many anecdotal reports suggest that individuals who are in high levels of aerobic fitness are able to deal with psychological stress more effectively than their less-fit counterparts. Specifically, it has been suggested that when compared to less-fit individuals, those who are in good aerobic fitness will show lower cardiovascular arousal when exposed to a stress and may be less prone to the depressions and illnesses that often follow periods of stress. It has also been suggested that aerobic exercise training may aid in the psychological as well as the physical rehabilitation of cardiac patients. In this chapter, I discuss research related to each of these possibilities.

This discussion is focused primarily on the research that has been conducted in my laboratory over the past few years. Focusing on that research program gives the discussion some coherence, and I think that our findings are generally representative of those in the field in general. However, in those instances in which our findings differ in some important respect from those obtained by other investigators, I point out the differences. It is important to note that in this chapter, I limit my comments to the *effects of fitness*, and I do not discuss the *effects of acute bouts of exercise* (i.e., the feelings and responses that occur immediately after a brief period of exercise). The effects of acute bouts of exercise are interesting and important, but that research is covered in Chapter 4 by Kim Tuson and David Sinyor. It should also be noted that whenever I refer to *fitness* or *exercise* in this chapter, I am referring to *aerobic* fitness or exercise and not to anaerobic fitness or exercise. The effects of anaerobic fitness and exercise are probably very different and are not within the purview of this chapter.

For some years, my colleagues and I had been studying the stress-reducing effects of strategies such as defense mechanisms, biofeedback, and meditation. Our results were interesting from a theoretical standpoint, but they usually suggested that the strategies we were studying had little practical utility. For example, in an early line of research, we found that the use of cognitive strategies such as *redefining the situation* (e.g., "This is not a test; it's a learning exercise") or *using distracting thoughts* during times of stress resulted in statistically reliable reductions in heart rate and blood pressure, but the magnitude of the effects was small and probably not of much practical importance (cf. Bennett & Holmes, 1975; Bloom, Houston, Holmes, & Burish, 1977; Houston & Holmes, 1974). The results of our more recent research on the effects of biofeedback and meditation were even less encouraging. Those procedures were effective for reducing arousal, but they were not more effective than simply sitting quietly for a comparable length of time (for reviews, see Holmes, 1981, 1984, 1985, 1987). Being somewhat disillusioned with those lines of research, we began looking elsewhere. Probably because most of us were distance runners, we began looking at the effects of exercise and fitness. As becomes apparent in the following sections, this has been a productive line of investigation, from both theoretical and practical standpoints.[1]

---

[1]It might be noted that at the beginning of our research program, we also examined the relationship between changes in aerobic fitness and changes in personality (see Jasnoski & Holmes, 1981; Jasnoski, Holmes, & Banks, 1988; Jasnoski, Holmes, Solomon, & Aguiar, 1981). We found that changes in fitness did indeed result in changes in personality, but the meaning and mechanism of those relationships were not clear to us, and because we believed that more basic work was necessary to elucidate them, we abandoned that line of research. Understanding the response to stress may someday lead us back to the relationship between fitness and personality.

# FITNESS AND CARDIOVASCULAR AROUSAL DURING STRESS

In our first investigation in this area, we simply identified 16 undergraduate women who were highly fit and 16 who were of low fitness, then we exposed them to a mild psychological stress and monitored their heart rates, blood pressures, and self-reported levels of arousal before, during, and following the stress (McGilley & Holmes, 1988). The stressor was the digits-backward-recall test in which the experimenter read six sets of five numbers, and after each set, it was the woman's task to repeat (recall) the set of numbers (digits) in reverse order (backward).

The results yielded four interesting findings.[2] First, the highly fit women showed lower baseline (prestress) heart rates and lower systolic blood pressures than women of low fitness. That simply confirmed the differences in fitness. Second, during the stress period, the women showed increases in arousal, as measured by heart rates, blood pressures, and self-report measures, thus confirming that the stressor was effective. Third and most important, during the stress period, the highly fit women showed smaller increases in heart rate, systolic blood pressure, diastolic blood pressure, and self-reported arousal than did the women with low fitness levels. That is, not only did the highly fit women come to the test with lower baseline levels of arousal, but also the highly fit women were less reactive to the stressor than were the women with low fitness levels. Fourth, there were no differences in arousal between the highly fit women and the women with low fitness levels during the recovery period that followed the stress period. The findings concerning heart rate and systolic blood pressure are presented in Figures 2.1 and 2.2

It is important to note that in addition to being statistically reliable, the differences in arousal during the stress period were of considerable magnitude. For example, the difference in heart rate was 29.0 beats per minute (bpm), and the difference in systolic blood pressure was 13.8 millimeters of mercury (mmHg). (The differences were 11.8 bpm and 11.5 mmHg, respectively, when baseline differences were eliminated.) Those substantial differences were all the more noteworthy because they were obtained in comparisons of individuals who fell within the normal range of fitness for undergraduate students. That is, they were not obtained from comparisons of elite athletes with sedentary sluggards.

In a second investigation, we used a submaximal bicycle ergometer test to identify 10 highly fit students and 10 students with low fitness levels

---

[2]All of the effects reported in this chapter are statistically significant/reliable ($p <$ .05) unless otherwise indicated. The specific statistical techniques that were used are not discussed because their understanding is irrelevant to the points being made. For discussions of the technical issues, the reader is referred to the original articles.

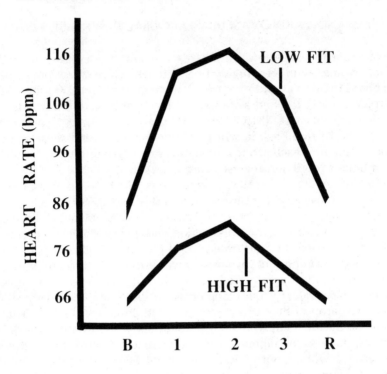

**Figure 2.1.** Highly fit women showed lower baseline heart rates and smaller increases in heart rate in response to psychological stress than did women of low fitness. (Adapted from McGilley & Holmes, 1988, Figure 3, p. 136.)

(Holmes & Roth, 1985). As was done in the earlier investigation, the students were then exposed to a mild stressor (digits-backward-recall task). Heart rates and subjective responses were assessed before, during, and following the stress. Similar to the earlier findings, the results indicated that when compared to students of low levels, the highly fit students (a) tended to have lower baseline heart rates ($p = .08$), (b) showed smaller heart-rate responses to the stress, such that there was a 19-bpm difference in heart rate during the stress, and (c) tended to have lower heart rates during the recovery period that followed the stress ($p = .09$). Unlike the earlier findings, the highly fit students and the students with low fitness levels did not report different levels of subjective arousal.

These findings linking fitness to a lower cardiovascular arousal during stress lead us to ask whether fitness might offset some of the heightened arousal during stress that is often found in individuals who have a family history of hypertension. There is a large body of data indicating that *nor-*

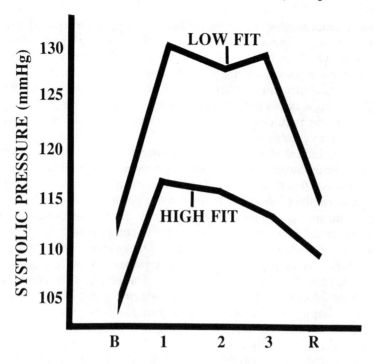

**Figure 2.2.** Highly fit women showed lower baseline systolic blood pressure and smaller increases in pressure in response to psychological stress than did women of of low fitenss. (Adapted from McGilley & Holmes, 1988, Figure 1, p. 135.)

*motensive individuals* (i.e., those with normal blood pressure) who have a *family history of hypertension* (at least one parent diagnosed as having essential hypertension) show greater *cardiovascular arousal* (heart rate and blood pressure) during stress than do individuals who do not have a family history of hypertension. Those elevated responses are of concern because they are considered to be precursors of essential hypertension and atherosclerosis. The questions we sought to answer were (a) Among individuals with a family history of hypertension, would those who are aerobically fit show lower levels of arousal during stress? and (b) Would the lower levels of arousal shown by the fit individuals who had a family history of hypertension be like the levels of arousal shown by individuals who did not have a family history of hypertension?

To answer those questions, we identified three groups of normotensive students: (1) 10 who had a family history of hypertension and who were in good aerobic condition, (2) 11 who had a family history of hypertension and who were in poor aerobic condition, (3) 21 who did not have a family history of hypertension (Holmes & Cappo, 1987). All of the students participated in a session in which their heart rates and blood pressures were assessed during a baseline period and during two stress periods. During the stress periods, the students did a serial-subtraction task (rapidly subtracting 7s from 2194) and a color/word-naming task (similar to the Stroop color-naming task, but requiring the opposite behavior—that is, reading color names that were printed in different colors).

The results indicated first that during the stress periods, the students who had a family history of hypertension and who were highly fit showed levels of arousal (heart rate, systolic blood pressure, diastolic blood pressure) that were like those of subjects who did not have a family history of hypertension, and second that the students in both of those groups showed levels of arousal that were lower than those of students who had a family history of hypertension and who had low fitness levels. In other words, aerobic fitness offset the genetic factor linking parental hypertension to high cardiovascular responsiveness in offspring. The results concerning heart rate and systolic blood pressure are presented in Figures 2.3 and 2.4.

We were happy and impressed with our findings linking fitness to cardiovascular arousal during psychological stress, but there was a problem with the findings, in that they were only correlational in nature (i.e., we had simply compared the responses of highly fit subjects and subjects having low fitness levels), and therefore, a conclusion concerning the *causal* relationship between fitness and lower arousal during stress could not be drawn. Furthermore, from the data we had collected to that point, it was not possible to determine what amount of training would be necessary to achieve the level of fitness that would result in the lower level of arousal during stress. Could the required level of fitness be achieved in a typical aerobic-conditioning class, or would it require years of intensive training to achieve the required level of fitness?

To answer the question of whether there was a causal link between fitness and arousal during stress, and to determine how much training was necessary to achieve the level of fitness that would lead to lower arousal during stress, we conducted two experiments in which we manipulated aerobic fitness and assessed the effects on arousal during stress. In the first of those experiments, 19 highly fit women and 18 women having low fitness levels participated in a training condition that involved attending an aerobic exercise class (two 50-minute meetings per week for 13 weeks), whereas 15 highly fit women and 15 women with low fitness levels participated in a no-training condition that did not involve an exercise class (Holmes & McGilley, 1987). The women's heart rates and subjective responses to stress (digits-backward-recall test) were assessed before and after the 13-week training/no-training period.

Figure 2.5 shows the heart-rate data that were collected during the stress

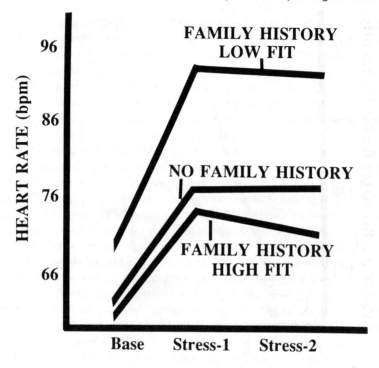

**Figure 2.3.**   Students who did not have a family history of hypertension and students who had a family history of hypertension but were highly fit showed comparable levels of heart rate during stress, and those levels were lower than the heart-rate level of students who had a family history of hypertension and had low fitness levels. (Adapted from Holmes & Cappo, 1987, Figure 1, p. 603.)

periods that occurred in the testing sessions that were conducted before and after the 13-week training/no-training period. Data are presented separately for women in the training and no-training conditions who were initially identified as highly fit or of low fitness levels. Four things are noteworthy about the findings in that figure. First, when tested before training, women with low fitness levels had higher stress-period heart rates than highly fit women, a finding that replicated our earlier finding, linking fitness to arousal during stress. Second, the women in all of the conditions had somewhat lower heart rates during the second stress session than the first, an effect that is probably simply due to the fact that the women had been through the test before, and the stressor was less stressful the second time. Third and most important, the women with low fitness levels, in the exercise condition, showed greater before-to-after training reductions in

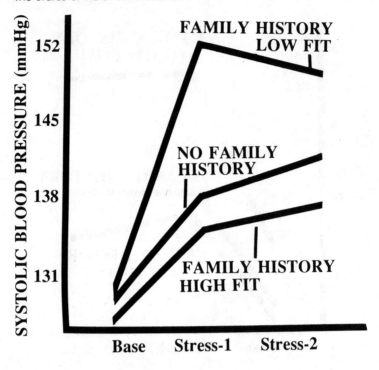

**Figure 2.4.** Students who did not have a family history of hypertension and students who had a family history of hypertension but were highly fit showed comparable levels of systolic blood pressure during stress, and those levels were lower than the blood-pressure levels of students who had a family history of hypertension and had low fitness levels. (Adapted from Holmes & Cappo, 1987, Figure 3, p. 603.)

heart rates than did the women in any other condition. That is, the aerobic training was effective for reducing heart rates during stress for women who were originally in poor aerobic condition, thereby confirming the causal relationship between fitness and arousal during stress. Finally, among highly fit women, those in the exercise condition did not show greater before-to-after training reductions in heart rates than did the women in the no-treatment condition. That was not surprising because it would not be expected that 13 weeks of mild exercise would influence the fitness (and hence the response to stress) of women who were already in good condition.

The results of the preceding experiment clearly indicated that cardiovascular arousal during stress could be reduced with a relatively brief period of exercise training, but the question arose, Is exercise training more,

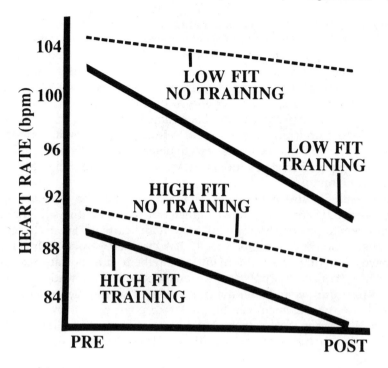

**Figure 2.5.**   Women with low fitness levels who participated in an aerobic training program showed greater before-training to after-training reductions in heart rate during stress than did women in other conditions. (Adapted from Holmes & McGilley, 1987, Figure 1, p. 371.)

equally, or less effective than other more traditional psychological interventions, such as training in relaxation and the use of mental imagery? To test the relative effectiveness of exercise versus more traditional psychological interventions, a more elaborate second experiment was conducted (Holmes & Roth, 1988). In that experiment, male and female college students who had experienced high degrees of life stress in the preceding year were assigned to one of three conditions: (1) exercise training, (2) relaxation training, and (3) no treatment. The two training conditions were structured as one-credit-hour college courses that met for a 1/2 hour 3 days per week over an 11-week period. Both courses were taught by the same instructor, who was trained in both clinical psychology and exercise physiology. Students in the exercise condition received individualized training programs that were based on pretest Balke treadmill tests, and the exercise was designed so that heart rate was maintained at approximately 75% of pre-dicted maximum. By the end of the class, most of the students were running continuously for at least 2 miles. Students in the relaxation condition were initially given training in progressive muscle relaxation (Bernstein & Given, 1984) but were also given training in other techniques, such as mental imagery (Lazarus, 1977). The students in the no-treatment condition were not seen except for testing at the beginning and the end of the 11-week period. Before and after the 11-week training/no-treatment period, stu-dents were given Balke treadmill tests to determine their fitness levels, and they were exposed to stress (digits-backward-recall test) while their heart rates were monitored.

The results of this experiment revealed first that the students in the exercise-training condition showed greater increases in fitness (higher esti-mated oxygen consumption and lower exercise heart rates) than students in the other conditions, thus indicating that the exercise manipulation was effective in altering fitness. More important, the results indicated that after the training period, students in the exercise condition showed lower heart rates before, during, and after the stress period than did the students in the relaxation or no-treatment conditions. At no point were there statistically reliable differences between the heart rates of students in the relaxation training and the no-treatment conditions. These results are presented in Figure 2.6.

Before concluding this section, some comment should be made con-cerning consistencies and inconsistencies between these findings and those reported by other investigators. Consistent with the findings in my labora-tory, a number of other investigators have also reported that during stress highly fit persons show lower cardiovascular arousal than do persons with low fitness levels (cf. Hull, Young, & Zeigler, 1984; Lake, Suarez, Schneiderman, & Tocci, 1984, but only for Type A individuals; Light, Obrist, James, & Strogatz, 1987; Roth, 1989, $p$ = .08). However, some investigators did not find the differences in arousal *during the stress period*, but instead found that highly fit persons showed lower arousal than persons with low fitness levels during a *recovery period* that occurred immediately following the stress period (Cantor, Zillman, & Day, 1978; Cox, Evans, & Jamieson, 1979; Hollander & Seraganian, 1984; Sinyor, Golden, Steinert, & Seraganian, 1986; Sinyor, Schwartz, Peronnet, Brisson, & Seraganian, 1986). That is, in this latter group of investigations, fitness did not offset arousal during the stress but hastened the recovery from the stress. At present, it is not clear why some investigations found the effects of fitness during the stress pe-riod, whereas other investigations found these effects during the recovery period. One possibility is that fitness is effective for reducing arousal during moderate but not high levels of stress, and it is effective for aiding in the recovery from high but not from moderate levels of stress. This remains to be tested.

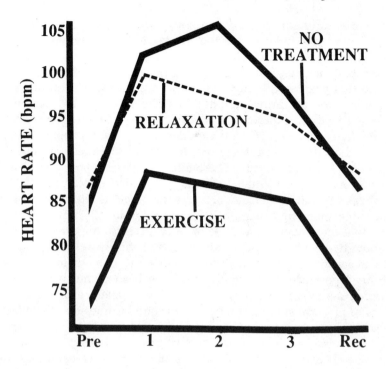

**Figure 2.6.** Students who had participated in an aerobic training program showed lower heart rates before, during, and following stress than did students who had participated in a relaxation training program or a no-treatment control condition. (Adapted from Holmes & Roth, 1988, Figure 1, p. 472.)

One other minor inconsistency in the findings related to arousal during stress should also be noted. In some investigations, it was found that the difference in arousal between highly fit individuals and persons with low fitness levels stemmed from the fact that the highly fit individuals *carried forward their lower baseline* levels of arousal *and* showed *smaller increases* in arousal during the stress, whereas in other investigations, the differences stemmed only from the fact that the highly fit individuals carried forward their lower baseline levels of arousal. These differences can be seen, for example, in comparisons of Figures 2.1 and 2.6. At present, the reason for the difference in findings is not clear. However, it might be speculated that individuals with very high levels of fitness might carry forward their low baseline levels of arousal and show less responsiveness, whereas those with only moderate levels of fitness might only carry forward their low baseline levels of arousal. This inconsistency in responsiveness and the inconsistency noted earlier concerning when the differences in arousal will occur (i.e., during either stress or recovery) do not in any way negate the effects of fitness; they simply indicate that the effects can be manifested in different ways and at different times.

Taken together, the results of these experiments provide considerable evidence that exercise training and fitness are associated with lower cardiovascular arousal during periods of psychological stress. The levels of stress used in these experiments was relatively mild and were probably comparable to the levels of stress experienced by many people during the course of their daily lives. Therefore, it appears that these findings have considerable external validity. These effects have also been found with a wide variety of individuals, a factor that also contributes to their generalizability. Finally, it is important to note that the effects were often of considerable magnitude (e.g., differences of almost 30 bpm), thus suggesting that they may very well be of some practical importance.

Although the effects we found were statistically reliable, consistent across experiments and populations, and large enough to be of some practical importance, they should not have been of much surprise. By definition, aerobically fit individuals show smaller cardiovascular responses to physical stress (exercise), and if one assumes that the effects of physical and psychological stress are comparable (e.g., elevated heart rate and blood pressure), then the effects of fitness during psychological stress should have been expected. Probably the only surprise is that it took investigators so long to begin investigating the relationship between aerobic fitness and arousal during psychological stress. With these findings as background, we can go on to examine the relationship between fitness and depression.

## FITNESS AND DEPRESSION

A second way in which the influence of fitness on stress has been tested is through the examination of the effects of fitness on depression. There are two ways in which stress can be linked to depression (one psychological and one physiological), and in each case, there are reasons to believe that exercise can serve to moderate the stress–depression relationship. First, stress (such as failure) can lead to lowered self-esteem, and the low self-esteem can lead to depression. Exercise may help to offset the development of low self-esteem because exercise can lead to tangible achievements, such as running a particular distance or improving body configuration.

Second, depression can result from low levels of certain neurotransmitters, most notably norepinephrine, in the hypothalamus. The low levels of norepinephrine can be due to genetic factors, a spontaneous breakdown in the system, or prolonged physical or psychological stress (see review by Holmes, 1991). Exercise may be effective for reducing physi-

ologically based depressions because exercise leads to increases in the production of norepinephrine in the central nervous system (see review by
Ransford, 1982).

Because of the effects that exercise can have on the self-concept and on
the levels of neurotransmitters, and because of the anecdotal reports of
"feeling good" after an acute bout of exercise, it was widely speculated that
exercise might be an effective treatment for depression. A number of well-
designed experiments have now been reported that provide support for the
antidepressant effects of aerobic exercise (see review by Simons, McGowan,
Epstein, & Kupfer, 1985).

In one of the first of those experiments, we identified 45 very depressed
undergraduate women (mean Beck depression scores of 15.53), and randomly assigned them to three conditions: (1) exercise, (2) placebo, and (3) no
treatment (McCann & Holmes, 1984). Women who were assigned to the
exercise condition were then enrolled in a rhythmical aerobic exercise class
that met for 1 hour twice per week. Those women were also required to
exercise outside of class, with the goal of achieving (including class exercise)
a total of 30 aerobic points per week (Cooper, 1968). Women in the placebo
condition were given instructions for progressive muscle relaxation, were
instructed to practice it 20 minutes per day 4 days a week, and were told that
each relaxation session should be preceded by a leisurely walk of at least 5
minutes duration. The women in both the exercise and the placebo conditions were told that the findings of recent research provided support for the
treatment they were receiving. Women who were assigned to the no-
treatment condition were told that openings were not available in the
treatment conditions, and that their treatment would have to be temporarily
postponed.

The results of this experiment indicated first that the women in the
exercise condition showed greater improvement in aerobic capacity than
did the women in the other conditions, thus providing evidence that the
exercise treatment was effective in altering fitness. Second, the results indicated that women in the exercise condition showed greater reductions in
depression than did women in either the placebo or the no-treatment conditions, and that women in the placebo and no-treatment conditions did not
differ in the degree to which their depression decreased. Notably, the
exercise-based reductions in depression were achieved by the midpoint in
treatment (i.e., after only 5 weeks). These effects are presented in Figure 2.7.
It should be noted that the greater improvement in depression in the exercise than in the placebo condition cannot be attributed to differential expectations concerning the effects of treatments because questionnaire responses
of the women indicated that the women in the two conditions had comparable expectations concerning the effectiveness of the treatments they
were undergoing.

The results of that experiment were strong and encouraging, but the

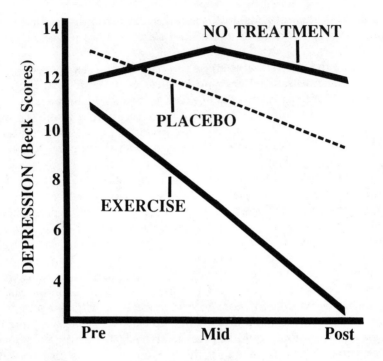

**Figure 2.7.** Among depressed women, those who participated in an aerobic-exercise training condition showed greater reductions in depression than did those who participated in relaxation exercises or in a no-treatment control condition. (Adapted from McCann & Holmes, 1984, Figure 1, p. 1145.)

experiment suffered from a problem, in that in addition to the exercise, the women in the exercise condition had a shared social and success experience (the exercise class and the physical improvements they underwent), whereas the women in the placebo condition did not, and it might be argued that the antidepressant effect was due to the social support and success experience rather than to the exercise per se. To overcome that problem and provide a better test of the effects of exercise on depression, we conducted a second experiment (Roth & Holmes, 1987). In that experiment, male and female students who had undergone high levels of life stress were assigned to (a) an aerobic-exercise training condition, (b) a relaxation-training condition, or (c) a no-treatment condition. The specific training/no-training procedures used in these conditions were described earlier, when we discussed their effects on the response to stress (see Holmes & Roth, 1988, discussed in the section, "Fitness and Cardiovascular Arousal During Stress"). Depression was assessed before, halfway through, immediately after, and 8 weeks after the 11-week training/no-treatment period.

The results of these procedures on depression are presented in Figure 2.8. Analyses of the data indicated that after participating in the program for 5 weeks (the midpoint of the program), the students in the exercise condition reported lower levels of depression than the students in the relaxation or no-treatment conditions, and that there were no differences in the levels of depression reported by students in relaxation and no-treatment conditions. The differences in depression between the exercising and nonexercising groups diminished and were no longer reliable at the end of the program, but they tended to reemerge ($p$ = .07) at the 8-week follow-up. With regard to these findings, it is particularly interesting to note that when students' expectations and impressions of the effects of the treatments were examined at the midpoint of the experiment, the students in the relaxation-training condition consistently rated their treatment higher than did the students in the exercise condition. It appears that the psychological intervention may

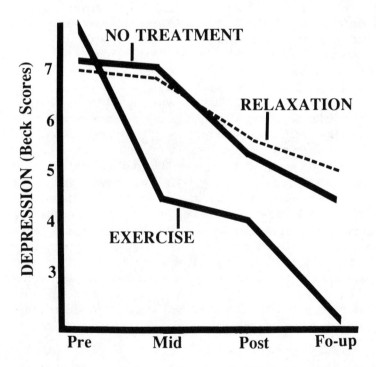

**Figure 2.8.** Among students who were experiencing high degrees of life stress, those who participated in an aerobic-exercise training program showed greater reductions in depression than did those who participated in relaxation training or in a no-treatment control condition. (Adapted from Roth & Holmes, 1987, Figure 1, p. 362.)

have had more face validity for the students, but it was the exercise intervention that actually had the greatest effect. Overall, this experiment provides strong additional evidence that aerobic exercise is associated with reductions in depression.

The results of the preceding experiments provide evidence that aerobic exercise can be an effective *treatment for depression,* but it might also be asked whether aerobic fitness is effective for *preventing the onset of depression* following prolonged psychological stress. To test that possibility, we conducted an investigation in which we identified students who either had or had not gone through a period of high life stress and who either were or were not in good aerobic fitness (Roth & Holmes, 1985). This resulted in the formation of four groups: (1) high life stress, highly fit; (2) high life stress, of low fitness levels; (3) low life stress, highly fit; and (4) low life stress, of low fitness levels. Nine weeks later, we examined the levels of depression that developed in these groups. The results indicated that the only students who developed depression were those who had experienced high life-stress and were in poor aerobic fitness. Those who had experienced high life stress and were in good aerobic fitness showed lower levels of depression, which were like those shown by students who had not experienced high life stress. The results of this investigation are presented in Figure 2.9. These findings suggest that aerobic fitness can serve a prophylactic function and can moderate the relationship between stress and depression.

These experiments, in combination with the others that have been reported (see review by Simons et al., 1985), provide consistent support for the antidepressant effects of exercise. However, it is important to recognize that although the results strongly imply that the effects of exercise on depression are mediated in large part by exercise-induced changes in the levels of neurotransmitters, at present, there is no direct evidence that the exercise increased the levels of neurotransmitters, which in turn reduced the depression. The reason we lack this evidence stems from the difficulty of measuring central nervous system neurotransmitter levels in humans. Demonstrating the exercise–neurotransmitter–mood chain is an important step that must be taken by future investigators. Having established the relationship between fitness and arousal during stress, and having demonstrated the relationship between exercise and mood, we can go on to an important practical application of fitness training: the use of fitness training in the rehabilitation of cardiac patients.

## FITNESS TRAINING IN THE REHABILITATION OF CARDIAC PATIENTS

Aerobic exercise programs are now widely used in the rehabilitation of patients following myocardial infarctions and coronary bypass surgery. The

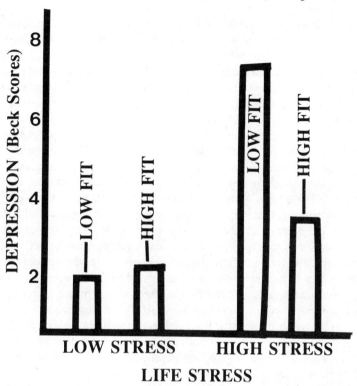

**Figure 2.9.** Follow-up data indicated that students who underwent high levels of life stress but were highly fit showed low levels of depression, which were like the levels of students who did not undergo high levels of life stress. (Adapted from Roth & Holmes, 1985, Figure 2, p. 170.)

main goals of the exercise treatment usually revolve around the rehabilitation of the cardiovascular system, but it is also possible that the treatment could have psychosocial benefits as well. Surprisingly, although exercise treatments are widely used, and there are many claims concerning their effects on a wide range of variables, evidence for their effects is minimal, and reliance on much of the existing evidence is hazardous because the investigations have been fraught with methodological problems (cf., Kentala, 1972; Mayou, 1983; McPherson et al., 1967; Naughton, Bruhn, & Lategola, 1968; Ott et al., 1983; Rechnitzer, Pickard, Paiva, Yuhasz, & Cunningham, 1972; Shaw, 1981; Stern & Cleary, 1982; Vermeulen, Lie, & Durrer, 1983). For example, (a) many of the investigations lacked controlled conditions, so comparisons could not be made; (b) biases were introduced because patients chose whether they wanted to exercise, and there were differential dropout rates across conditions; (c) in most cases, we do not know whether patients actually got the prescribed treatments because levels of exercise in the exercise and control conditions were not monitored; (d) in many cases, the exercise was not of sufficient intensity or duration to achieve the desired effects; and (e) outcome measures were often of questionable reliability and validity.

In an attempt to provide a better test of the effects of an exercise rehabilitation program on cardiac patients, we conducted an experiment in which cardiac patients were assigned to either an exercise-based rehabilitation program condition or a routine-care condition (Roviaro, Holmes, & Holmsten, 1984). The 27 patients in the exercise condition were enrolled in a 3-month program that required that they come to the hospital 3 days per week and participate in individually prescribed exercise regimens that involved walking, jogging, bicycling, and swimming. The activities were closely monitored by a cardiologist, cardiac nurses, and physical therapists. In contrast, the 19 patients who were assigned to the routine-care condition received standard medical care during the 3-month period, were given an exercise prescription but were not brought in for supervised exercise. The patients in both conditions had their levels of cardiovascular, psychological, and social functioning assessed before and after the 3-month training/care period, and their levels of psychological and social functioning were assessed again 4 months later.

The results of this investigation were quite striking and provided clear and consistent support for the beneficial impact of an exercise-based rehabilitation program on cardiac patients. Specifically, when compared to the patients in the routine-care condition, those in the exercise condition showed more efficient cardiovascular functioning, as measured by resting heart rate, resting diastolic blood pressure, treadmill performance, exercise heart rate, and exercise systolic blood pressure. Furthermore, the patients in the exercise condition evidenced more positive self-perceptions concerning health, body concept, self-concept, and progress toward personal goals. They also showed better psychosocial functioning, as reflected in decreased employment-related emotional stress, increased household activities, more frequent sexual activity, and more strenuous physical activities.

Unfortunately, the picture was not as positive 6 years later when we collected follow-up data on 26 of the patients from the original group (McGilley, Holmes, & Holmsten, 1991). Specifically, during the follow-up period, the patients in the exercise condition showed decreases in treadmill performance, decreases in body concept, decreases in ratings of current health, decreases in expected future health, increases in the degree to which they were overweight, and increases in depression. As a consequence of these changes, the initial benefits of the program were eliminated, and after the 6-year follow-up period, the patients in the exercise condition were functioning at levels like or *below* those of patients in a routine-care condition. Had the exercise program not had an effect, or worse—had it actually had long-term negative effects? The answer to both questions is, "no." The changes in functioning were due to the fact that during the 6-year follow-up period, the patients in the exercise condition reduced the frequency, duration, and intensity of their exercise, whereas those in the routine-care condition tended to increase their exercise. The mistake we made was not in treating our patients with exercise, but in presenting the exercise as a *time-limited treatment* rather than as a *change in life-style* that had to be maintained. At the end of the treatment period, the patients in the exercise condition considered themselves "cured" and stopped exercising, just as one would stop taking medication at the end of a treatment period. From these investigations, we learned that exercise was effective for overcoming the problems of cardiac patients, but we also learned an important lesson about how to present exercise to the patients.

## EXERCISE, THE IMMUNE SYSTEM, AND ILLNESS

Numerous investigators have reported that a high level of life stress often precedes the onset of physical illness (see reviews by Dohrenwend & Dohrenwend, 1974, and Jemmott & Locke, 1984). This relationship appears to be due to the fact that psychological stress reduces the functioning of the immune system (e.g., reduces the production of disease-fighting lymphocytes), and the reduced functioning of the immune system leaves the individual at increased risk for developing a physical illness. There are two reasons why aerobic fitness and exercise may moderate the stress–illness relationship. First, if fitness reduces the response to stress (see earlier discussion), then highly fit individuals would experience less stress; consequently, the functioning of their immune systems would be less likely to be reduced, and the individuals would be less likely to become ill than less fit individuals. Second, there is some evidence to suggest that aerobic exercise increases the functioning of the immune system (e.g., Edwards et al., 1984; Hedfors, Holm, Ivansen, & Wahren, 1983; Landmann et al., 1984). That is, an acute bout of strenuous aerobic exercise will increase the levels of the various lymphocytes that are crucial in fighting disease, and therefore, exercising individuals would be less likely to become ill.

To examine the role that fitness plays in the stress–illness relationship, we conducted two investigations. In the first investigation, we identified individuals who either had or had not recently experienced high degrees of life stress, and who either were or were not in good aerobic condition (Roth & Holmes, 1985). This resulted in the formation of four groups: (1) high life stress, highly fit; (2) high life stress, with low fitness levels; (3) low life stress, highly fit; and (4) low life stress, low levels of fitness. We then examined the incidence of subsequent physical illnesses in those four groups of individuals. The results were clear: Psychological stress was related to high levels of physical illness, but only among individuals with low fitness levels. Indeed, individuals who had experienced high degrees of life stress but who were in good aerobic condition did not show higher levels of physical illness than did individuals who had not experienced high degrees of life stress. These results are presented in Figure 2.10.

Buoyed by these findings, we conducted a second investigation, in which we experimentally manipulated fitness, in an attempt to intervene in the stress–illness relationship (Roth & Holmes, 1987). That is, we wanted to determine whether an increase in the fitness levels of individuals who were

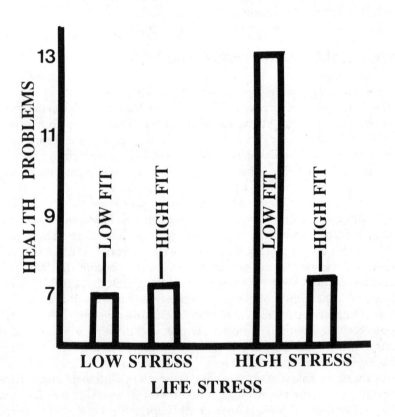

Figure 2.10.    Follow-up data indicated that students who underwent high levels of life stress but were highly fit showed low levels of physical illness, which were like those of students who did not undergo high levels of life stress. (Adapted from Roth & Holmes, 1985, Figure 1, p. 169.)

undergoing stress could reduce their subsequent levels of illness. In this experiment, we randomly assigned individuals who had recently undergone a high degree of life stress to one of three conditions: (1) aerobic exercise training, (2) relaxation training, or (3) no treatment. (For a discussion of the procedures used in these conditions, see the earlier discussion of Roth & Holmes, 1987, in the section on "Fitness and Depression.") The results indicated that when compared to the individuals in the relaxation and the no-treatment conditions, those in the exercise condition showed greater improvements in fitness, a reduction in the cardiovascular response to stress, and a reduction in depression, but they did *not* show lower levels of physical illnesses. That is, although exercise training had all of the other expected effects, it did not reduce the level of physical illness. There are two possible explanations for the lack of effect on illness. First and most likely, fitness may serve a prophylactic function but not a treatment function. That is, if the effects of stress are to be warded off, the individual must be in good condition when the stress occurs. Getting in shape after the onset of stress may be like closing the gate after the horse has escaped. The second possible explanation is that the relationship between fitness and wellness following stress is due to some third variable, such as diet. We could not find evidence for a mediating variable, but that does not preclude the existence of one. Overall, then, it appears that aerobic fitness may moderate the relationship between psychological stress and physical illness, but for that to occur, the individual must be in good shape when the stress occurs. In view of the costs associated with illness and the other positive side effects of aerobic fitness, this line of investigation deserves additional attention.

## SUMMARY AND COMMENTS

The research that I have reviewed here provides consistent evidence that aerobic fitness plays an important role in determining the way in which humans respond to stress. Specifically, it indicates that (a) fitness is associated with lower levels of cardiovascular arousal during and following psychological stress, (b) relatively brief exercise training programs can be effective for reducing arousal during psychological stress, (c) relatively brief exercise training programs can be effective for reducing depression, (d) fitness is associated with lower levels of depression following prolonged life stress, (e) exercise training programs can be effective for improving the cardiovascular and psychosocial functioning of cardiac patients, and (f) fitness is associated with lower levels of physical illness following prolonged life stress.

The breadth and consistency of these findings is impressive, but even more impressive is the magnitude of the findings. In addition to being statistically reliable (significant), the effects are generally large. As I pointed out in the introduction to this chapter, in my laboratory we have studied a variety of stress-reducing strategies, including traditional defense mechanisms, other cognitive-coping techniques, biofeedback, and meditation. The effects of those strategies pale when compared to the effects of aerobic fitness and exercise training. There is no doubt that aerobic fitness and exercise play a crucial role in reducing the effects of stress, and the challenge before us now is to implement what we know.

## REFERENCES

Bennett, D., & Holmes, D. S. (1975). Influence of denial (situation redefinition) and projection on anxiety associated with threat to self-esteem. *Journal of Personality and Social Psychology, 32,* 915–921.

Bernstein, D., & Given, B. (1984). Progressive relaxation: Abbreviated methods. In R. Woolfolk & P. Lehrer (Eds.), *Principles and practice of stress management.* New York: Guilford Press.

Bloom, L. J., Houston, B. K., Holmes, D. S., & Burish, T. (1977). The effectiveness of attentional diversion and situation redefinition for reducing stress due to a nonambiguous threat. *Journal of Research in Personality, 11,* 83–94.

Cantor, J. R., Zillmann, D., & Day, K. D. (1978). Relationship between cardiorespiratory fitness and physiological response to films. *Perceptual and Motor Skills, 46,* 1123–1130.

Cooper, K. C. (1968). *Aerobics.* New York: Bantom Books.

Cox, J. P., Evans, J. F., & Jamieson, J. L. (1979). Aerobic power and tonic heart rate response to psychosocial stressors. *Personality and Social Psychology Bulletin, 5,* 160–163.

Dohrenwend, B. S., & Dohrenwend, B. P. (1974). *Stressful life events.* New York: Wiley.

Edwards, A. J., Bacon, T. H., Elms, C. A., Veradi, R., Felder, M., & Knight, S. C. (1984). Changes in the populations of lymphoid cells in human peripheral blood following physical exercise. *Clinical and Experimental Immunology, 58,* 420–427.

Hedfors, E., Holm, G., Ivansen, M., & Wahren, J. (1983). Physiological variation of blood lymphocyte reactivity: T-cell subsets, immunoglobulin production, and mixed lymphocyte reactivity. *Clinical Immunology and Immunopathology, 27,* 9–14.

Hollander, B. J., & Seraganian, P. (1984). Aerobic fitness and psychophysiological reactivity. *Canadian Journal of Behavioral Science, 16,* 257–261.

Holmes, D. S. (1981). The Uue of biofeedback for treating patients with migraine headaches, Raynaud's disease and hypertension: A critical evaluation. In L. Bradley & C. Prokop (Eds.), *Medical psychology: A new perspective* (pp. 423–437). New York: Academic Press.

Holmes, D. S. (1984). Meditation and somatic arousal reduction: A review of the experimental evidence. *American Psychologist, 39,* 1–10.

Holmes, D. S. (1985). Self-control of somatic arousal: An examination of meditation and biofeedback. *American Behavioral Scientist, 28,* 486–496.

Holmes, D. S. (1987). The influence of meditation versus rest on physiological arousal: A second examination. In M. West (Ed.), *The psychology of meditation* (pp. 81–103). Oxford, England: Oxford University Press.

Holmes, D. S. (1991). *Abnormal psychology*. New York: HarperCollins.

Holmes, D. S., & Cappo, B. M. (1987). Prophylactic effect of aerobic fitness on cardiovascular arousal among individuals with a family history of hypertension. *Journal of Psychosomatic Research, 31*, 601–605.

Holmes, D. S., & McGilley, B. M. (1987). Influence of a brief aerobic training program on heart rate and subjective response to stress. *Psychosomatic Medicine, 49*, 366–374.

Holmes, D. S., & Roth, D. L. (1985). Association of aerobic fitness with pulse rate and subjective responses to psychological stress. *Psychophysiology, 22*, 525–529.

Holmes, D. S., & Roth, D. L. (1988). Effects of aerobic exercise training and relaxation training on cardiovascular activity during psychological stress. *Journal of Psychosomatic Research, 32*, 469–474.

Houston, B. K., & Holmes, D. S. (1974). Effectiveness of avoidant thinking and reappraisal in coping with threat involving temporal uncertainty. *Journal of Personality and Social Psychology, 30*, 382–388.

Hull, E. M., Young, S. H., & Zeigler, M. G. (1984). Aerobic fitness affects cardiovascular and catecholamine responses to stressors. *Psychophysiology, 21*, 353–360.

Jasnoski, M., & Holmes, D. S. (1981). Influence of initial aerobic fitness, aerobic training, and changes in aerobic fitness on personality functioning. *Journal of Psychosomatic Research, 25*, 553–556.

Jasnoski, M., Holmes, D. S., & Banks, D. (1988). Changes in personality associated with changes in aerobic and anaerobic fitness in women and men. *Journal of Psychosomatic Research, 32*, 273–276.

Jasnoski, M., Holmes, D. S., Solomon, S., & Aguiar, C. (1981). Exercise, changes in aerobic capacity, and changes in self-perception: An experimental investigation. *Journal of Research in Personality, 15*, 460–466.

Jemmott, J. B., & Locke, S. E. (1984). Psychosocial factors, immunologic mediation, and human susceptibility to infectious diseases: How much do we know? *Psychological Bulletin, 95*, 78–108.

Kentala, E. (1972). Physical fitness and feasibility of physical rehabilitation after myocardial infarction in men of working age. *Annals of Clinical Research, 4.,1*.

Lake, B. W., Suarez, E. C., Schneiderman, N., & Tocci, N. (1985). The Type A behavior pattern, physical fitness, and psychophysiological reactivity. *Health Psychology, 4*, 169–187.

Landmann, R. M., Muller, F. B., Perini, C., Wesp, M., Erne, P., & Buhler, R. R. (1984). Changes of immunoregulatory cells induced by psychological and physical stress: Relationship to plasma catecholamines. *Clinical and Experimental Immunology, 58*, 127–135.

Lazarus, A. (1977). *In the mind's eye: The power of imagery for personal enrichment*. New York: Guilford Press.

Light, K. C., Obrist, P. A., James, S. A., & Strogatz, D. S. (1987). Cardiovascular responses to stress: II. Relationships to aerobic exercise patterns. *Psychophysiology, 24,* 79–86.

Mayou, R. (1983). A controlled trial of early rehabilitation after myocardial infarction. *Journal of Cardiac Rehabilitation, 3,* 397–402.

McCann, I. L., & Holmes, D. S. (1984). Influence of aerobic exercise on depression. *Journal of Personality and Social Psychology, 46,* 1142–1147.

McGilley, B. M., & Holmes, D. S. (1988). Aerobic fitness and response to psychological stress. *Journal of Research in Personality, 22,* 129–139.

McGilley, B. M., Holmes, D. S., & Holmsten, D. (1991). *The effects of an exercise-based cardiac rehabilitation program on cardiac patients: A seven-year follow-up.* Manuscript submitted for publication.

McPherson, B., Paivo, A., Ynasz, M., Rechnitzer, P., Pickard, H., & Lefcoe, N. (1967). Psychological effects of an exercise program for postinfarct and normal adult men. *Journal of Sports Medicine and Physical Fitness, 7,* 95–102.

Naughton, J., Bruhn, J., & Lategola, M. (1968). Effects of physical training of physiological and behavioral characteristics of cardiac patients. *Archives of Physical Medicine and Rehabilitation, 49,* 131–137.

Ott, C., Sivarajan, E., Newton, K., Almes, M., Bruce, R., Bergner, M., & Gilson, B. (1983). A controlled randomized study of early cardiac rehabilitation: The Sickness Impact Profile as an assessment tool. *Heart & Lung, 12,* 162–170.

Ransford, C. P. (1982). A role for amines in the antidepressant effects of exercise: A review. *Medicine and Science in Sports, 14,* 1–10.

Rechnitzer, P., Pickard, H., Paivo, A., Yuhasz, M., & Cunningham, D. (1972). Long-term follow-up study of survival and recurrence rates following myocardial infarction in exercise and control subjects. *Circulation, 45,* 853–857.

Roth, D. L. (1989). Acute emotional and psychophysiological effects of aerobic exercise. *Psychophysiology, 26,* 593–602.

Roth, D. L., & Holmes, D. S. (1985). Influence of physical fitness in determining the impact of stressful life events on physical and psychological health. *Psychosomatic Medicine, 47,* 164–173.

Roth, D. L., & Holmes, D. S. (1987). Influence of aerobic exercise training and relaxation training on physical and psychological health following stressful life events. *Psychosomatic Medicine, 49,* 355–365.

Roviaro, S., Holmes, D. S., & Holmsten, D. (1984). Influence of a cardiac rehabilitation program on the cardiovascular, psychological, and social functioning of cardiac patients. *Journal of Behavioral Medicine, 7,* 61–81.

Shaw, L. (1981). Effects of a prescribed supervised exercise program on mortality and cardiovascular morbidity in patients after a myocardial infarction. *American Journal of Cardiology, 48,* 39–46.

Simons, A. D., McGowan, C. R., Epstein, L. H., & Kupfer, D. J. (1985). Exercise as a treatment for depression: An update. *Clinical Psychology Review, 5,* 553–568.

Sinyor, D., Golden, M., Steinert, Y., & Seraganian, P. (1986). Experimental manipulation of aerobic fitness and the response to psychosocial stress: Heart rate and self-report measures. *Psychosomatic Medicine, 48,* 324–337.

Sinyor, D., Schwartz, S. G., Peronnet, F., Brisson, G., & Seraganian, P. (1983). Aerobic fitness level and reactivity to psychosocial stress: Physiological, biochemical, and subjective measures. *Psychosomatic Medicine, 45,* 205–217.

Stern, M., & Cleary, P. (1982). The National Exercise and Heart Disease Project: Long-term psychosocial outcome. *Archives of Internal Medicine, 142,* 1093–1097.

Vermeulen, A., Lie, K., & Durrer, D. (1983). Effects of cardiac rehabilitation after myocardial infarction: Changes in coronary risk factors and long-term prognosis. *American Heart Journal, 105,* 798–801.

# 3

# Conceptualization and Quantification of Aerobic Fitness and Physical Activity

STEPHEN H. BOUTCHER

The relationship between aerobic fitness and psychological processes is currently receiving increased attention from psychophysiologists and exercise and health psychologists. The results of research examining the effect of fitness on phenomena such as cardiac reactivity to stressors (van Doornen, de Geus, & Orlebeke, 1988), affect (Boutcher & Landers, 1986), and personality (Dienstbier, 1984), however, are equivocal. Much of this equivocality appears to have been created by conceptualization and quantification issues regarding aerobic fitness and physical activity (Boutcher, 1990). Consequently, the first section of this chapter discusses aspects of physical fitness, physical activity, and physiological fitness that should be considered when examining exercise and psychological relationships. The second section outlines the strengths and weaknesses of laboratory and field measures of aerobic power and of questionnaire assessments of physical activity.

## CONCEPTUAL ISSUES

Past research examining exercise and psychological phenomena has generally focused on the aerobic component of fitness. For instance, researchers examining the influence of cardiac reactivity to psychological stressors have wondered whether fitter individuals possess less cardiac reactivity to psychological stressors, compared to their unfit counterparts. Typically, researchers have assessed subjects' aerobic fitness (usually inadequately; see next section) and have then compared the cardiac responses of fit and unfit groups. Unfortunately, these researchers, like others in related areas, have failed to consider the complexity of aerobic fitness. The major problems across areas have been the failure to address a number of important characteristics of aerobic fitness (e.g., the influences of training and of heredity on aerobic power) and the use of inappropriate fitness-assessment techniques. Thus, past research has not considered what aspect of aerobic fitness may cause fitter subjects to display different psychological or behavioral responses. Furthermore, in studies that have shown that fitter subjects do exhibit different responses, the specific physiological mechanisms underlying these changes have not been examined (see Boutcher, 1990). Finally, the most valid and reliable ways of assessing aerobic fitness and physical activity have generally not been utilized. These types of problems emerge in all areas of exercise-psychology research that focuses on aerobic fitness as a variable of interest. To throw light on some of these issues, the characteristics of physical fitness, physical activity, and physiological fitness are briefly described, after which suggestions for future research are outlined.

### Physical Fitness

*Physical fitness* is a complex phenomenon that is generally viewed as the ability to perform muscular work (Bouchard, Shephard, Stephens, Sutton, & McPherson, 1990). Components of overall physical fitness include flexibility, body composition, muscular strength and endurance, anaerobic ability, and aerobic ability (Skinner, Baldini, & Gardner, 1990). *Aerobic fitness*, which is the focus of this chapter, is the capability to consume oxygen and is determined by the integrated performance of the cardiovascular, pulmonary, vascular, and muscular systems (for a review of other components, see

McArdle, Katch, & Katch, 1986). *Aerobic power* is the largest volume of oxygen the body can utilize per minute and is expressed as maximal oxygen uptake or $\dot{V}O_2$ max. Although cardiovascular, metabolic, and respiratory changes accompany repetitive bouts of aerobic exercise, the biggest influence on aerobic power appears to be heredity. Thus, inheriting an efficient cardiovascular system that is suitable for high levels of aerobic work is a prerequisite for those individuals aspiring to be elite middle- and long-distance runners. The training and heredity components of aerobic power should be considered when selecting subjects and identifying underlying mechanisms that may be influencing the phenomenon of interest.

The influence of hereditary factors on aerobic fitness has largely been ignored in past research. For instance, examination of identical twins has shown that heredity alone can account for more than 90% of the observed differences in aerobic power, as measured by $\dot{V}O_2$ max (Klissouras, 1971; Klissouras, Pirnay, & Petit, 1973). Although a 1986 study has indicated that these twin studies may represent the upper limits of genetic influence (Bouchard et al.), the research in this area overall indicates that aerobic power is significantly influenced by heredity (Bouchard & Lortie, 1984; Bouchard & Malina, 1983). Thus, subjects assessed as aerobically fit through $\dot{V}O_2$ max testing may possess high genetic aerobic power but may not have physiologically adapted to aerobic exercise. Therefore, an untrained individual with a high $\dot{V}O_2$ max may be able to run a similar length of time on the treadmill as a trained runner possessing a similar $\dot{V}O_2$ max, but the untrained subject would not be able to run at the same intensity in longer exercise situations (e.g., a 10-km race) because such a person's slow-twitch fibers are not metabolically adapted to more lengthy, submaximal aerobic exercise. Consequently, aerobic fitness assessment by $\dot{V}O_2$ max alone confounds physiological status and exercise participation. If adaptation responses to aerobic exercise are the research foci, then examining untrained, genetically fit individuals may be inappropriate. Of course, hereditary influences on aerobic fitness are an important area of research in their own right (see Malina & Bouchard, 1984).

A 1990 study from my laboratory underscores the issue of heredity and training for cardiac-reactivity research (Boutcher, Nugent, & Weltman). This study compared the cardiac responses to physiological stressors among three groups of subjects: (1) 10 trained male runners possessing low resting heart rates (HRs), (2) 10 untrained males with inherently low resting HRs, and (3) 10 unconditioned males with normal resting HRs. All subjects completed a $\dot{V}O_2$ max test and on a separate occasion also completed easy and hard mental arithmetic and the Stroop task. It was hypothesized that although the runners and the low-inherent-HR group possessed similar low resting HRs, the runners would exhibit less of a cardiac response during the stressors and a quicker poststress recovery. Thus, possessing resting bradycardia (HR less than 60 beats per minute) as a result of both training and heredity would provide a greater buffer to the cardiac response to stressors than just bradycardia brought about by heredity influences alone. Surprisingly, the results indicated that both the runners and the low-inherent-HR groups had practically identical stressor responses. Both groups had significantly lower absolute HR responses during and when recovering from stressors, in comparison to the control group. Thus, both trained bradycardia and inherently untrained bradycardia appear to significantly reduce absolute HR response to psychological stressors. Interestingly, the $\dot{V}O_2$ max of the inherent group was substantially higher than that expected for sedentary males of this age. Consequently, low resting HR in healthy, asymptomatic males may reflect a more efficient cardiovascular system, which in turn may be responsible for a higher-than-average $\dot{V}O_2$ max. These data suggest that both the training and the heredity components of aerobic fitness can influence cardiac reactivity to psychological stressors and should be considered when examining these kinds of relationships.

A related issue is the breadth of physiological adaptations occurring through exposure to regular aerobic exercise. For most aerobic activities, major adaptations occur in the oxygen transport system, in the oxidative potential of the exercising musculature, and in the autonomic and endocrine systems. As $\dot{V}O_2$ max is mostly influenced by the increase in stroke volume accompanying training, many noncardiac adaptations are not assessed by $\dot{V}O_2$ max. Also, other physiological changes occurring through regular exercise can occur independently of $\dot{V}O_2$ max. For instance, decrease in blood pressure (Seals & Hagberg, 1984) and improvement in glucose tolerance (Bjorntorp, 1976) have been observed in training studies without changes in $\dot{V}O_2$ max. The important point is that $\dot{V}O_2$ max alone may not provide a full picture of the training effect. Thus, the effects of a wide range of central and peripheral adaptations on psychological and behavioral variables should be examined to better understand the aerobic fitness–psychology relationship.

Also, few researchers have attempted to examine the underlying mechanisms common to both aerobic adaptation and the psychological phenomenon of interest. Instead, researchers have attempted to correlate aerobic fitness with phenomena such as reduced autonomic reactivity. Van Doornen and coworkers (van Doornen, de Geus, & Orlebeke, 1988) have argued that research should focus on measurement of complex response patterns instead of isolated parameters. They have also called for a reevaluation of assumptions concerning aerobic exercise and phenomena such as cardiovascular reactivity to psychological stress by pointing out that the physiological response to aerobic exercise and psychological stress share only a superficial similarity. Thus, the identification and integration of mechanisms involved in the training adaptation response with psychological and behavioral phenomena is an important challenge for future research.

## Physical Activity

Performance of activities such as running, cycling, and swimming are termed *aerobic*, as they involve the use of large muscles and depend on the body's ability to use oxidative energy systems. In contrast, activities such as weight lifting, football, and sprinting are described as *anaerobic*, as they are usually performed at maximal intensity over short periods of time and are not dependent on oxidative energy systems (Piehl, 1974). *Physical activity* involves any aerobic or anaerobic movement that results in energy expenditure. Physical activity can occur during occupation or leisure time; thus, individuals can be relatively active yet record comparatively low aerobic fitness levels. In contrast, because of the large hereditary component of aerobic fitness, some people can be sedentary yet record relatively high levels of aerobic power. Consequently, to differentiate between these kinds of individuals, researchers must validly assess both the physical activity patterns of subjects and their aerobic fitness.

Level of physical adaptation to aerobic exercise is another factor that should be considered. Major cardiovascular and metabolic adaptations occur with regular aerobic exercise, such as running and cycling (Karvonen, 1949). However, these adaptations will only occur at or above a certain intensity, frequency, and duration of exercise. The American College of Sports Medicine (1978) has suggested that the minimum aerobic exercise training program needed to bring about significant physiological changes resulting in increased $\dot{V}O_2$ max is a regimen consisting of 3–5 sessions per week, at an intensity of 60–75% maximum, for longer than 20 minutes, for a duration of 15 to 20 weeks. In the exercise-psychology literature, researchers using cross-sectional designs have typically examined individuals involved in low to moderate aerobic and anaerobic exercise. The disadvantages of using individuals engaged in low-intensity aerobic or anaerobic exercise (e.g., light jogging, golf, weight lifting) is that these activities are unlikely to bring about physiological adaptations to aerobic exercise (American College of Sports Medicine, 1978).

Thus, the major differences between those individuals who exercise at very low intensity levels and sedentary persons are likely to be body composition and psychological factors such as attitude, motivation, and personality disposition. Consequently, the influence of physiological adaptation to aerobic exercise cannot be examined unless subjects have undergone a moderately intensive aerobic program.

The advantage of using trained individuals as subjects for research (e.g., elite runners) is that they have typically undergone major physiological changes as a result of exercise programs that may have been in progress for many years. The disadvantages are that results could be influenced by self-selecting variables such as personality dispositions, attitude, and socioeconomic background. For instance, appraisal processes and coping strategies of trained athletes and sedentary individuals may differ. Thus, trained athletes may try harder during testing because they may adopt a more competitive attitude and they also may possess more efficient coping strategies developed from the experience of athletic competition. Consequently, a cross-sectional design may not differentiate between the effect of appraisal and coping and that of increased fitness.

A training experiment eliminates the self-selection problem if subjects are randomly assigned to treatments and there is no substantial attrition rate. Although, the attrition rate for nonexercisers involved in a training program for the first time is typically high (Dishman, 1988), motivational strategies have been used to prevent dropout in recent training studies (Sinyor, Golden, Steinert, & Seraganian, 1986; Stein & Boutcher, 1990). However, if significant subject attrition does occur, it could negatively affect randomization. It is also difficult to obtain a genuine random sample, as subjects who volunteer to participate in an exercise program may differ from nonvolunteers in many ways. Randomly assigning a sample of volunteer exercisers to either a control or an exercise group eliminates problems with volunteer self-selection. However, as nonvolunteers cannot be coerced into participating in the exercise program, samples will be biased toward the characteristics of those individuals who are motivated to volunteer. In this situation, extensive biometric information (e.g., weight, height, socioeconomic status, level of motivation, and personality disposition) would help to assess the generalizability of the results.

The length of the training program used poses another issue. Past research using either longitudinal or training studies to examine the influence of fitness on psychological variables has typically conducted shorter exercise programs (varying from 5 to 10 weeks) at light to moderate intensity. Thus, training programs of less than 10 weeks and of low intensity may not be adequate to bring about significant physiological adaptations. Also, absolute posttraining $\dot{V}O_2$ max of previously untrained individuals in short-term training programs are typically substantially lower than $\dot{V}O_2$ max of athletes who have exercised intensively for many years. Thus, level of adaptation to exercise and its corresponding effect on psychological and behavioral variables is another important consideration for future research.

## Physiological Fitness

*Physiological fitness* refers to other biological systems that may or may not be affected by physical activity. Variables include blood pressure, glucose tolerance, blood lipoprotein levels, body composition, and fat distribution (Williams & Wallace, 1989). The important point is that active or fit individuals are not necessarily healthy. Thus, even highly trained athletes may have elevated blood pressures or high blood lipid levels. In some areas of exercise-psychology research, the physiological fitness of the subjects may be an important variable to consider.

It can be seen from these definitions that clear differences exist among physical activity, physical fitness, and physiological fitness. Unfortunately, researchers examining exercise/psychology phenomena have typically failed to differentiate among these different aspects. For example, numerous studies have used a single measure of aerobic fitness, such as a single submaximal fitness test, to differentiate between fit and unfit individuals. Unfortunately, individuals recording high fitness levels on such tests need not necessarily be physically active because as already discussed, the hereditary component of aerobic fitness is high. As mentioned previously, subjects classified as fit may be highly adapted to aerobic exercise or may not possess any physiological adaptations at all. Furthermore, subjects' physiological fitness and health may also influence psychological processes and consequently should be considered. Other individual characteristics that also could influence the relationship between exercise and psychological phenomena are life-style habits (e.g., smoking and diet) and personal factors (e.g., gender, socioeconomic status, age, and psychological characteristics).

Figure 3.1 illustrates the possible relationships and kinds of factors that should be considered when conducting research into exercise/psychological phenomena. This figure implies that although physical activity, physical fitness, and physiological fitness are related, each component has unique characteristics that should be considered. Furthermore, these components

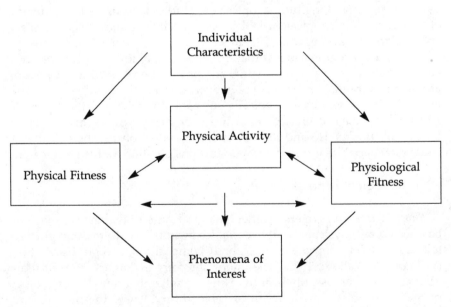

**Figure 3.1.** Potential relationships among aspects of aerobic fitness, individual differences, and the phenomena of interest.

can be influenced by heredity, levels of physical adaptation, type of fitness assessment, and individual characteristics. The implications of these inter- acting components for exercise/psychology research is that researchers must fine-tune their question of interest and must be cognizant of other factors that may confound their results.

Thus, any examination of the exercise/psychology relationship must carefully consider which aspect of the physical activity, physical fitness, and physiological fitness relationship is to be studied. For example, if the re- search question focuses on physiological adaptations to training, then a longitudinal training study should be the preferred method of investiga- tion. If a cross-sectional design is used instead, then physiological adapta- tions to the exercise stimulus should be documented. For instance, aerobic power, activity patterns, and resting bradycardia of fit subjects could be assessed (see Boutcher, 1990). Finally, individual characteristics that may affect the phenomenon (Figure 3.1) under examination should be assessed. Thus, especially in cross-sectional designs, individual factors such as diffi- culty of task, pre- and posttask anxiety and affect levels, and psychological characteristics should be measured.

## Summary

Physical fitness, physical activity, and physiological fitness are phenom- ena that possess unique characteristics. Consequently, these factors should be viewed as interacting components of the total exercise/psychology pic- ture. The effect of heredity, both as an underlying mechanism and as a confounding variable, should be considered. Also, the nature and kind of physiological adaptation to the exercise stimulus should be taken into ac- count. Finally, the influence of individual characteristics on the phenom- enon of interest should also be considered.

## QUANTIFICATION OF AEROBIC FITNESS

Aerobic fitness can be assessed by a variety of methods, such as labo- ratory, field, and questionnaire assessment. As the validity and reliability of these measures differ, not all are suited for exercise-psychology research. The following discussion describes the major techniques of assessing aerobic fitness and physical activity, including the relative strengths and weaknesses of each.

### Maximal Oxygen Uptake ($\dot{V}O_2$ max)

$\dot{V}O_2$ *max* (maximal oxygen uptake) is the standard measure of aerobic fitness and is typically quantified in milliliters of oxygen consumed per minute, adjusted for body size. For example, the $\dot{V}O_2$ max of sedentary males typically ranges from 35 to 50 mL/kg/minute (McArdle, Katch, & Katch, 1986), whereas the $\dot{V}O_2$ max of elite male runners generally exceeds 70 mL/kg/minute. Measuring $\dot{V}O_2$ max involves determining pulmonary ventilation and the concentration of $O_2$ and $CO_2$ in the expired air of subjects who have been exercised to exhaustion (for full descriptions of the $\dot{V}O_2$max test, see American College of Sports Medicine, 1986; Wasserman, Hansen, Sue, & Whipp, 1987). The $\dot{V}O_2$ max can be determined using various forms of exercise, although treadmill walking or running or bicycle ergometry are usually employed. The $\dot{V}O_2$ max is routinely assessed in exercise laboratories, and the interfacing of computers with treadmills has made the procedure relatively straightforward.

Directly measured $\dot{V}O_2$ max is a reliable and valid measure of aerobic power and is considered by many exercise physiologists to be the "gold standard" of aerobic fitness assessment. As mentioned previously, one shortcoming of the direct $\dot{V}O_2$ max test concerns the high genetic influence on aerobic power. As genetic inheritance has been estimated to account for approximately 60–93% of aerobic power (Bouchard & Lortie, 1984; Klissouras, 1971; Klissouras, Pirnay, & Petit, 1973), one administration of the test cannot differentiate between hereditary and training influences on $\dot{V}O_2$ max.

## Lactate Threshold

Although $\dot{V}O_2$ max is typically viewed as the best measure of cardiovascular fitness other researchers have argued that lactate threshold is a better measure of physiological adaptation to aerobic exercise (Weltman, Snead, Seip, Schurer, Levine, & Rogol, 1987; Yoshida, Chida, Ichioka, & Suda, 1987; Yoshida, Suda, & Takeuchi, 1982). Because $\dot{V}O_2$ max primarily measures central changes to aerobic training (Saltin, 1985, 1988), it is possible that $\dot{V}O_2$max is not sensitive to specific local adaptations in active skeletal muscle (Farrell, Wilmore, Coyle, Billing, & Costill, 1979; Weltman, 1989). This notion is supported by a number of studies that have indicated that lactate threshold, compared to $\dot{V}O_2$ max, is a better predictor of endurance performance (Allen, Seals, Hurley, Ehsani, & Hagberg, 1985; Costill, Thomason, & Roberts, 1973; Coyle et al., 1983).

Much controversy exists regarding the definition, terminology, measurement, and mechanisms underlying lactate threshold (see Brooks, 1985; Weltman, 1989). For instance, some research groups define *lactate threshold* as the highest velocity or workload that is attained during an incremental work task and is not associated with an increase in blood lactate above baseline (Weltman, 1989). In contrast, other groups have suggested that the *lactate threshold* occurs at an absolute (i.e., fixed) blood lactate concentration of 2.5 millimoles (mM) (Hagberg, 1986). Other groups have defined the onset of blood lactate accumulation (OBLA) as a fixed blood-lactate concentration of 4.0 mM (Karlsson & Jacobs, 1982).

Whatever the definition, the *lactate threshold* is achieved when the accumulation of lactate in the blood increases through greater exercise intensity. Blood-lactate accumulation with incremental increases in exercise is probably due to the inability of oxidative metabolism to remove or resynthesize lactate (Brooks, 1985). Lactic acid begins to accumulate in the blood at about 55% of the untrained person's $\dot{V}O_2$ max (Dodd, Powers, Callender, & Brooks, 1984). For trained endurance athletes, however, lactate threshold may not occur until 80–90% of $\dot{V}O_2$ max (Conley, Krahenbuhl, Burkett, & Millar, 1981).

Lactate threshold is typically assessed by taking multiple blood samples during continuous incremental running or cycling protocols (Weltman, 1989). The method is costly and requires the capability to sample and analyze lactate in blood (for overview of technique see Weltman, 1989). However, because the influence of central (cardiovascular) and peripheral (local muscles) adaptations on psychological variables is unclear, there is potential for fruitful research in this area despite the cost and invasiveness of the technique.

## Submaximal Tests

Measuring $\dot{V}O_2$ max and lactate threshold requires expensive equipment; therefore, a less costly, more easily administered substitute would be desirable. Submaximal tests can be used to estimate $\dot{V}O_2$ max, which require less equipment than direct $\dot{V}O_2$ max assessment. Treadmill walking and running, bicycle ergometry, and bench stepping have all been used as submaximal exercise modalities. Because HR is linearly related to $O_2$ uptake, HRs collected at submaximal workloads can be used to estimate $\dot{V}O_2$ max. Maximum HR is similar for untrained and trained individuals of the same age; however, at any given submaximal load, the trained individual will have a lower HR (Blair, 1984). Thus, with assumptions concerning the efficiency of the exerciser's body to perform work, together with formulas developed for estimating $O_2$ uptake for various activities, $\dot{V}O_2$ max can be estimated from submaximal exercise (McArdle, Katch, & Katch, 1986). Submaximal tests do not require the subject to work to exhaustion and only require electrocardiograph (ECG) monitoring; they therefore have potential for mass testing in field settings (Blair, 1984).

Unfortunately, however, studies examining the relationship between directly measured $\dot{V}O_2$ max and submaximal estimated $\dot{V}O_2$ max have produced only moderate correlations (Gutin, Fogle, & Stewart, 1976; Jessup, Terry, & Landiss, 1975; Woynarowska, 1980). Kasch (1984) has suggested that submaximal tests may not be an adequate substitute for the direct $\dot{V}O_2$ max test and suggests that the results of submaximal tests should be interpreted with caution.

## Field Testing

Cooper (1968) has developed the 12-minute walk–run field test, which has become the most popular field test for estimating $\dot{V}O_2$ max. The test can be performed on any measured course and requires subjects to run or walk as far as they can in 12 minutes. The rationale of this test is that the distance an individual can run in the 12-minute period is determined by maximum aerobic power. An alternative, the 1.5-mile test (Hockey, 1989), is sometimes preferred to the 12-minute run test because it is easier to administer; this test involves running 1.5 miles in the shortest time possible. Unfortunately, $\dot{V}O_2$ max is not the only determining factor of running performance in either of these tests, as body weight, running efficiency, percentage of aerobic power achieved without lactic-acid buildup, and motivational factors all contribute to running performance. The modest correlations between 12-minute run performance and $\dot{V}O_2$ max have led several authors to suggest that field tests are too unreliable for research purposes and even in field situations should be used with caution (Katch, Pechar, McArdle, & Weltman, 1973; Maksud, Cannistra, & Dublinski, 1976; Maksud & Coutts, 1971; Shephard, 1984).

## Assessment of Physical Activity

Maximal and submaximal testing have largely been confined to laboratory situations. However, in epidemiological research, the need to obtain some measure of the fitness of large numbers of subjects makes these techniques impractical. Consequently, researchers have developed such methods as questionnaire, observation, movement assessment, and estimates of energy expenditure of physical activity patterns (Montoye & Taylor, 1984). For exercise-psychology research, where researchers typically are interested in knowing whether their subjects have been physically active or sedentary, questionnaire assessment is probably the easiest and quickest way to assess past and present physical-activity patterns.

The physical-activity questionnaire is the most widely used method of assessing physical activity of large numbers of individuals (Montoye & Taylor, 1986). The basic assumption behind such tests is that more active persons have higher aerobic fitness. Most physical-activity questionnaires require subjects to recall specific physical activities or general activity level either immediately (in diary form) or retrospectively over time periods ranging from days to years. Retrospective recall has been the preferred technique, due to the burden of keeping a daily diary. A variety of physical-activity questionnaires in the form of self-administered inventories and structured interviews exist and mostly differ in the amount of completion time, detail, time frame of the physical activity examined, and kind of physical activity assessed. (For overviews of physical-activity questionnaires, see Blair, 1984; Washburn & Montoye, 1986).

For instance, the Tecumeh questionnaire (Reiff, Montoye, & Remington, 1967) takes between 60 and 90 minutes to complete and asks subjects to recall their physical activity over the preceding year. In contrast, the Harvard Alumni Survey (Paffenbarger, Wing, & Hyde, 1978) takes between 10 and 15 minutes to complete and focuses on the kinds and lengths of activities carried out during the preceding 7 days. Generally, adequate validation and reliability of physical-activity questionnaires has not been achieved because of the lack of acceptable criterion measures and variations in subjects' activity levels (Washburn & Montoye, 1986). According to Washburn and Montoye (1986), physical-activity questionnaires as a method of assessing the physical-activity patterns of large numbers of individuals will remain as the method of choice for epidemiological research. In research that involves the active manipulation of variables, however, the physical-activity questionnaire may only be suited as one of a combination of strategies to assess subjects' exercise patterns and aerobic fitness.

Other forms of physical-activity assessment include time–motion analysis, pedometers, electronic counters, and actometers. These kinds of assessment are of more interest to epidemiologists examining the relationship between physical activity and health. For an overview of these methods, see Montoye and Taylor (1984).

## SUMMARY

At present, the most valid test for the assessment of aerobic fitness is $\dot{V}O_2$ max. However, a single $\dot{V}O_2$ max will only measure aerobic power at that particular time; consequently, a large component of this measure may be genetic. If the test is administered before and after a training program, then this is currently one of the best methods for assessing aerobic fitness improvement. Assessing lactate threshold during continuous exercise, however, appears to be a better assessment of peripheral adaptation to aerobic exercise. If a cross-sectional design is used in conjunction with the $\dot{V}O_2$ max test, and the influence of physiological adaptation is the focus of research, then the individual's activity patterns should also be assessed, through physical-activity questionnaires. Submaximal and field tests do not correlate well with direct measurement of $\dot{V}O_2$ max and, thus, are not accurate enough for research purposes.

## ACKNOWLEDGMENTS

Parts of this chapter are a version of an article in the *Journal of Sports and Exercise Psychology, 12,* 235–247. Reproduced with permission of the Editor.

## REFERENCES

Allen, W. K., Seals, D. R., Hurley, B. F., Ehsani, A. A., & Hagberg, J. M. (1985). Lactate threshold and distance running performance in young and old endurance athletes. *Journal of Applied Physiology, 58,* 1281–1284.

American College of Sports Medicine. (1978). Position statement on the recommended quantity and quality of exercise for developing and maintaining fitness in healthy adults. *Medicine and Science in Sports and Exercise, 10,* vii–x.

American College of Sports Medicine. (1986). *Guidelines for exercise testing and prescription.* Philadelphia: Lea & Febiger.

Bjorntorp, P. (1976). Effect of exercise and physical training and carbohydrate and lipid metabolism in man. *Advances in Cardiology, 18,* 158–164.

Blair, S. (1984). Assessment of physical fitness. In J. D. Mattarazzo, S. M. Weiss, J. A. Herd, N. E. Miller, & S. M. Weiss (Eds.), *Behavioral health* (pp. 424–442). New York: Wiley.

Bouchard, C., Lesage, R., Lortie, G., Simoneau, J., Hamel, P., Boulay, M., Perusse, L., Thriault, G., & LeBlanc, C. (1986). Aerobic performance in brothers, dizygotic and monozygotic twins. *Medicine and Science in Sports and Exercise, 18,* 639–646.

Bouchard, C., & Lortie, G. (1984). Heredity and endurance performance. *Sports Medicine, 1,* 38–64.

Bouchard, C., & Malina, R. M. (1983). Genetics of physiological fitness and motor performance. *Exercise and Sport Sciences Reviews, 11,* 275–305.

Bouchard, C., Shephard, R. J., Stephens, T., Sutton, J. R., & McPherson, B. D. (1990). *Exercise, fitness, and health.* Champaign, IL: Human Kinetics.

Boutcher, S. H. (1990). Aerobic fitness: Measurement and issues. *Journal of Sport Psychology, 12,* 76–85.

Boutcher, S. H., & Landers, D. M. (1986). The effects of vigorous exercise on anxiety, heart rate, and alpha activity of runners and nonrunners. *Psychophysiology, 25,* 696–702.

Boutcher, S. H., Nugent, F. W., & Weltman, A. L. (1990, May). *The effect of resting bradycardia on cardiac reactivity to psychological stress.* Paper presented at the annual meeting of the American College of Sports Medicine, Salt Lake City.

Brooks, G. A. (1985). Anaerobic threshold: Review of the concept and directions for future research. *Medicine and Science in Sports and Exercise, 17,* 22–29.

Conley, D. L., Krahenbuhl, G. S., Burkett, L. N., & Millar, A. L. (1981). Physiological correlates of female road racing performance. *Research Quarterly for Exercise and Sport, 52,* 441–448.

Cooper, K. (1968). *Aerobics.* New York: Evans.

Costill, D. L. (1986). *Inside running: Basics of sports physiology.* Indianapolis: Benchmark Press.

Costill, D. L., Thomason, H., & Roberts, E. (1973). Fractional utilization of the aerobic capacity during distance running. *Medicine and Science in Sports and Exercise, 5,* 248–252.

Coyle, E. F., Martin, W. H., Ehsani, A. A., Hagberg, J. M., Bloomfield, S. A., Sinacore, D. R., & Holloszy, J. O. (1983). Blood lactate threshold in some well-trained ischemic heart disease patients. *Journal of Applied Physiology, 54,* 18–23.

Dienstbier, R. A. (1984). The effect of exercise on personality. In M. L. Sachs & G. W. Buffone (Eds.), *Running as therapy* (pp. 253–272). Lincoln: Nebraska Press.

Dishman, R. K. (1988). *Exercise adherence* (pp. 1–13). Champaign, IL: Human Kinetics.

Dodd, S., Powers, S. K., Callender, T., & Brooks, E. (1984). Blood lactate disappearance at various intensities of recovery exercise. *Journal of Applied Physiology, 57,* 1462–1471.

Farrell, P. A., Wilmore, J. H., Coyle, E. F., Billing, J. E., & Costill, D. L. (1979). Plasma lactate accumulation and distance running performance. *Medicine and Science in Sports and Exercise, 11,* 338–349.

Gutin, B., Fogle, R. K., & Stewart, K. (1976). Relationship among submaximal heart rate, aerobic power, and running performance in children. *Research Quarterly,* 536–539.

Hagberg, J. M. (1986). Physiological implications of the lactate threshold. *International Journal of Sports Medicine, 5,* 106–109.

Hockey, R. V. (1989). *Physical fitness.* St. Louis: Times Mirror.

Jessup, G. T., Terry, J. W., & Landiss, C. W. (1975). Prediction of workload for the Astrand Rhyming Test using stepwise multiple linear regression. *Journal of Sports Medicine and Physiology of Fitness, 15,* 37–42.

Karlsson, J., & Jacobs, I. (1982). Onset of blood lactate accumulation during muscular exercise as a threshold concept. *International Journal of Sports Medicine, 3,* 190–201.

Karvonen, M. J. (1949). The effects of training on heart rate: A longitudinal study. *Annals of Medical Experimental Biology, 35,* 305.

Kasch, F. W. (1984). The validity of the Astrand and Sjostrand submaximal tests. *The Physician and Sportsmedicine, 12,* 47–51.

Katch, F. I., Pechar, G. S., McArdle, W. D., & Weltman, A. L. (1973). Relationship between individual differences in steady pace endurance running performance and maximal oxygen intake. *Research Quarterly, 44,* 206–215.

Klissouras, V. (1971). Heritability of adaptive variation. *Journal of Applied Physiology, 31,* 338–344.

Klissouras, V., Pirnay, F., & Petit, J. (1973). Adaptation to maximal effort: Genetics and age. *Journal of Applied Physiology, 35,* 288–293.

Maksud, M. G., Cannistra, C., & Dublinski, D. (1976). Energy expenditure and $\dot{V}O_2$ max of female athletes during treadmill exercise. *Research Quarterly, 47,* 692–697.

Maksud, M. G., & Coutts, K. D. (1971). Application of the Cooper twelve-minute run–walk to young males. *Research Quarterly, 42,* 54–61.

Malina, R. M., & Bouchard, C. (1984). Sport and human genetics. Champaign, IL: Human Kinetics.

McArdle, W. D., Katch, F. I., & Katch, V. L. (1986). *Exercise physiology: Energy, nutrition, and human performance* (pp. 167–187). Philadelphia: Lea & Febiger.

Montoye, H. J., & Taylor, H. L. (1984). Measurement of physical activity in population studies: A review. *Human Biology, 56,* 131–146.

Montoye, H. J., & Taylor, H. L. (1986). The assessment of physical activity by questionnaire. *American Journal of Epidemiology, 123,* 563–576.

Paffenbarger, R. S., Wing, A. L., & Hyde, R. T. (1978). Physical activity as an index of heart attack risk in college alumni. *American Journal of Epidemiology, 108,* 161–175.

Piehl, K. (1974). Glycogen storage and depletion in human skeletal muscle fibers. *Acta Physiologica Scanda* (Suppl.), *402,* 1–33.

Reiff, G. G., Montoye, H. J., & Remington, R. D. (1967). Assessment of physical activity by questionnaire and interview. *Journal of Sports Medicine and Physical Fitness, 7,* 135–142.

Saltin, B. (1985). Hemodynamic adaptations to exercise. *The American Journal of Cardiology, 55,* 42D–47D.

Saltin, B. (1988). Capacity of blood flow delivery to exercising skeletal muscle in humans. *The American Journal of Cardiology, 62,* 30E–35E.

Seals, D. R., & Hagberg, J. M. (1984). The effect of exercise training on human hypertension. *Medicine and Science in Sports and Exercise, 16,* 207–215.

Shephard, R. J. (1984). Tests of maximum oxygen uptake: A critical review. *Sports Medicine, 1,* 99–124.

Sinyor, D., Golden, M., Steinert, Y., & Seraganian, P. (1986). Experimental manipulation of aerobic fitness and response to psychosocial stress: Heart rate and self-report measures. *Psychosomatic Medicine, 48,* 324–337.

Skinner, J. S., Baldini, F. S., & Gardner, A. W. (1990). Assessment of fitness. In C. Bouchard, R. J. Shephard, T. Stephens, J. R. Sutton, & B. D. McPherson (Eds.), *Exercise, fitness, and health* (pp. 109–115). Champaign, IL: Human Kinetics.

Stein, P. K., & Boutcher, S. H. (1990, May). *A comparison of cardiovascular responses to psychological and exercise stressors in sedentary middle-aged men.* Paper presented at the annual meeting of the North American Society for the Psychology of Sport and Physical Activity, Houston, TX.

van Doornen, L. J. P., de Geus, E. J. C., & Orlebeke, J. F. (1988). Aerobic fitness and the physiological stress response: A critical review. *Sociological Scientific Medicine, 26,* 303–307.

Washburn, R. A., & Montoye, H. J. (1986). The assessment of physical activity by questionnaire. *American Journal of Epidemiology, 123,* 563–576.

Wasserman, K., Hansen, J. E., Sue, D. Y., & Whipp, B. J. (1987). *Principles of exercise testing and interpretation.* Philadelphia: Lea & Febiger.

Weltman, A. (1989). The lactate threshold and endurance performance. In W. A. Grana, J. A. Lombardo, B. J. Sharkey, & J. A. Stone (Eds.), *Advances in sports medicine and fitness* (pp. 91–109). Chicago: YearBook Medical.

Weltman, A., Snead, D., Seip, R., Schurer, R., Levine, S., & Rogol, A. (1987). Prediction of lactate threshold and fixed blood lactate concentrations from 3200-m running performance in male runners. *International Journal of Sports Medicine, 8,* 401–406.

Williams, R. S., & Wallace, A. G. (1989). Biological effects of physical activity. Champaign, IL: Human Kinetics.

Woynarowska, B. (1980). The validity of indirect estimations of maximal oxygen uptake in children 11–12 years of age. *European Journal of Applied Physiology, 43,* 19–23.

Yoshida, T., Chida, M., Ichioka, M., Suda, Y. (1987). Blood lactate parameters related to aerobic capacity and endurance performance. *European Journal of Applied Physiology, 56,* 7–11.

Yoshida, T., Suda, Y., & Takeuchi, N. (1982). Endurance training regimen based on arterial blood lactate: Effects on anaerobic threshold. *European Journal of Applied Physiology, 49,* 223–230.

# 4

# On the Affective Benefits of Acute Aerobic Exercise: Taking Stock After Twenty Years of Research

**KIM M. TUSON AND DAVID SINYOR**

Since the early 1970s, we have witnessed a dramatic increase in the public's participation in a variety of physical-exercise activities, such as jogging, cycling, swimming, and aerobic-exercise classes. Perhaps the most important reason for this change has been the wealth of evidence that has emerged suggesting that physical fitness may serve to promote and maintain physical health. For example, physical fitness has been found to reduce the risk for heart attack (Oberman, 1985), lower blood pressure (Blair,

Goodyear, Gibbons, & Cooper, 1984), and improve the metabolism of carbohydrates (Lennon et al., 1983) and fats (Rosenthal, Haskell, Solomon, Widstrom, & Reavan, 1983). More recently, a second reason for engaging in exercise has surfaced—the belief that exercise is associated with psychological benefits. One source contributing to this belief has been the multitude of anecdotal reports indicating that people commonly feel better after they exercise (Morgan, 1985). Some people even report that they experience altered states of consciousness, or what is called a "runner's high" during exercise (Carmack & Martens, 1979). Another, more systematic source for this belief has been empirical research linking exercise to such psychological benefits as decreased levels of anxiety (Bahrke & Morgan, 1978) and depression (Doyne, Chambless, & Beutler, 1983), as well as to improved levels of cognitive functioning (Tomporowski & Ellis, 1986) and self-concept (Folkins & Sime, 1981). These psychological benefits of exercise have been propagandized by the popular press and are now widely accepted by the public. However, among researchers, there is less agreement concerning such benefits of exercise, with some suggesting that this view is overly optimistic (e.g., Hughes, 1984; Wilfley & Kunce, 1986).

Among the various psychological benefits that have been investigated by researchers, the possibility that exercise may lead people to experience improved affect[1] has received the greatest attention. Interest in the influence of exercise on affective states seems to have emerged for two primary reasons. First, there was a need to empirically substantiate the numerous subjective claims that exercise leads to positive affect, and to understand the parameters necessary for such effects to take place. Second, the idea that exercise might lead to improved affect carried intriguing implications for mental health; it was speculated that perhaps exercise could be used in a therapeutic manner, as a treatment for affective disorders such as depression or as a method for managing anxiety (McCann & Holmes, 1984; Martinsen, Hoffart, & Solberg, 1989).

Research examining the influence of exercise on affective states has followed two basic approaches. One approach has focused on the *chronic* effects of exercise—that is, the effects associated with extended training or long-term exercise participation. The other approach has limited its focus to the *acute* effects of exercise, or the effects associated with a single bout of exercise. Typically, studies examining the chronic effects have compared the affect that subjects reported at the completion of a training program to that which they reported prior to engaging in the program. Thus, this type of research is concerned primarily with the effect of training on people's

---

[1]Throughout the exercise literature, the terms *psychological benefits, mood states, feelings,* and *affect* have been used interchangeably. For the sake of consistency, we use the term *affect* throughout this chapter.

affect. The implicit assumption that seems to underlie these studies is that repeated bouts of exercise are required in order to bring about changes in affect. By contrast, studies examining the acute effects of exercise seem to follow the implicit assumption that changes in affect can occur after a single session of exercise (although it is acknowledged that these effects may differ for trained and untrained individuals). As such, studies of this type have compared the affect that subjects reported following a single session of exercise to that which they reported immediately before the session.

In this chapter, we summarize and critically evaluate the research examining the acute effects of exercise on affective states. Our goal is not only to provide a comprehensive review of the relevant studies and their findings, but also to discuss this research in terms of important theoretical and methodological considerations that we feel should be given to this field of inquiry. Accordingly, the chapter is divided into two main sections. The first section is devoted to a review of the literature. We begin by outlining the criteria that were used in selecting the studies to be included in this review. Next, we describe the three principal research designs that have been used by researchers in this area, in order to highlight the relative strengths and weaknesses of each approach and thereby prepare the reader for our critical review of the literature, which follows. The literature review is structured around three fundamental questions: (1) Is acute exercise associated with improvements in affective states? (2) If so, under what conditions do these effects hold; that is, what are the variables that moderate these effects? (3) What psychological or physiological process(es) have been proposed to mediate these effects? Research relevant to each question is reviewed and evaluated.

The second section of the chapter is devoted to a discussion of theoretical and methodological issues that we feel should be given consideration when examining the influence of acute exercise on affective states. We have identified three issues that seem to be especially crucial to this field of research at present: (1) the need to adopt a theoretical conceptualization of affective change to guide research, (2) based on this theoretical framework, the need to postulate and directly test specific mediating processes that may lead to changes in affect, and (3) the need to explore the possible role that psychological variables may play in both moderating and mediating the impact of exercise on affective states. The purpose of this discussion is to stimulate consideration of new approaches for future research.

## LITERATURE REVIEW

### Selection of Studies

A literature search spanning the years 1960 to 1991 was conducted, to identify published articles describing the acute effects of exercise on either self-reported indices of affective states or psychophysiological correlates of affective states. These articles were acquired through a computer search (PSYCLIT), inspection of reference lists in published articles, and hand searches of relevant journals. Case studies were eliminated from the list of articles retained, as they were considered to be seriously undermined by their lack of generalizability beyond the particular individual under investigation. Also excluded were studies published solely in the form of conference abstracts. In total, 45 studies met the inclusion criteria.[2]

## Description of Research Designs Employed

Research that has evaluated the impact of acute exercise on affective states can be grouped into three broad categories, according to the research design employed. These categories are referred to as "nonexperimental," "quasi-experimental," and "true experimental" designs (Campbell & Stanley, 1963). A brief description of the three designs and the typical protocols followed in each is presented here, with the primary goal being to familiarize the reader with the relative strengths and weaknesses of each approach. Because the value of any research finding is largely dependent on the quality of the strategy employed to obtain the finding, it is hoped that, armed with this background information, the reader will be in a better position to critically evaluate the findings and interpretations that follow in our subsequent review of the literature.

*Nonexperimental studies* consist of the one group pretest–posttest type, where measures of affect sampled prior to and following an exercise bout are compared, in order to determine whether the exercise bout was associated with improved affect. The major limitation of studies of this type is that they lack a control group. Without such a comparison group, it becomes impossible to determine whether changes in affect observed following exercise are attributable to the exercise itself, as opposed to one or more other variables. As a result, several plausible rival hypotheses present themselves. For example, subjects in these studies are often regular exercisers who may have certain expectations regarding the affective benefits of exercise, and these expectations, rather than the exercise itself, may have influenced their self-reports. Similarly, the preexercise measure of affect may have been tainted by subjects' apprehensions concerning the test situation, such that any improvements in affect observed following the exercise may have simply reflected a sense of relief in having completed the session. In spite

---

[2]Two articles obtained in the literature search (Felts, 1989; Goldfarb, Hatfield, Sforzo, & Flynn, 1987) were excluded from the review because they reported findings that represented a segment of larger research projects. The results of these larger projects were presented in more complete form in publications already included in the review (Felts & Vaccaro, 1988; Hatfield, Goldfarb, Sforzo, & Flynn, 1987).

of these potential problems, we have included nonexperimental studies in our review for the sake of comprehensiveness, and because they may contribute, albeit in a modest way, to our understanding of the influence of acute exercise on affective states.

*Quasi-experimental studies* consist of the nonequivalent control-group type, where a group of regular exercisers is compared to a group of subjects participating in some nonexercise activity of the same duration, such as a hobby class or a college lecture. All subjects complete self-report measures of affect prior to and following their treatment condition, with pre–post changes in affect being compared between the exercise and the no-exercise groups. This comparison is intended to demonstrate that exercise is associated with improved affect, whereas the no-exercise activity is not. The inclusion of a no-exercise control group in quasi-experimental designs represents an important improvement over nonexperimental designs, in that it affords greater control over the potential effects of such variables as subjects' motivation or expectancies for an activity (which are presumably equivalent across the groups), the passage of time, or the effects of socializing with other individuals who share similar interests. Furthermore, these studies have typically been conducted in natural settings and therefore possess a high degree of external validity. Nevertheless, the fact that the subject, rather than the experimenter, selects the activity to be performed presents a serious problem in interpreting the findings. Specifically, it is possible that subjects who choose to exercise differ in some systematic way from those who choose to participate in a hobby or lecture class, and that it is this difference that may be accounting for the observed changes in affect following the activity.

*True experimental studies* are primarily of the pretest–posttest control-group type, where subjects who exercise are compared to subjects who quietly rest or read for the same duration of time. Typically, exercise is performed under controlled laboratory conditions, either on a motorized treadmill or on a stationary bicycle ergometer. Although this allows the experimenter to control, with greater precision, the intensity at which the exercise is performed, it can be argued that this procedure limits the external validity of the findings. Both between- and within-subject designs have been used, with the former including the requisite random assignment of subjects to treatment conditions, and the latter employing counterbalancing techniques to control for sequencing effects.

While it may be argued that any research, regardless of design, can contribute to our understanding, it is generally accepted that the true experimental approach is the most rigorous, and that findings obtained through this approach can be regarded with somewhat greater confidence than those obtained through the other two approaches. The superiority of the true experimental approach lies in the fact that it includes appropriate control conditions, as well as the assignment of subjects to treatment conditions by the experimenters, rather than through self-selection by subjects. That is, by randomly assigning subjects to an exercise or a control condition, the experimenter has presumably distributed subject characteristics evenly across the groups, such that the sole difference between them is in whether or not exercise is performed. Thus, any differences in affect observed between the groups following exercise can be attributed, with greater certainty, to the exercise itself.

Of the 45 studies included in our review, 18 were nonexperimental, 6 were quasi-experimental, and 21 were true experimental.

## IS ACUTE EXERCISE ASSOCIATED WITH IMPROVED AFFECT?

With the foregoing methodological considerations in mind, we now survey the relevant studies to address the first question of whether an acute bout of aerobic exercise is associated with improvements in affective states. Of the 45 studies included in this review, 34 studies used self-report measures as an index of subjects' affective state, 8 studies used psychophysiological measures (i.e., electromyograph—EMG or electroencephalograph —EEG) as correlates of affective state, and 3 studies used both self-report and psychophysiological measures. As no strong evidence exists, to date, for a direct relation between self-reported affective states and psychophysiological measures, it was decided to focus our efforts primarily on studies presenting self-report data. Nonetheless, we briefly discuss the psychophysiological data in a separate section.

### Self-Report Measures

A summary of those studies that examined the effects of acute exercise on self-reported affective states is presented in Table 4.1. The studies have been organized into three separate categories, according to the research design that was employed.[3] The primary purpose of the summary table is to pro-

---

[3]Several studies classified as nonexperimental in Table 4.1 actually represent true experimental designs when considered in their entirety. However, the primary question addressed by these studies was somewhat different from that posed here, and therefore we focused on that segment of the study that bore directly on our question. In limiting our focus, these studies, which had originally satisfied the criteria for true experimental research, were effectively reduced to nonexperimental designs. Specifically, although these studies employed control conditions appropriate to their research question, none of them had a no-exercise condition. Because this condition represents, for our purposes, the critical comparison, we were forced to classify these as nonexperimental studies. These studies are identified by the superscript letter "c" in Table 4.1.

**TABLE 4.1 SUMMARY OF STUDIES EXAMINING THE EFFECTS OF ACUTE EXERCISE ON SELF-REPORTED AFFECTIVE STATES**

| Authors | N | Mean age | Sex | Fitness level |
|---|---|---|---|---|
| | | Subject characteristics | | |
| **Nonexperimental studies** | | | | |
| Allen & Coen (1987) | 12 | 21 | M | Trained |
| Farrell, Gustafson, Garthwaite, Kalkhoff, Cowley, & Morgan (1986) | 8 | 24.2 | M | Trained |
| Farrell, Gustafson, Morgan, & Pert (1987) | 7 | 27.4 | M | Trained |
| Fillingim, Roth, & Haley (1989) | 60 | Students | F | Untrained |
| Grossman, Bouloux, Price, Drury, Lam, Turner, Thomas, Besser, & Sutton (1984) | 6 | 18–31 | M | Untrained |
| Hatfield, Goldberg, Sforzo, & Flynn (1987) | 16 | 26.1 & 66.0 | M | Untrained |
| Janal, Colt, Clark, & Glusman (1984) | 12 | 38.8 | M | Trained |
| Kraemer, Dzewaltowski, Blair, Rinehardt, & Castracane (1990) | 23 | 30.1 | MF | Trained/ untrained |
| Markoff, Ryan, & Young (1982) | 15 | 36.8 | MF | Trained |
| McMurray, Berry, Hardy, & Sheps (1988) | 11 | 19–48 | M | Trained |
| McMurray, Berry, Vann, Hardy, & Sheps (1988) | 8 | 21–41 | M | Trained |
| Morgan, Roberts, & Feinerman (1971, Exp. 1) | 120 | Professors | M | — |
| Nowlis & Greenberg (1979) | 18 | 17–55 | MF | Trained |
| Steptoe & Cox (1988) | 32 | 20 | F | Trained/ untrained |

| | Methodology | | | | |
|---|---|---|---|---|---|
| Exercise type | Exercise intensity | Exercise duration[a] | Control condition[b] | Measure(s) | Outcome |
| Treadmill | 50–75% $\dot{V}O_2$ | 45 | None | POMS, VAS—euphoria | Improved—globally[c] |
| Bicycle ergometer | 70% $\dot{V}O_2$ | 30 | None | POMS—anxiety only | Improved[c] |
| Treadmill | 40%, 60%, 80% $\dot{V}O_2$ | 80 40 | None | POMS—anxiety only | Improved—at 60% & 80% $\dot{V}O_2$[c] |
| Bicycle ergometer | 50 rpm at 49 watts | 10 | None | POMS | High distraction worsened, low distraction improved—Anx[c] |
| Bicycle ergometer | 40%, 80% $\dot{V}O_2$ | 20 | None | VAS—euphoria | No change[c] |
| Bicycle ergometer | To $\dot{V}O_2$ max | — | None | MAACL | No change |
| Running | 85% $\dot{V}O_2$ | 44(avg) | None | VAS—euphoria | Improved[c] |
| Treadmill | 80% HR max | 30 | None | POMS | Improved—Anx, Dep, Ang, Confusion |
| Running | Self-selected | 99(avg) | None | POMS | Improved—Anx, Dep, Ang[c] |
| Treadmill | 70% $\dot{V}O_2$ | 10 miles | None | GAS | Improved—globally[c] |
| Treadmill, outdoor run | 70% $\dot{V}O_2$ | 10 miles | None | GAS | Improved—globally[c] |
| Bicycle or treadmill | 150, 160, 170, or 180 bpm | — | None | DACL | No differences between groups[c] |
| Running | Self-selected | 12 miles | None | MACL | Improved—Pleasantness |
| Bicycle ergometer | 25, 100 watts | 8 | None | POMS | High intensity worsened—Anx; low intensity improved—Vigor |

TABLE 4.1 (continued)

| Authors | N | Mean age | Sex | Fitness level |
|---|---|---|---|---|
| | | **Subject characteristics** | | |
| Wildmann, Kruger, Schmole, Niemann, & Matthaei (1986) | 21 | 29.8 | M | Trained |
| Wood (1977) | 106 | Students | MF | — |
| **Quasi-experimental studies** | | | | |
| Berger & Owen (1983) | 100 | 22.3 | MF | Trained/ untrained |
| Berger & Owen (1988) | 170 | 22.4 | MF | — |
| Dyer & Crouch (1987) | 59 | 18–24 | MF | Trained/ untrained |
| Lichtman & Poser (1983) | 64 | 25.6 | MF | Trained/ untrained |
| Weinberg, Jackson, & Kolodny (1988) | 183 | Students | MF | — |
| Wilson, Berger, & Bird (1981) | 42 | 21–27 | MF | Trained/ untrained |
| **True experimental studies** | | | | |
| Abood (1984) | 42 | 18–22 | F | — |
| Bahrke & Morgan (1978) | 75 | 51.9 | M | Trained |
| Bahrke & Smith (1985) | 65 | 10.6 | MF | — |
| Boutcher & Landers (1988) | 30 | 28.3 | M | Trained/ untrained |
| Ewing, Scott, Mendez, & McBride (1984) | 52 | 22.4 | MF | Trained |
| Farrell, Gates, Maksud, & Morgan (1982) | 6 | 30 | MF | Trained |
| Felts & Vaccaro (1988) | 24 | 18–28 | F | Trained/ |
| Flory & Holmes (1991) | 18 | Students | F | Trained |

| | Methodology | | | | |
|---|---|---|---|---|---|
| Exercise type | Exercise intensity | Exercise duration[a] | Control condition[b] | Measure(s) | Outcome |
| Running | Self-selected | 39(avg) | None | Adjective Checklist | No change |
| Running | Self-selected | 12 | None | STAI | High anxious improved, low anxious worsened |
| Swimming | Self-selected | 40 | College lecture | POMS | Improved—Anx, Dep, Ang, Vigor, Confusion |
| Swimming | Self-selected | 40 | College lecture | POMS, STAI | Improved—Anx, Dep, on first of 3 days |
| Running | Self-selected | | College lecture | POMS | Improved—Anx, Dep, Ang, Confusion |
| Exercise class | Self-selected | 45 | Hobby class | POMS, MACL | Improved—Anx,[d] Dep,[d] Ang, Fatigue |
| Swimming or jogging class | 60% HR max | 30 | Resting or massage | POMS, STAI, AD ACL | Improved—Anx,[d] Dep,[d] Ang[d] Vigor[d] |
| Running or exercise class | Self-selected | 40 | Eating lunch | STAI | Improved[d] |
| Bench step | 30 steps/min | 5 | Resting | STAI | High anxious no change; low anxious worsened |
| Treadmill | 70% HR max | 20 | Meditation or resting | STAI | Improved[d] |
| Run–walk | Self-selected | 15 | "Busywork" or quiet rest | STAI | High anxious improved[d] |
| Treadmill | 80–85% HR max | 20 | Reading | POMS, STAI | Improved for trained Ss on STAI only |
| Treadmill | 65–70% HR max | 5 | Reading | POMS | Improved—globally |
| Treadmill | Self-selected, 60%, 80% $\dot{V}O_2$ | 30 | Resting | POMS | No change |
| Bicycle | 30%, 60% | 25 | Relaxation | STAI | Improved[d] |
| Exercise class | 60–80% of HR max | 40 | No exercise | MAACL, POMS | Improved—Vigor |

**TABLE 4.1** *(continued)*

| Authors | N | Mean age | Sex | Fitness level |
|---|---|---|---|---|
| | | | Subject characteristics | |
| McGowan, Robertson, & Epstein (1985) | 12 | 21–29 | M | — |
| Morgan, Roberts & Feinerman (1971, Exp. 2) | 36 | Students | MF | — |
| Raglin & Morgan (1987, Exp. 1) | 15 | 34.2 | M | Trained |
| Raglin & Morgan (1987, Exp. 2) | 15 | 60.5 | M | Trained |
| Roth (1989) | 80 | 20.8 | MF | Trained/ untrained |
| Roth, Bachtler, & Fillingim (1990) | 57 | 20.5 | F | Untrained |
| Thayer (1987) | 18 | 19–38 | MF | — |

*Note.* AD ACL = Activation–Deactivation Adjective Checklist; DACL = Depression Adjective Checklist; GAS = General Affect Scale; IPAT = Institute for Personality & Ability Testing; MAACL = Multiple Affect Adjective Checklist; MACL = Mood Adjective Checklist; POMS = Profile of Mood States; STAI = Spielberger State–Trait Anxiety Inventory (state form); VAS = Visual Analogue Scale; Anx = Anxiety/tension, Dep = Depression, Ang = Anger/hostility (POMS subscales). $VO_2$ = Volume of oxygen uptake; $VO_2$ max = Maximum oxygen uptake. HR max = Maximum heart rate.

[a]In minutes unless otherwise specified.

[b]Refers to a no-exercise control condition.

[c]Technically, this study represents a true experimental design, but for our purposes it has been classified within the nonexperimental design category, as it does not include a no-exercise condition.

[d]This outcome was also demonstrated by the control condition(s) and therefore was not unique to the exercise condition(s).

| | Methodology | | | | |
|---|---|---|---|---|---|
| Exercise type | Exercise intensity | Exercise duration[a] | Control condition[b] | Measure(s) | Outcome |
|---|---|---|---|---|---|
| Bicycle ergometer | 40, 55, 70% $\dot{V}O_2$ | 15 | Cognitive task | Addiction Research Centre Inventory | No change |
| Treadmill | 0% or 5% grade | 17 | Resting | DACL, IPAT Anxiety Battery | No differences between groups |
| Various sports | Self-selected | 40 | Resting | STAI | Improved |
| Running, bicycle ergometer, treadmill | Self-selected | 40 | Reading | STAI | Improved[d] |
| Bicycle ergometer | 115–135 bpm | 20 | Resting | POMS | Improved—Anx |
| Bicycle ergometer | 50 watts | 10 | Resting | POMS | Improved—Anx, Vigor |
| Walking | Self-selected | 10 | Sugar snack | AD ACL | Improved |

vide the reader with an overview of the types of subject characteristics, exercise parameters, and outcome measures that have been used by researchers. As can be seen, there exists considerable diversity among the studies. Some researchers have studied the effects of exercise with trained individuals, whereas others have studied these effects with untrained individuals. A wide range of exercise activities, intensities, and durations have been used. Finally, several different self-report measures have been used for assessing affective changes, the Profile of Mood States (POMS) and the state form of the Spielberger State–Trait Anxiety Inventory (STAI) being the two most frequently used. Such diversity could be considered a strength to the field if, despite the different parameters used, all studies yielded similar findings. However, such is not the case, and unfortunately, this diversity has proven to be a considerable problem for the field, in that it makes comparisons across studies exceedingly difficult. This problem becomes even more troublesome given the absence of direct replications.

As shown in Table 4.1, each study was assigned an outcome of "improved," "no change," or "worsened." An improved outcome was assigned to those studies in which one or more measures of affect demonstrated changes in a positive direction following exercise (e.g., reduced anxiety, increased vigor). This outcome was assigned independent of whether corresponding changes were also observed in the control group(s). We opted for this admittedly liberal approach because it allowed us to standardize the outcome variable across studies that did or did not include a control group(s). However, we have identified with a superscript letter "d" those studies in which both the exercise and the control condition(s) showed improved affect. An examination of study outcomes reveals that the majority of studies found exercise to be associated with some improvement in affect, although a sizable number found no changes in affect, and a select few even found that exercise was associated with a worsening of affect. These outcomes should be viewed with caution, however, given that many of the studies are plagued by methodological problems. These problems are discussed at various points throughout this chapter. In addition, it should be noted that numerous studies sampled several affective states but found improvement on only a subset of these.

To further examine the influence of exercise on specific affective states, self-report measures assessing similar constructs were grouped together, yielding five separate affective categories, which were labeled as "anxiety," "depression," "anger," "vigor," "fatigue," and "confusion." Table 4.2 presents the number of studies within each category that demonstrated improved, no change, or worsened outcomes, as well as a summed total for each outcome across the five affective categories. As can be seen, with the possible exception of anxiety, studies conducted to date have not found acute exercise to be reliably associated with improved affective states. Over-

**TABLE 4.2    FREQUENCY COUNT OF STUDY OUTCOMES ACROSS SELF-REPORTED AFFECTIVE STATES**

| Affective states | Improved | No change | Worsened |
|---|---|---|---|
| Anxiety | 21 | 14 | 4 |
| Depression | 9 | 13 | 0 |
| Anger | 6 | 5 | 1 |
| Vigor | 6 | 9 | 0 |
| Fatigue | 3 | 9 | 1 |
| Confusion | 3 | 9 | 0 |
| Total | 48 | 59 | 6 |

all, there were more instances of no change and worsening in affective states (65) than there were of improvement (48).[4]

Of course, we recognize that a frequency count of outcomes does not take into consideration the quality of the research designs used to obtain these. Given our stated concern with the importance of considering the relative strengths and weaknesses of the research design employed, we decided to select and closely examine those studies that were more rigorous in their design and methodology, and whose findings could therefore be viewed with greater confidence. The criteria used to select these studies included the use of (a) a true experimental design, (b) standardized measures of affect, (c) adequate sample sizes, (d) a suitable control group(s), (e) appropriate statistics, (f) an exercise duration sufficient to qualify it as aerobic (i.e., a minimum of 20 minutes; American College of Sports Medicine, 1980), and (g) an exercise protocol that allowed for some standardization and specification of workload. Only five studies satisfied these criteria. These studies, along with their findings, are described next.

Bahrke and Morgan (1978), in an often-cited paper, compared changes in state anxiety following an acute bout of exercise to those observed following practiced relaxation or quiet rest. Using a between-groups design, they randomly assigned 75 trained men to 20 minutes of one of the following: (a) walking on a motorized treadmill at 70% of maximum heart rate (HR max), (b) practicing a passive relaxation technique, or (c) resting quietly in a

---

[4]Occasionally, there was more than one outcome reported for a particular affective state within a single study, because different conditions sometimes resulted in differing outcomes. In addition, some studies employed more than one measure of a particular affective state (e.g., STAI, POMS—Anxiety Subscale) and did not find consistent results across these measures. Thus, the number of outcomes reported for some affective states may exceed the number of studies actually employing relevant measures.

reclining chair. Subjects completed the STAI prior to, immediately following, and 10 minutes after treatment. Results indicated that subjects in all three conditions reported significant reductions in state anxiety at both posttreatment sampling points, as compared to their pretreatment levels. The authors concluded that all three conditions were equally effective in reducing state anxiety and speculated that the similar reductions observed may have reflected a common underlying process, namely a distraction or a "time-out" from life stresses and worries. However, it is also conceivable that all three treatments were actually ineffective in affecting anxiety per se, and that the observed reductions were in fact artifactual. That is, other possibilities may have accounted for the observed reductions, such as the effects of repeatedly completing the STAI, the biasing of responses through subjects' expectancies regarding the experimental hypothesis, or the influence of subjects' pretreatment apprehension regarding the upcoming session, which may have diminished by session end. Because it is impossible to distinguish between these possibilities and the interpretation offered by the authors (which has never been directly tested), their conclusion regarding the effectiveness of acute exercise in reducing anxiety should be regarded as speculative.

Boutcher and Landers (1988) examined the impact of acute exercise on state anxiety, as well as on depression, anger, vigor, fatigue, and confusion. They used a within-subject design, in which 15 trained and 15 untrained men ran for 20 minutes on a motorized treadmill at 80–85% of HR max, and on a separate occasion, sat quietly and read for the same period of time. The order of sessions was counterbalanced across subjects. The STAI was administered at four points (5 and 13 minutes before, and at the same intervals after treatment), and the POMS was administered immediately prior to and 17 minutes after treatment. The only significant effect that emerged was for trained subjects in the exercise condition, with these subjects reporting significantly lower STAI scores at both sample points following exercise, in comparison to untrained subjects in the exercise condition. The authors interpreted this finding as supportive of the anxiety-reducing effects of exercise. However, it was not clear from the data presentation whether trained subjects in the exercise condition reported less anxiety than when in the reading condition. Moreover, no effects were seen on any of the affective states assessed by the POMS, one of which was a measure of anxiety.

Felts and Vaccaro (1988) extended this work by examining the influence of aerobic fitness level and exercise intensity on state anxiety following an acute bout of exercise. A within-subject design was used, in which 24 women who differed in aerobic fitness participated in each of three conditions. The two exercise conditions consisted of pedaling for 25 minutes on a bicycle ergometer at 30% and 60% of HR max, while the control condition consisted of listening to a relaxation tape containing environmental sounds.

The order of these treatment conditions was randomized across subjects. The STAI was administered once prior to, and twice following treatment (the precise sampling times were not specified). Results indicated that all treatment conditions were associated with reductions in anxiety, relative to pretreatment levels, although the time course of the effects differed between the exercise and the control conditions. Specifically, while significant reductions in anxiety were observed at the first posttreatment sampling point in the control condition, it was not until the final posttreatment sampling point that significant reductions were observed in the exercise conditions. At this final sampling point, there were no differences in anxiety levels among the three conditions. Fitness level did not influence the results. These findings were taken as evidence for the effectiveness of exercise in reducing anxiety. However, given the equivalent reductions observed in all conditions by the final sampling point, it would seem that the same caution offered in reviewing Bahrke and Morgan's (1978) study may also apply here.

Roth (1989) randomly assigned 40 trained and 40 untrained subjects of both genders to either 20 minutes of pedaling on a bicycle ergometer at approximately 60–70% of HR max or to a quiet rest condition. The POMS was administered approximately 20–30 minutes prior to treatment, and again 15 minutes following treatment. The findings revealed reductions in anxiety following exercise and increases in confusion following rest. No effects emerged on any of the other POMS subscales (i.e., depression, anger, vigor, and fatigue). Neither fitness level nor gender influenced these results.

Finally, in a recent study, Flory and Holmes (1991) examined the impact of exercise performed in a naturalistic setting on anxiety, depression, vigor, and fatigue. A within-subject design was used, in which 18 women either participated or did not participate in a 40-minute aerobic dance class performed at 60–80% of HR max. Subjects had been regularly attending these classes during the previous month. In the exercise condition, subjects were asked to attend the dance class prior to arriving at the laboratory, whereas in the no-exercise control condition, subjects were asked to miss the dance class prior to their arrival. The order of conditions was counterbalanced across subjects. The laboratory testing session consisted of a 40-minute study period, at the end of which the subject was asked to complete selected subscales of the POMS, as well as the Multiple Affect Adjective Checklist (MAACL), based on how she felt during the study period. The only significant finding obtained was that of greater vigor following the exercise condition, as compared to the no-exercise condition. Exercise was not found to influence anxiety, depression, or fatigue.

Taken together, the results of these five studies seem quite consistent with the pattern of findings that emerged in Table 4.2, although the effect found for anxiety was somewhat more positive than is implied by the table. Four of the five studies revealed reductions in self-reported anxiety following exercise. Of the three studies that assessed affective states other than anxiety, none revealed effects on depression, anger, fatigue, or confusion, although one study reported increased vigor following exercise (i.e., Flory & Holmes, 1991).

With respect to anxiety reduction, it is noteworthy that this effect was not always unique to exercise, but was also observed in the comparison group(s) for two of the five studies. More generally, when examining the outcome of all studies (15) that included a comparison group(s) and that demonstrated reductions in anxiety, it was found that approximately half (7) reported equivalent reductions in both the exercise and the control condition(s).[5] Most researchers have interpreted this finding in line with the interpretation offered by Bahrke and Morgan (1978): That all treatments were equally effective in reducing anxiety, and that this finding may be due to the effects of distraction or "time-out" (e.g., Felts & Vaccaro, 1988; Raglin & Morgan, 1987, Experiments 1 and 2; Wilson, Berger, & Bird, 1981). We would argue, however, that such an interpretation may be premature, given that the role of distraction has never been directly tested. As a result, it becomes impossible to rule out the previously mentioned alternative explanations for the findings. Nevertheless, assuming that the observed effects are not artifactual, the finding that reductions in anxiety are often observed following both exercise and nonexercise conditions suggests that such reductions may not be unique to exercise.

Even if acute exercise affords no unique benefits in the overall reduction of anxiety, it is conceivable that the onset or duration of these reductions may differ for the exercise and the no-exercise conditions. To investigate this possibility, we examined those studies that sampled anxiety at more than one point following treatment. There were five such studies. Two of these studies found equivalent reductions in anxiety across both the exercise and the no-exercise conditions, immediately and at 10 minutes posttreatment (Bahrke & Morgan, 1978; Bahrke & Smith, 1985). The other two studies found that whereas anxiety was significantly reduced immediately following the control condition, it was not until 15–20 minutes later that anxiety reduction was seen in the exercise condition (Felts & Vaccaro, 1988; Raglin & Morgan, 1987, Experiment 2). The reliability of this finding is

---

[5]It should be noted that in four of the eight studies that reported reductions in anxiety following exercise (but not following control condition[s]), the effects were either statistically questionable or apparently not reliable. In one of these studies, the conclusion was based on the results of post hoc tests, even though the results of the analysis of variance (ANOVA) did not warrant their use (Berger & Owen, 1983); in another study, separate one-way ANOVAs rather than a more appropriate two-factor model was applied to the data (Raglin & Morgan, 1987, Experiment 1); and in the remaining two studies, a significant effect was found on only one of the two measures of anxiety (Berger & Owen, 1988; Boutcher & Landers, 1988).

strengthened by the fact that one of these studies used two exercise intensities, both of which showed this differential effect in the time course of anxiety reduction. Finally, the fifth study reported a significant reduction in anxiety following exercise in comparison to a control condition of quiet rest (Raglin & Morgan, 1987, Experiment 1). It was found that, whereas anxiety was not significantly reduced immediately postexercise, it was reduced 20 minutes following the exercise bout.

### Psychophysiological Measures

Table 4.3 provides a summary of the 11 studies that examined the effects of acute exercise on psychophysiological measures of affective states. Researchers examining this question have typically not specified the affective state under investigation, although their use of terms such as "stress," "relaxation," and "tranquilizer effect" presumably implies that of anxiety. The majority (9) of these studies employed one of two measures of spinal motor neuron activity, as determined by EMG recordings at one of several muscle sites, such as the frontalis or biceps muscles. The first measure assesses the spontaneous firing rate of these neurons, while the second measure assesses their excitability in response to electrical or mechanical stimulation of a reflex arc in which they reside. Both of these measures are considered to reflect central nervous system arousal, with reductions in firing rate or excitability implying reduced arousal (Hatfield & Landers, 1987). Eight of these studies employed true experimental designs, comparing a bout of exercise with a no-exercise control condition consisting of quiet rest or reading. Six studies demonstrated significant reductions in the spontaneous or evoked firing rate of these neurons following exercise (Bulbulian & Darabos, 1986; deVries, 1968; deVries & Adams, 1972; deVries, Simard, Wiswell, Heckathorne, & Carabetta, 1982; deVries, Wiswell, Bulbulian, & Moritani, 1981; Russell, Epstein, & Erickson, 1983), whereas two studies failed to demonstrate any effects of exercise (Felts & Vaccaro, 1988; McGowan, Robertson, & Epstein, 1985). Finally, there was one nonexperimental study conducted using EMG measures, which also did not find any effects of exercise (Balog, 1983).

The remaining two studies examined changes in brain-wave activity, measured by the EEG, that were associated with an acute bout of exercise. Both of these studies demonstrated increases in the percentage of alpha waves following exercise (Boutcher & Landers, 1988; Pineda & Adkisson, 1961). An increase in alpha waves is generally thought to reflect reduced arousal and a state of relaxation (Carlson, 1991).

We should point out that we have not reviewed psychophysiological data derived from skin conductance or cardiovascular measures, as it is even less clear how these measures are related to affective states. For a more detailed discussion of the effects of acute exercise on a variety of psycho-

## TABLE 4.3 SUMMARY OF STUDIES EXAMINING THE EFFECTS OF ACUTE EXERCISE ON PSYCHOPHYSIOLOGICAL MEASURES

| Authors | N | Subject characteristics | | |
| | | Mean age | Sex | Fitness level |
|---|---|---|---|---|
| **Nonexperimental studies** | | | | |
| Balog (1983) | 20 | Students | MF | — |
| Pineda & Adkisson (1961) | 16 | 22–36 | — | — |
| **Experimental studies** | | | | |
| Boutcher & Landers (1988) | 30 | 28.3 | M | Trained/untrained |
| Bulbulian & Darabos (1986) | 10 | 28.7 | MF | Trained |
| deVries (1968) | 29 | 19–39 | MF | — |
| deVries & Adams (1972) | 10 | 52–70 | M | — |
| deVries, Simard, Wiswell, Heckathorne, & Carabetta (1982) | 6 | 25.5 | MF | — |
| deVries, Wiswell, Bulbulian & Moritani (1981) | 10 | 27.3 | MF | — |
| Felts & Vaccaro (1988) | 24 | 18–28 | F | Trained/untrained |
| McGowan, Robertson, & Epstein (1985) | 12 | 21–29 | M | — |
| Russell, Epstein, & Erickson (1983) | 12 | 18–30 | M | Untrained |

[a] In minutes.

[b] Refers to a no-exercise control condition.

[c] Although the authors interpreted their ANOVA results as indicating exercise-related changes in EMG scores, the absence of post hoc tests did not allow for confirmation of this claim.

| | Methodology | | | | |
|---|---|---|---|---|---|
| Exercise type | Exercise intensity | Exercise duration[a] | Control condition[b] | Measure(s) | Outcome |
| Bicycle ergometer | To 150 bpm | 30 | None | EMG-frontalis | No change |
| Treadmill | To exhaustion | 50 | None | EEG-alpha waves | Increased |
| Treadmill | 80–85% HR max | 20 | Reading | EEG-alpha waves | Increased |
| Treadmill | 40%, 75% $\dot{V}O_2$ | 20 | No exercise | EMG-H/M ratio | Reduced |
| Bench step | 30 steps/minute | 5 | Rest | EMG-biceps, quadriceps | Reduced in biceps only |
| Treadmill | 100, 120 bpm | 15 | Reading, tranquilizer | EMG-biceps | Reduced at 100 bpm |
| Bicycle ergometer | 40% HR max | 20 | Reading | EMG-H/M ratio EMG-achilles tendpm tap | Reduced |
| Bicycle ergometer | 40% HR max | 20 | Reading | EMG-H/M ratio | Reduced |
| Bicycle ergometer | 30%, 60% HR max | 25 | Relaxation | EMG-frontalis, elbow flexor | No change |
| Bicycle ergometer | 40, 55, 70% $\dot{V}O_2$ | 15 | Cognitive task | EMG-frontalis, biceps, sternomastoid | No change |
| Bicycle ergometer | 60% HR max | 20 | Smoking, vigilance task | EMG-frontalis | Reduced?[c] |

physiological measures, the reader is referred to a review paper by Hatfield and Landers (1987) on this issue.

## Summary

Studies using self-report measures to address the question of whether an acute bout of exercise is associated with improved affective states have revealed only a modest anxiety-reducing effect of exercise. No reliable effects were found for any of the other affective states examined, specifically depression, anger, vigor, fatigue, or confusion. The apparent beneficial effect found for anxiety is consistent with the results of a recent meta-analysis in which a small but significant effect size was found for the anxiolytic effects of acute exercise (Petruzzello, Landers, Hatfield, Kubitz, & Salazar, 1991). It remains unclear, however, as to whether exercise affords unique benefits in the reduction of anxiety, or whether such reductions also follow other, nonexercise activities (e.g., quiet rest, meditation, hobby class). Nevertheless, there was some tentative suggestion that exercise may differ from these other treatments in the time course of its effects. In several studies, reductions in anxiety were seen immediately following the nonexercise condition(s), but did not emerge until 15–20 minutes following the exercise condition(s).

Studies using psychophysiological measures as correlates of affect also appear to lend support to the notion that acute exercise is associated with reduced anxiety. The majority of studies demonstrated exercise-related changes on EMG or EEG measures, indicative of reduced central nervous system arousal. While suggestive, these findings must be tempered by an important caveat, namely that it has not been conclusively established that changes in EMG or EEG measures actually reflect changes in anxiety states.

## WHAT VARIABLES MODERATE THE EFFECTS OF ACUTE EXERCISE ON AFFECT?

Given the apparent, albeit modest effects of acute exercise on anxiety, an important next question to ask is whether particular subject or exercise variables reliably moderate (i.e., enhance or lessen) these effects. The subject variables that have been examined include age, gender, fitness level, and preexercise anxiety; the exercise variables include exercise type and intensity. In addressing this question, we examined those studies that incorporated different levels of these variables in their research design and that also provided the appropriate statistical comparisons to allow for an evaluation of their impact. Given the relatively small pool of studies that met these criteria, we have included studies from all three design categories in the following discussion.

## Subject Variables

**Age.**   It is difficult to examine the possible moderating effects of age on anxiety reductions following exercise because most studies in this area have used college students as subjects. Only one study compared anxiety reductions in groups of younger and older males who exercised on a bicycle ergometer, with results indicating no significant age-group differences following exercise (Hatfield, Goldberg, Sforzo, & Flynn, 1987).

**Gender.**   An acute bout of exercise does not appear to differentially influence the anxiety levels of males and females. Although a number of studies included subjects of both genders, only seven of these provided separate analyses of their data by gender, and none of these revealed any gender differences (Bahrke & Smith, 1985; Berger & Owen, 1983, 1988; Kraemer, Dzewaltowski, Blair, Rinehardt, & Castracane, 1990; Morgan, Roberts, & Feinerman, 1971, Experiment 2; Roth, 1989; Wood, 1977).

**Fitness Level.**   Likewise, a subject's fitness level does not appear to differentially influence levels of anxiety reported following acute exercise. Although six studies (Boutcher & Landers, 1988; Dyer & Crouch, 1987; Felts & Vaccaro, 1988; Kraemer et al., 1990; Roth, 1989; Steptoe & Cox, 1988) provided comparisons between trained and untrained subjects, only one (Boutcher & Landers, 1988) found a difference between these groups. This one study found that trained subjects reported lower levels of anxiety following exercise in comparison to untrained subjects who also exercised. It is important to emphasize that the exercise workloads in these studies were tailored to subjects' fitness levels, so that all subjects within a particular study exercised at the same relative workload.

**Preexercise Anxiety.**   Finally, although several investigators have proposed that exercise may be especially beneficial for subjects who experience high levels of anxiety, the literature does not provide any empirical evidence for this suggestion. Four studies to date have examined this possibility by comparing the impact of exercise in subjects with high levels of anxiety to those with low levels. Two of these studies found reductions in state anxiety for high anxious subjects only, although this effect emerged following both the exercise and the control conditions (Bahrke & Morgan 1978; Bahrke & Smith, 1985). The third study found that state anxiety decreased for high anxious subjects following exercise, whereas it increased for low anxious subjects (Wood, 1977). However, this study did not include a no-exercise control condition, and therefore, it is impossible to rule out statistical regression toward the mean as a possible explanation for the findings. Finally, Abood (1984) found that whereas high anxious females showed no change in state anxiety following exercise, low anxious females reported increases in anxiety.

### Exercise Variables

In examining the possible influence of exercise variables on anxiety levels following exercise, we were interested in those studies that compared different exercise types, intensities, and durations. Because no studies have compared the impact of different exercise durations, we only present findings related to exercise type and intensity.

**Exercise Type.**    Only three studies have compared the effects of different types of exercise on anxiety (Berger & Owen, 1988; Weinberg, Jackson, & Kolodny, 1988; Wilson, Berger, & Bird, 1981). One of these studies compared anxiety levels in subjects who ran on an indoor track for 40 minutes to those of subjects who participated in an exercise class for the same duration and found that both groups showed pre- to postexercise reductions in anxiety (Wilson et al., 1981). A second study compared 30 minutes of jogging to an equivalent period of swimming and found anxiety reductions only with jogging, although this effect emerged on just one of two measures of anxiety (Weinberg et al., 1988). A third study compared anxiety levels following swimming, body conditioning, yoga, and fencing; however, because swimming was the only activity that could be confidently designated as aerobic, this precluded any meaningful comparisons (Berger & Owen, 1988).

**Exercise Intensity.**    Six studies compared the impact of different exercise intensities on anxiety, but only three of these found an effect. Among these three studies, one reported a greater anxiety-reducing effect for two higher intensities, as compared to a lower intensity (Farrell, Gustafson, Morgan, & Pert, 1987); one reported a worsening of anxiety for the higher intensity but no change for the lower intensity (Steptoe & Cox, 1988), and a third reported similar anxiety reductions for two intensities of exercise (Felts & Vaccaro, 1988). The reader can refer to Table 4.1 for the actual intensities or workloads; they are not included here, as the different methods used to establish them do not allow for any meaningful comparisons across studies.

### Summary

It is difficult to arrive at any strong statements regarding the potential moderating impact of particular subject and exercise variables on the anxiety-reducing effects of exercise because these have, for the most part, not been systematically investigated *within* single studies. Furthermore, comparisons *across* studies were not feasible given the serious confounds presented by the diverse methodologies employed. Nonetheless, we are able to tentatively suggest that gender, fitness level, and prior levels of state anxiety do not appear to moderate the effects of exercise on anxiety. There was little meaningful information available regarding the influence of age, exercise type, intensity, or duration as potential moderators of exercise effects.

## WHAT PROCESSES MEDIATE THE EFFECTS OF ACUTE EXERCISE ON AFFECT?

Several processes or mechanisms have been proposed to underlie the impact of acute exercise on affect. These are referred to as the endorphin, monoamine, thermogenic, distraction, and mastery hypotheses.

### Endorphin Hypothesis

The endorphin hypothesis proposes that the effects of acute exercise on affect, specifically euphoria, are the result of the release and subsequent binding of endogenous opioids, notably ß-endorphin, to receptor sites in the brain (Steinberg & Sykes, 1985). This hypothesis appeared shortly after the discovery of the endorphins and continues to be promoted by several investigators. Twelve of the studies included in our review tested this hypothesis through one of two strategies. The first strategy involves correlating the levels of circulating ß-endorphin, usually sampled during an exercise bout, with affective measures, usually sampled subsequent to the exercise bout (Farrell, Gates, Maksud, & Morgan, 1982; Farrell et al., 1987; Hatfield, Goldfarb, Sforzo, & Flynn, 1987; Kraemer et al., 1990; McMurray, Berry, Vann, Hardy, & Sheps, 1988; Wildmann, Kruger, Schmole, Niemann, & Matthaei, 1986). The second strategy compares affective responses following exercise in a group of subjects administered opiate receptor antagonists (naloxone or naltrexone) to the responses of subjects who receive saline (Allen & Coen, 1987; Farrell et al., 1986; Grossman et al., 1984; Janal, Colt, Clark, & Glusman, 1984; Markoff, Ryan, & Young, 1982; McMurray, Berry, Hardy, & Sheps, 1988). Only one of the correlational studies (Wildmann et al., 1986) and two of the opiate-antagonist studies (Allen & Coen, 1987; Janal et al., 1984) supported the endorphin hypothesis. Thus, although this hypothesis possesses a high degree of face validity, given the anecdotal reports of an opiate-like "runner's high" associated with exercise, direct tests of this hypothesis have generally failed to support it.

### Monoamine Hypothesis

The monoamine hypothesis proposes that the affective benefits of exercise may derive from increased levels of central monoamine neurotransmitters accompanying exercise, specifically norepinephrine (Ransford, 1982). This hypothesis is intuitively appealing, given the well-established relationship between deficits in monoamine activity and depression. Nevertheless, the lines of evidence that are cited in its support are weak in terms of addressing causality. Other than the admittedly compelling arguments related to the monoamine–depression link, the only line of evidence that supports this hypothesis is the demonstration that the primary metabolite of norepinephrine (i.e., 3-methoxy-4-hydroxyphenolglycol—MHPG) reliably appears in urine or plasma following an acute bout of exercise (see Morgan & O'Connor, 1988). However, there have been no systematic attempts to relate this physiological response to affective changes. Thus, this hypothesis remains tenable but largely unsubstantiated.

## Thermogenic Hypothesis

The thermogenic hypothesis maintains that it is the elevation in body temperature accompanying exercise that contributes to affective changes associated with exercise. This hypothesis draws only indirect support from the observation that both acute exercise and passive heating (sauna) are associated with changes on EMG measures that reflect reduced central nervous system arousal (Bulbulian & Darabos, 1986; deVries, Beckman, Huber, & Dieckmeir, 1968). However, to date, there have been no direct tests of this hypothesis, and although it has received some attention from researchers (Hatfield, 1991; Morgan & O'Connor, 1988), it remains largely in the realm of speculation.[6]

## Distraction Hypothesis

The distraction hypothesis proposes that it is not acute exercise per se that is responsible for improved affect, but rather the temporary respite from life stresses or worries that it provides (Morgan, 1985). This suggestion is based on the finding of several studies that exercise was no more effective than nonexercise conditions, such as meditation or quiet rest, in reducing anxiety (e.g., Bahrke & Morgan, 1978; Felts & Vaccaro, 1988). However, this hypothesis has only been proposed in a post hoc fashion and has never been empirically verified. In addition, it is inconsistent with other studies, which have found reductions in anxiety following exercise, but not following quiet rest (e.g., Roth, 1989; Roth, Bachtler, & Fillingim, 1990).

---

[6]Two recent journal abstracts related to this issue were not included in the literature review, given our selection criteria, but they are mentioned here, as they represent the first direct tests of the thermogenic hypothesis (Petruzzello, Landers, & Salazar, 1991; Youngstedt, Dishman, Cureton, Peacock, Wells, Fluech, & Hinson, 1991). Both studies manipulated ambient temperature during exercise, and neither study found any impact of these manipulations on postexercise anxiety levels. Thus, the thermogenic hypothesis was not supported.

## Mastery Hypothesis

The mastery hypothesis suggests that exercise may increase people's sense of mastery or accomplishment and thereby lead to improved affect (e.g., Brown, 1991; Norris, Carroll, & Cochrane, 1990; Simons, McGowan, Epstein, Kupfer, & Robertson, 1985). Several lines of research in other areas, including the work of Bandura (1989) on self-efficacy, Deci and Ryan (1985) on perceived competence, and Rodin (1986) on perceived control, all point to the potential influence that perceived mastery may have on affective states. As with the distraction hypothesis, the notion of mastery has only been mentioned in passing and has not been empirically tested. Nonetheless, given that several lines of research point to its potential importance, it may prove to be a promising topic for future research.

## Summary

There is currently no strong support for any of the hypotheses proposed with respect to possible mechanisms underlying the impact of acute exercise on affect. There has been virtually no direct testing of these hypotheses, with the exception of the endorphin hypothesis, which has received little support. It is noteworthy that little consideration has been given to psychological processes that may mediate the effects of exercise. In general, it seems that researchers have chosen to concentrate their efforts on demonstrating that changes in affect are indeed associated with exercise, without exploring the underlying basis for such changes.

## RESEARCH IN OUR LABORATORY

As can be seen, there is a dearth of psychological variables that have been proposed and tested as possible mechanisms underlying the effect of acute exercise on affective states. Because it is conceivable that the phenomenon in question is largely psychological—namely, changes in affective states—the failure to consider psychological variables may explain why researchers in this area have had difficulty in reliably demonstrating effects of exercise.

Recently, we conducted a study to test the influence of two psychological variables that we hypothesized may play an important role in determining affective states experienced following an acute bout of exercise (Tuson, Sinyor, & Pelletier, in press). First, we postulated that *perceived* exercise intensity, as opposed to actual exercise intensity, would be a better predictor of postexercise affective states, specifically those related to positive affect (PA). Traditionally, exercise intensity has been determined using objective methods, such as maintaining exercise workload during the exercise bout at a specific level based on subjects' $\dot{V}O_2$max. However, evidence is growing within the psychological literature that people's perceptions, rather than the actual situation, may be a more important determinant of psychological consequences (e.g., Langer, 1975). Accordingly, we assessed subjects' PA following light, moderate, or intense exercise, as established objectively by maintaining exercise workload at one of three levels of $\dot{V}O_2$max (25%, 50%, and 75% $\dot{V}O_2$max, respectively), and we compared these results to those obtained using these same subjects' subjective ratings of whether the exercise was perceived to be light, moderate, or intense, using Borg's Ratings of Perceived Exertion (RPE; Borg, 1977). With respect to the subjective exercise intensities, we further hypothesized that subjects would only report increased PA following exercise bouts perceived to be of *moderate* intensity but not following exercise bouts perceived to be light or intense. Our rationale for this prediction was that exercise bouts perceived to be of moderate intensity would create situations of optimal challenge, whereas exercise bouts perceived to be light or intense would create situations of boredom or stress, respectively.

The second psychological variable that we considered to play an important role in determining postexercise affect was that of *pre*exercise affect, a variable that has typically been relegated to the role of a dependent rather than independent variable in this area of research. We believe that this may have been an important oversight when considering the impact of exercise on affect. Our reasoning is as follows. As mentioned, we predicted that only those exercise intensities perceived to be moderate would be followed by increases in PA. However, this prediction must be qualified in terms of subjects' initial affect. In keeping with the theory of optimal stimulation (Csikszentmihalyi, 1982), we hypothesized that subjects who report low initial PA would report increases in PA following a bout of exercise perceived to be of moderate intensity but would maintain their low levels of PA following bouts perceived to be light or intense. Conversely, we hypothesized that subjects who report a high initial PA would maintain these levels following a bout of exercise perceived to be of moderate intensity but would report a decrease in PA following bouts perceived to be light or intense. This distinction becomes very important when testing for significant pre–post changes in affective states. For instance, if a subject reports high initial PA and then proceeds to exercise at a perceived moderate intensity, a significant change in affect should not be expected to occur. Similarly, if a subject reports low initial PA and then exercises at intensities perceived to be either light or intense, there should be little reason to expect a significant change in affect.

Thus, we postulated that consideration of the interaction between initial affect and subjective perceptions of exercise intensity may yield a clearer understanding of the process by which exercise exerts its influence on postexercise affect. To test our hypotheses, we randomly assigned 65 university students (32 women and 33 men, ages 19–30) to 30 minutes of exercise on a motorized treadmill at 25, 50, or 75% of their estimated $\dot{V}O_2$max, or to a no-exercise control group of quiet rest. These conditions constituted our objective measure of exercise intensity. We also collected ratings of perceived exercise intensity, using the RPE, at three points during the exercise bout, which were then averaged to establish a global rating of intensity. These ratings, which were classified as reflecting either light, moderate, or intense exercise, constituted our subjective measure of exercise intensity (analysis of the heart rate data confirmed that, regardless of the method used to establish intensity, subjects in the different groups were exercising at significantly different intensities). Self-reported affect, assessed by the Multiple Affect Adjective Checklist—Revised (MAACL-R; Zuckerman & Lubin, 1985), was sampled prior to and 5, 17, and 30 minutes following the exercise bout. Based on initial affect scores, two groups (low initial PA and high initial PA) were formed through a median split of scores on the PASS subscale of the MAACL-R; the PASS subscale represents a composite measure of positive affect.

Our discussion of affective changes following exercise centers around the affect scores obtained 30 minutes following the exercise bout, as this was the time at which the effect began to appear. To test our predictions regarding the impact of initial affect and exercise intensity on postexercise affect, planned contrasts were performed comparing subjects' preexercise affect to their postexercise affect for each exercise condition. The results of these analyses are presented separately for the low and high initial PA groups for both the perceived and objective definitions of exercise intensity in Figure 4.1.

In general, our predictions were supported. Comparisons across the perceived and objective exercise conditions in the figure reveals that a different pattern of results emerged, depending on the method used to establish exercise intensity. As can be seen, the conventional method of establishing exercise intensity, or the objective definition, was not associated with any pre–post affective changes, save for what appears to be a spurious reduction of affect in subjects with high initial PA in the control condition. By contrast, when we analyzed the data according to these same subjects' perception of exercise intensity, we found results that were as we predicted. Specifically, subjects who reported a low initial PA did not show significant affective changes when the exercise was perceived to be light or intense but did show significant improvements in affect when the exercise was perceived to be of moderate intensity. In a similar fashion, subjects who reported a high initial PA did not show significant affective changes when the exercise was perceived to be of moderate intensity but did show significant reductions in affect when the exercise was perceived to be intense and a tendency in the same direction when the exercise was perceived to be light. These results, although preliminary, provide some support for our

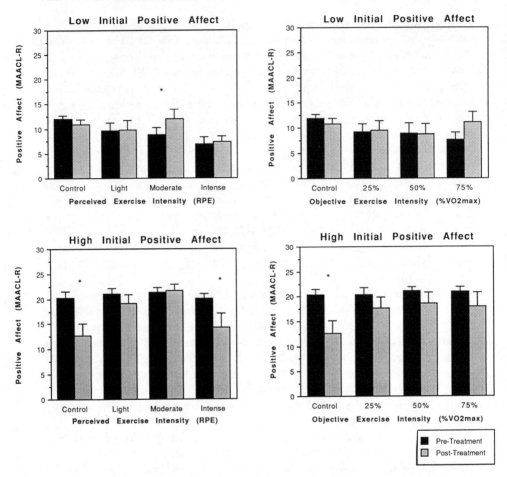

**Figure 4.1.**   Mean pre- and postexercise affect scores as a function of low versus high initial positive affect (PA), and perceived versus objective exercise intensity. Panels on the left present PA scores for low (upper panel) and high (lower panel) initial PA, with exercise intensity defined by ratings of perceived exertion (RPE). Panels on the right present PA scores for low (upper panel) and high (lower panel) initial PA, with exercise intensity defined by objective workload as a percentage of $\dot{V}O_2$ max.

position that examination of psychological processes as determinants of affective changes following exercise may be a constructive approach for addressing the issue of affective changes related to exercise.

## SUMMARY OF PREVIOUS RESEARCH

Our review of the literature suggests that an acute bout of exercise may be associated with reductions in anxiety but does not appear to influence other affective states, specifically depression, anger, vigor, fatigue, or confusion. The anxiety-reducing effects, although modest, emerged on both self-report measures and psychophysiological indices. It remains unclear whether this effect is unique to exercise because it was also evident in a number of nonexercise comparison groups. With respect to gender, fitness level, and prior levels of anxiety, none of these were found to moderate the effects of exercise on anxiety; there was little information regarding the impact of age or exercise parameters. As for possible mechanisms mediating the effects of exercise on affective states, only the endorphin hypothesis has been directly tested, and it has received minimal support. There is currently little basis for drawing any conclusions regarding the other hypotheses—the monoamine, thermogenic, distraction, and mastery hypotheses—although they all remain tenable. We have noted the relative absence of inquiry regarding psychological variables that may moderate or mediate the effects of exercise, and we have conducted some preliminary work to explore the impact of such variables. Our research suggested that both preexercise affect and perceived, as opposed to objective, exercise intensity may be important predictors of the affective response to exercise.

Overall, our conclusions regarding the impact of acute exercise on affective states appear to be at odds with the popular belief that exercise improves affect, as well as with the more encouraging conclusions that have been offered by other investigators who have reviewed this literature (e.g., Hatfield, 1991; Morgan, 1985; Morgan & O'Connor, 1988). There are two important points to consider in accounting for the apparent discrepancy between our conclusions and those of other reviewers. First, these reviewers often included, and gave equal weighting to, poorly designed studies, journal abstracts, and unpublished manuscripts in arriving at their conclusions. Second, they have usually emphasized the positive findings and generally overlooked the failure of other affective measures to demonstrate improvements. This may have led to an overestimation of the overall impact of exercise on affective states. In fact, it may be that the discrepancy between our conclusions and those offered in previous reviews is more cosmetic than substantive. Although the message conveyed by most of these reviews is that acute exercise possesses considerable benefits for affective states in general, this view is often based on outcomes that are specific to anxiety. In this way, the conclusions reached by previous reviewers may not differ markedly from our own, although they may not be qualified to the same extent.

## THEORETICAL AND METHODOLOGICAL ISSUES

In reviewing the research examining the influence of acute exercise on affective states, three striking features of this literature emerged. First, research conducted in this area has been largely atheoretical; that is, it has not been embedded within a conceptual framework incorporating a clear definition of affect and affective change. Second, few studies have hypothesized and tested, in an a priori manner, specific processes that may mediate the impact of acute exercise on affective states. Finally, in their focus on the distinctly physical nature of exercise, researchers have paid little attention, other than in passing, to the role that psychological variables may play in moderating or mediating the effects of exercise on affective states. Each of these issues is addressed, in turn, in the following section.

### The Need for Definition: What Is Affect and How Does It Change?

An important ingredient that should be included for a meaningful analysis of any research problem is the presentation of a clear definition of the phenomenon under investigation. Therefore, it would seem that a necessary first step for researchers examining the influence of acute exercise on changes in affective states would be to specify the definition or conceptualization of *affect* that they will use to guide their research. Outlining a specific definition of *affect* is crucial because it will determine, among other things, (1) the boundaries of what does and does not constitute affect, (2) the attributes or criteria essential to affect, and (3) the types of processes and variables that should be studied. What follows is a brief discussion of these definitional issues. The ideas presented are based largely on the kinds of problems that researchers studying emotion have been debating for years. We should point out that in presenting these problems, we have not taken a particular stance on how they should be resolved. This, we feel, is a matter to be determined by the individual researcher. Instead, our goal is simply to raise awareness that such issues may be important to consider when formulating a conceptual framework for studying affective changes related to exercise.

**The Boundaries of What Constitutes Affect.**   Research conducted in the area of exercise and affective change has explored the impact of exercise on a number of constructs, such as anxiety, depression, anger, vigor, fatigue, confusion, pleasantness, and euphoria. The question that arises, however, is whether these different constructs all belong under the rubric of *affect*. For many researchers working in the area of emotion, only some of these constructs are viewed as true examples of affect, with others being viewed as merely affect-related (e.g., Johnson-Laird & Oatley, 1989; Lazarus, 1991; Ortony & Clore, 1989). Lazarus (1991) for example, would argue that of those constructs listed, only anxiety, anger, and euphoria represent true affect. The others, he would claim, are either an admixture of several types of affect (depression), or are only affect-related (fatigue, confusion, vigor, pleasantness). We have raised this issue of distinguishing between what does and does not constitute *affect* because we feel its consideration is germane to the formulation of a conceptual model of affective change. Because any model must delineate the underlying mechanism(s) responsible for affective change, it would stand to reason that the affective constructs incorporated in the model be influenced by one or more common underlying mechanisms. It is conceivable, however, that the various affective constructs that have been examined within the exercise literature may not be influenced by similar underlying mechanisms, and consequently, their indiscriminate inclusion may have confounded the findings, contributing to the present state of confusion in this area.

A more general problem related to the issue of defining *affect* concerns researchers' use of inconsistent and ill-defined terms. Throughout the exercise literature, the terms *psychological benefits, mood states, feelings,* and *affect* have been used interchangeably to refer to a wide range of variables, including anxiety, depression, fatigue, and confusion. This diversity in terminology begs the question of whether these terms should be considered synonymous. According to some researchers, they should not. For instance, Lazarus (1991) would argue that *mood* and *affect* do not represent the same thing, and that *mood* represents a transient state, whereas *affect* (or emotion) is somewhat more enduring. As another example, "psychological benefits" could refer to improvements in affective states but could also refer to improvements in other affect-related constructs or even nonaffective constructs such as cognitive functioning. At first blush, these distinctions may seem quite trivial. However, such distinctions could come to have significance when considering the processes leading to affective change. Take, for example, the implication of Lazarus's distinction between transient mood states and enduring affect. It seems reasonable to suppose that these two kinds of affect may not be similarly influenced by the two principal classes of exercise (i.e., acute and chronic), such that acute exercise may be expected to have a greater impact on transient mood states and chronic exercise may be expected to have a greater impact on more enduring affect.[7] Thus, there

---

[7]We have implied here that there are different mechanism(s) underlying the impact of acute and chronic exercise on affective states. We recognize that this contrasts with the suggestions of other researchers, who argue that because chronic exercise consists of repeated single bouts of exercise, the affective changes accompanying acute exercise may accumulate to produce chronic effects (Haskell, 1987; Morgan, 1976). However, discussion of this issue is outside the scope of this paper.

is a need for researchers to present a clear description of what is intended by the terms they have chosen to use.

**Attributes Essential to Affect and Affective Change.**    Another issue related to the problem of defining affect concerns the specific attributes or criteria that are essential to affect. Two commonly debated questions are (1) Is physiological change necessary to experience affect? and (2) Is cognition (or the subjective meaning attributed to a situation) necessary to experience affect? While some researchers would argue that physiological change is the most important defining attribute of affect (e.g., Levenson, 1988; Mason, 1975), others would argue that it is insufficient for the experience of affect and that the cognitive appraisal or subjective meaning that a person attaches to a situation is the key determinant of affect (e.g., Lazarus, 1991; Schachter, 1964).[8] More specifically, researchers in the first camp maintain that each type of affect is defined by its own unique pattern of physiological change, whereas it is the contention of researchers in the second camp that the empirical basis for such a position is sparse and that the more plausible explanation is that once physiological arousal is experienced, the affect that follows will depend on the type of appraisal made regarding the arousal (Petri, 1991). This debate is clearly an important one for researchers to consider in conceptualizing the influence of exercise on affect, as these different frameworks may point to different processes that should be the central focus of study.

**Mediating Processes of Affective Change.**    The suggestion that emerges from the preceding discussion is that the way in which one chooses to define or conceptualize *affect* will largely determine the kinds of processes and variables that will be the focus of research. Presumably, if one supports a physiological basis for affective change, the focus will be on identifying those physiological qualities that are critical to the affect of interest and then measuring how these respond to a session of exercise. By contrast, if one supports a more cognitive or psychological basis for affective change, the focus will be on identifying the types of appraisals that may be relevant to the experience of engaging in a session of exercise and then verifying their influence. These different theoretical frameworks may also point to a separate class of variables that might be expected to moderate the influence of exercise on affect. It can be seen, then, that working from a well-specified

---

consists of repeated single bouts of exercise, the affective changes accompanying acute exercise may accumulate to produce chronic effects (Haskell, 1987; Morgan, 1976). However, discussion of this issue is outside the scope of this paper.

[8]We should point out that both Lazarus and Schachter incorporate physiological changes in their theories and that they differ from other researchers largely in the emphasis and central focus of their research.

theoretical framework has the advantage of directing attention to those underlying processes and moderating variables that could be key to understanding how exercise may influence affect.

## The Need for Direct Testing of Hypothesized Mediating Processes

Perhaps owing to the relative absence of theoretical frameworks guiding research efforts, there has been virtually no direct testing of possible processes mediating affective changes associated with acute exercise. Instead, such processes have been proposed almost exclusively in a post hoc fashion. At present, the only mediating process that has been posited and tested in an a priori manner pertains to the release of endorphins. The thermogenic, monoamine, distraction, and mastery hypotheses all remain largely in the realm of speculation. With respect to the distraction hypothesis, it is particularly noteworthy that this mechanism was first proposed more than a decade ago (Bahrke & Morgan, 1978), and although it continues to be promoted by a number of researchers (e.g., Bahrke & Smith, 1985; Felts & Vaccaro, 1988; McGowan, Robertson, & Epstein, 1985; Wilson, Berger, & Bird, 1981), it has never been empirically tested. This state of affairs causes concern, given that it is only through the direct testing of hypothesized processes that we can gain a clearer understanding of the way in which exercise may influence affective states. It is our opinion that unless researchers begin to make a concerted effort to incorporate such direct tests into their research designs, any advancement in knowledge is likely to be limited and tentative.

## The Need to Consider Psychological Variables

As previously mentioned, there has been a preponderance of attention devoted to non-psychological variables thought to play a role in determining affective states following acute exercise. Perhaps researchers have found it intuitively appealing to consider such consequences as being largely physically based, given that a vigorous bout of exercise represents a significant departure from physiological homeostatis. It is understandable, then, that they have generally tried to identify physiological mechanisms, such as changes in endorphin levels, as possible determinants of affective change, as well as physically related variables that may moderate this effect, such as fitness level or the intensity of the exercise bout. However, numerous studies examining such variables have not been able to reliably establish their role in determining postexercise changes in affect.

In their focus on the distinctly physical nature of exercise, researchers seem to have overlooked the fact that the phenomenon they are attempting to explain may be one that can be considered largely *psychological*. We suspect that the difficulty researchers have encountered in empirically demonstrating the link between exercise and improved affective states is due, in part, to their failure to consider possible psychological variables that may be playing a role. That is, quite conceivably it is not exercise per se that leads to changes in affect, but rather psychological variables related to the experience of engaging in exercise.

In particular, the reasons which lead people to engage in exercise and the appraisal or subjective meaning which they ascribe to the exercise experience may be the principal determinants of their affective responses. In our opinion, it is especially important to consider such motivational and cognitive processes in the study of affective changes associated with exercise, given their central role in several proposed models of affective change (e.g., Lazarus, 1991; Schachter, 1964; Weiner, 1985). In general, it has been argued that in order for a situation or experience to elicit an affective state, it must have significance or meaning to the individual, and that this significance or meaning is largely determined by a person's motivation or personal goals (e.g., Lazarus, 1991). Moreover, the type of affect that will be experienced is thought to depend on the nature of these personal goals and the extent to which the individual perceives them to be satisfied.

One implication of this position is that subjects participating in a study investigating the impact of exercise on affective states may arrive at the experimental session with particular motives or goals in mind. For instance, one subject's motive may be to physically challenge herself, another may hope to impress the experimenter with his physical prowess, while another may be seeking diversion from school stresses. The affective states experienced by these subjects following the exercise session may depend largely on the extent to which they perceive these goals as being achieved. In the case of the first subject, if she successfully completed the challenging exercise session, she may feel proud and masterful for having done so and consequently may experience an improved affective state; however, if she felt underchallenged and bored or overchallenged and hence inadequate, she may experience no change or even a worsening of affective state. In the case of the second subject, if he perceived his performance to be positively evaluated by the experimenter, then improvement in affect is likely to ensue; if not, he may feel disappointed or discouraged, and thus may experience a worsening of affective state. Finally, the third subject may experience an improvement in affect, but only if the exercise session succeeded in serving as a distraction from worries.

In the studies identified through our literature review, the potential role of motivational and cognitive processes was largely left unstudied. Therefore, such processes could have exerted an unforeseen confounding effect or even masked the relationship between exercise and improved affect. It would seem then, that examination of subjects' motivation or goals toward exercise, and their subsequent appraisals of whether these were realized, may prove to be a promising topic for future research. One strategy that researchers could employ in studying this question would be to obtain measures of both motivation and cognitive appraisals related to the exercise session and to correlate these with affective states following exercise. However, a preferred strategy would involve the experimental manipulation of these processes because this would provide a more definitive test of their possible causal role. For example, researchers interested in evaluating the influence of mastery-oriented goals or motives on affective states associated with exercise could adopt the following strategy. Subjects could be provided with a goal to achieve during an upcoming exercise bout, and their appraisal of whether or not that goal was achieved could be experimentally manipulated through success or failure feedback, regardless of whether that feedback was actually true. A manipulation check to verify the effectiveness of the feedback on subjects' appraisals of self-mastery could be performed, and the impact of such appraisals on subsequent affective states could then be evaluated. Conceivably, a similar approach could be adopted to explore the possible contribution of distraction-oriented motives on affective responses to exercise.

While we recognize that the foregoing ideas represent a departure from those traditionally explored in this area, we feel that a change of approach is timely, given the relatively modest success achieved by the existing approach. That is, it is our opinion that affective states following acute exercise cannot be predicted from a physiological standpoint alone, but that serious consideration must also be given to psychological processes that may be playing a role. At the very least, even if exercise researchers are not interested in directly studying such psychological processes, we believe it may be wise for them to ensure that their research has properly controlled for the influence of these processes.

## CONCLUDING REMARKS

The belief that a bout of exercise can positively influence affective states is longstanding and widespread. There is probably not a regular exerciser who would dispute the existence of such effects. Why, then, has it proven so difficult for researchers to reliably demonstrate these effects? Perhaps part of the answer lies in the approach that researchers have traditionally followed in addressing this question. In our opinion, this physically-based approach has led to a serious oversight—namely, the failure to consider the potential importance of psychological variables in determining affective changes associated with exercise. These variables include, among others, such things as affective states prior to exercise, motives for exercising, and the sense of accomplishment or mastery associated with performing exercise. We believe that examining the possible contribution of these variables offers promising directions for future research.

## ACKNOWLEDGMENTS

We wish to thank all the individuals who commented on earlier versions of this paper. We are especially grateful for the insightful suggestions of Luc G. Pelletier.

## REFERENCES

Abood, D. A. (1984). The effects of acute physical exercise on the state anxiety and mental performance of college women. *American Corrective Therapy Journal, 38,* 69–74.

Allen, M. E., & Coen, D. (1987). Naloxone blocking of running-induced mood changes. *Annals of Sports Medicine, 3,* 190–195.

American College of Sports Medicine. (1980). *Guidelines for graded exercise testing and exercise prescription* (2nd ed). Philadelphia: Lea & Febiger.

Bahrke, M., & Morgan, W. P. (1978). Anxiety reduction following exercise and meditation. *Cognitive Therapy and Research, 2,* 323–333.

Bahrke, M. S., & Smith, R. G. (1985). Alterations in anxiety after exercise and rest. *American Corrective Therapy Journal, 39,* 90–94.

Balog, L. F. (1983). The effects of exercise on muscle tension and subsequent muscle relaxation training. *Research Quarterly in Exercise and Sport, 54,* 119–125.

Bandura, A. (1989). Human agency in social cognitive theory. *American Psychologist, 44,* 1175–1184.

Berger, B. G., & Owen, D. R. (1983). Mood alteration with swimming: Swimmers really do "feel better." *Psychosomatic Medicine, 45,* 425–432.

Berger, B. G., & Owen, D. R. (1988). Stress reduction and mood enhancement in four exercise modes: Swimming, body conditioning, hatha yoga, and fencing. *Research Quarterly for Exercise and Sport, 59,* 148–159.

Blair, S. N., Goodyear, N. N., Gibbons, L. W., & Cooper, K. H. (1984). Physical fitness and incidence of hypertension in healthy normotensive men and women. *Journal of the American Medical Association, 252,* 487–490.

Borg, G. (1977). Simple rating methods for estimation of perceived exertion. In G. Borg (Ed.), *Physical work and effort.* New York: Pergamon Press.

Boutcher, S. H., & Landers, D. M. (1988). The effects of vigorous exercise on anxiety, heart rate, and alpha activity of runners and nonrunners. *Psychophysiology, 25,* 696–702.

Brown, J. D. (1991). Staying fit and staying well: Physical fitness as a moderator of life stress. *Journal of Personality and Social Psychology, 60,* 555–561.

Bulbulian, R., & Darabos, B. L. (1986). Motor neuron excitability: The Hoffman reflex following exercise of low and high intensity. *Medicine and Science in Sports and Exercise, 18,* 697–702.

Campbell, D. T., & Stanley, J. C. (1963). *Experimental and quasi-experimental designs for research.* Chicago: Rand McNally.

Carlson, N. R. (1991). *Physiology of behavior* (4th ed.). Toronto: Allyn & Bacon.

Carmack, M. A., & Martens, R. (1979). Measuring commitment to running: A survey of runners' attitudes and mental states. *Journal of Sport Psychology, 1*, 25–42.

Csikszentmihalyi, M. (1982). Toward a psychology of optimal experience. In L. Wheeler (Ed.), *Review of personality and social psychology* (Vol. 3, pp. 13–36). Beverly Hills, CA: Sage Publishers.

Deci, E. L., & Ryan, R. M. (1985). *Intrinsic motivation and self-determination in human behavior.* New York: Plenum Press.

deVries, H. A. (1968). Immediate and long term effects of exercise on muscle action potential level. *Journal of Sports Medicine and Physical Fitness, 8*, 2–11.

deVries, H. A., & Adams, G. M. (1972). Electromyographic comparison of single doses of exercise and meprobamate as to effects on muscular relaxation. *American Journal of Physical Medicine, 51*, 130–149.

deVries, H. A., Beckman, P., Huber, H., & Dieckmeir, L. (1968). Electromyographic evaluation of the effects of sauna on the neuromuscular system. *Journal of Sports Medicine, 8*, 61–69.

deVries, H. A., Simard, C. P., Wiswell, R. A., Heckathorne, E., & Carabetta, V. (1982). Fusimotor system involvement in the tranquilizer effect of exercise. *American Journal of Physical Medicine, 61*, 111–122.

deVries, H. A., Wiswell, R., Bulbulian, R., & Moritani, T. (1981). Tranquilizer effects of exercise: Acute effects of moderate aerobic exercise on spinal reflex activation level. *American Journal of Physical Medicine, 51*, 57–66.

Doyne, E. J., Chambless, D. L., & Beutler, L. E. (1983). Aerobic exercise as a treatment for depression in women. *Behavior Therapy, 14*, 434–440.

Dyer, J. B., & Crouch, J. G. (1987). Effects of running on moods: A time-series study. *Perceptual and Motor Skills, 64*, 783–789.

Ewing, J. H., Scott, D. G., Mendez, A. A., & McBride, T. J. (1984). Effects of aerobic exercise upon affect and cognition. *Perceptual and Motor Skills, 59*, 407–414.

Farrell, P. A., Gates, W. K., Maksud, M. G., & Morgan, W. P. (1982). Increases in plasma ß-endorphin/ß-lipotropin immunoreactivity after treadmill running in humans. *Journal of Applied Physiology, 52*, 1245–1249.

Farrell, P. A., Gustafson, A. B., Garthwaite, T. L., Kalkhoff, R. K., Cowley, A. W., & Morgan, W. P. (1986). Influence of endogenous opioids on the response of selected hormones to exercise in humans. *Journal of Applied Physiology, 61*, 1051–1057.

Farrell, P. A., Gustafson, A. B., Morgan, W. P., & Pert, C. B. (1987). Enkephalins, catecholamines and psychological mood alterations: Effects of prolonged exercise. *Medicine and Science in Sports and Exercise, 19*, 347–353.

Felts, W. M. (1989). Relationship between ratings of perceived exertion and exercise-induced decrease in state anxiety. *Perceptual and Motor Skills, 69*, 368–370.

Felts, W. M., & Vaccaro, P. (1988). The effect of aerobic exercise on post-exercise state anxiety and psychophysiological arousal as a function of fitness level. *Clinical Kinesiology, 42*, 89–96.

Fillingim, R. B., Roth, D. L., & Haley, W. E. (1989). The effects of distraction on the perception of exercise-induced symptoms. *Journal of Psychosomatic Research, 33*, 241–248.

Flory, J. D., & Holmes, D. S. (1991). Effects of an acute bout of aerobic exercise on cardiovascular and subjective responses during subsequent cognitive work. *Journal of Psychosomatic Research, 35,* 225–230.

Folkins, C. H., & Sime, W. E. (1981). Physical fitness training and mental health. *American Psychologist, 36,* 373–389.

Goldfarb, A. H., Hatfield, B. D., Sforzo, G. A., & Flynn, M. G. (1987). Serum ß-endorphin levels during a graded exercise to exhaustion. *Medicine and Science in Sports and Exercise, 19,* 78–82.

Grossman, A., Bouloux, P., Price, P., Drury, P. L., Lam, K. S., Turner, T., Thomas, J., Besser, G. M., & Sutton, J. (1984). The role of opioid peptides in the hormonal responses to acute exercise in man. *Clinical Science, 67,* 483–491.

Haskell, W. L. (1987). Developing an activity plan for improving health. In W. P. Morgan & S. E. Goldston (Eds.), *Exercise and mental health* (pp. 37–55). Washington, DC: Hemisphere.

Hatfield, B. D. (1991). Exercise and mental health: The mechanisms of exercise-induced psychological states. In L. Diamant (Ed.), *Psychology of sports, exercise, and fitness: Social and personal issues* (pp. 17–49). New York: Hemisphere Publishing.

Hatfield, B. D., Goldfarb, A. H., Sforzo, G. A., & Flynn, M. G. (1987). Serum beta-endorphin and affective responses to graded exercise in young and elderly men. *Journal of Gerontology, 42,* 429–431.

Hatfield, B. D., & Landers, D. M. (1987). Psychophysiology within exercise and sports research: An overview. *Exercise and Sports Science Reviews, 15,* 351–387.

Hughes, J. R. (1984). Psychological effects of habitual aerobic exercise: A critical review. *Preventive Medicine, 13,* 66–78.

Janal, M. N., Colt, E. W., Clark, W. C., & Glusman, M. (1984). Pain sensitivity, mood and plasma endocrine levels in man following long-distance running: Effects of naloxone. *Pain, 19,* 13–25.

Johnson-Laird, P. N., & Oatley, K. (1989). The language of emotions: An analysis of a semantic field. *Cognition and Emotion, 3,* 81–123.

Kraemer, R. R., Dzewaltowski, D. A., Blair, M. S., Rinehardt, K. F., & Castracane, V. D. (1990). Mood alteration from treadmill running and its relationship to beta-endorphin, corticotropin, and growth hormone. *Journal of Sports Medicine and Physical Fitness, 30,* 241–246.

Langer, E. J. (1975). The illusion of control. *Journal of Personality and Social Psychology, 32,* 311–328.

Lazarus, R. S. (1991). Progress on a cognitive-motivational-relational theory of emotion. *American Psychologist, 46,* 819–834.

Lennon, D., Stratman, F. W., Shrago, E., Nagle, F. J., Hanson, P. G., Maddon, M., & Spennetta, T. (1983). Total cholesterol and HDL-cholesterol changes during acute, moderate intensity exercise in men and women. *Metabolism, 32,* 244–249.

Levenson, R. W. (1988). Emotion and the autonomic nervous system: A prospectus for research on autonomic specificity. In H. Wagner (Ed.), *Social psychophysiology and emotion: Theory and clinical applications* (pp. 17–42). London: Wiley.

Lichtman, S., & Poser, E. G. (1983). The effects of exercise on mood and cognitive functioning. *Journal of Psychosomatic Research, 27,* 43–52.

Markoff, R. A., Ryan, P., & Young, T. (1982). Endorphins and mood changes in long-distance running. *Medicine and Science in Sports and Exercise, 14,* 11–15.

Martinsen, E. W., Hoffart, A., & Solberg, O. Y. (1989). Aerobic and non-aerobic forms of exercise in the treatment of anxiety disorders. *Stress Medicine, 50,* 115–120.

Mason, J. W. (1975). Emotion as reflected in patterns of endocrine integration. In L. Levi (Ed.), *Emotions: Their parameters and measurement* (pp. 143–181). New York: Raven.

McCann, I. L., & Holmes, D. S. (1984). Influence of aerobic exercise on depression. *Journal of Personality and Social Psychology, 46,* 1142–1147.

McGowan, C. R., Robertson, R. J., & Epstein, L. H. (1985). The effects of bicycle ergometer exercise at varying intensities on the heart rate, EMG and mood state responses to a mental arithmetic stressor. *Research Quarterly for Exercise and Sport, 56,* 131–137.

McMurray, R. G., Berry, M. J., Hardy, C. J., & Sheps, D. S. (1988). Physiologic and psychologic responses to a low dose of naloxone administered during prolonged running. *Annals of Sports Medicine, 4,* 21–25.

McMurray, R. G., Berry, M. J., Vann, R. T., Hardy, C. J., & Sheps, D. S. (1988). The effect of running in an outdoor environment on plasma beta endorphins. *Annals of Sports Medicine, 3,* 230–233.

Morgan, W. P. (1976). Psychological consequences of vigorous physical activity and sport. In M. G. Scott (Ed.), *Introduction to sport psychology* (pp. 15–30). St. Louis, MO: Mosby.

Morgan, W. P. (1985). Affective beneficence of vigorous physical activity. *Medicine and Science in Sports and Exercise, 6,* 422–425.

Morgan, W. P., & O'Connor, P. J. (1988). Exercise and mental health. In R. K. Dishman (Ed.), *Exercise adherence: Its impact on public health* (pp. 91–121). Champaign, IL: Human Kinetics.

Morgan, W. P., Roberts, J. A., & Feinerman, A. D. (1971). Psychological effect of acute physical activity. *Archives of Physical Medicine and Rehabilitation, 52,* 422–433.

Norris, R., Carroll, D., & Cochrane, R. (1990). The effects of aerobic and anaerobic training on fitness, blood pressure and psychological stress and well-being. *Journal of Psychosomatic Research, 34,* 367–375.

Nowlis, D. P., & Greenberg, N. (1979). Empirical description of effects of exercise on mood. *Perceptual and Motor Skills, 49,* 1001–1002.

Oberman, A. (1985). Exercise and the primary prevention of cardiovascular disease. *American Journal of Cardiology, 55,* 10D–20D.

Ortony, A., & Clore, G. L. (1989). Emotions, moods, and conscious awareness: Comment on Johnson-Laird and Oatley's "The language of emotions: An analysis of a semantic field." *Cognition and Emotion, 3,* 125–137.

Petri, H. L. (1991). *Motivation: Theory, research, and applications* (3rd ed.). Belmont, CA: Wadsworth Publishing.

Petruzzello, S. J., Landers, D. M., Hatfield, B. D., Kubitz, K. A., & Salazar, W. (1991). A meta-analysis on the anxiety-reducing effects of acute and chronic exercise. *Sports Medicine, 11,* 143–182.

Petruzzello, S. J., Landers, D. M., & Salazar, W. (1991). Exercise and anxiety reduction: Examination of the thermogenic hypothesis. *Medicine and Science in Sports and Exercise, 23,* (Abstract No. 245).

Pineda, A., & Adkisson, M. A. (1961). Electroencephalographic studies in physical fatigue. *Texas Reports of Biological Medicine, 19,* 332–342.

Raglin, J. S., & Morgan, W. P. (1987). Influence of exercise and quiet rest on state anxiety and blood pressure. *Medicine and Science in Sports and Exercise, 19,* 456–463.

Ransford, C. P. (1982). A role for amines in the antidepressant effect of exercise: A review. *Medicine and Science in Sports and Exercise, 14,* 1–10.

Rodin, J. (1986). Aging and health: Effects of the sense of control. *Science, 233,* 1271–1276.

Rosenthal, M., Haskell, W. L., Solomon, R., Widstrom, A., & Reavan, G. M. (1983). Demonstration of a relationship between level of physical training and insulin-stimulated glucose utilization in normal humans. *Diabetes, 32,* 408–411.

Roth, D. L. (1989). Acute emotional and psychophysiological effects of aerobic exercise. *Psychophysiology, 26,* 593–602.

Roth, D. L., Bachtler, S. D., & Fillingim, R. (1990). Acute emotional and cardiovascular effects of stressful mental work during aerobic exercise. *Psychophysiology, 27,* 694–701.

Russell, P. O., Epstein, L. H., & Erickson, K. T. (1983). Effects of acute exercise and cigarette smoking on autonomic and neuromuscular responses to a cognitive stressor. *Psychological Reports, 53,* 199–206.

Schachter, S. (1964). The interaction of cognitive and physiological determinants of emotional state. In L. Berkowitz (Ed.), *Advances in experimental social psychology* (Vol. 1). New York: Academic Press.

Simons, A. D., McGowan, C. R., Epstein, L. H., Kupfer, D. J., & Robertson, R. J. (1985). Exercise as a treatment for depression: An update. *Clinical Psychology Review, 5,* 553–568.

Steinberg, H., & Sykes, E. A. (1985). Introduction to symposium on endorphins and behavioral processes: Review of literature on endorphins and exercise. *Pharmacology, Biochemistry and Behavior, 23,* 857–862.

Steptoe, A., & Cox, S. (1988). Acute effects of aerobic exercise on mood. *Health Psychology, 7,* 329–340.

Thayer, R. E. (1987). Energy, tiredness, and tension effects of a sugar snack versus moderate exercise. *Journal of Personality and Social Psychology, 52,* 119–125.

Tomporowski, P. D., & Ellis, N. R. (1986). Effects of exercise on cognitive processes. *Psychological Bulletin, 99,* 338–346.

Tuson, K. M., Sinyor, D., & Pelletier, L. G. (in press). Acute exercise and affect: An investigation of psychological processes leading to changes in affect. *International Journal of Sport Psychology.*

Weinberg, R., Jackson, A., & o, K. (1988). The relationship of massage and exercise to mood enhancement. *The Sport Psychologist, 2,* 202–211.

Weiner, B. (1985). An attributional theory of achievement motivation and emotion. *Psychological Review, 92,* 548–573.

Wildmann, J., Kruger, A., Schmole, M., Niemann, J., & Matthaei, H. (1986). Increase of circulating beta-endorphin-like immunoreactivity correlates with the change in feeling of pleasantness after running. *Life Sciences, 38,* 997–1003.

Wilfley, D., & Kunce, J. T. (1986). Differential physical and psychological effects of exercise. *Journal of Counselling Psychology, 33,* 337–342.

Wilson, V. E., Berger, B. G., & Bird, E. I. (1981). Effects of running and of an exercise class on anxiety. *Perceptual & Motor Skills, 53,* 472–474.

Wood, D. T. (1977). The relationship between state anxiety and acute physical activity. *American Corrective Therapy Journal, 31,* 67–69.

Youngstedt, S., Dishman, R. K., Cureton, K., Peacock, L., Wells, W., Fluech, D., & Hinson, B. (1991). Does body temperature mediate anxiolytic effects of acute exercise? *Medicine and Science in Sports and Exercise, 23* (Abstract No. 244).

Zuckerman, M., & Lubin, B. (1985). *Manual for the MAACL-R. The Multiple Affect Adjective Checklist Revised.* San Diego: Educational and Industrial Testing Service (EdITS).

# 5

# Meta-Analytic Techniques in Exercise Psychology

WALTER SALAZAR, STEVEN J. PETRUZZELLO,
DANIEL M. LANDERS, JENNIFER L. ETNIER,
AND KARLA A. KUBITZ

With the continued increase of research studies in the exercise and sport sciences, the need for good literature reviews has also increased. Until the end of the 1970s, narrative reviews were the only source of summarized information available. This situation started to change with Glass's (1976, 1977) publication of a methodology he called "meta-analysis," which is basically a quantitative technique used to summarize research findings across many studies.

The purposes of this chapter are to (a) present the historical background of meta-analysis within the statistical sciences; (b) describe the common steps followed in order to conduct a meta-analysis; (c) illustrate how meta-analysis has been used in the sport sciences; (d) show how meta-analysis has provided insights into the relationship between exercise and certain psychological variables; (e) describe some common criticisms and misconceptions regarding meta-analysis; and (f) indicate future directions for the use of meta-analytic techniques in sport science.

## THE DEVELOPMENT OF META-ANALYTIC TECHNIQUES

When Glass (1976, 1977) coined the term "meta-analysis," many people thought that the methodology involved was also new. However, the underlying statistical theory was not new, having first been developed during the 1930s. As discussed by Hedges and Olkin (1982), two distinct approaches have been developed in order to combine research evidence. Both of these approaches are derived from a methodology that was originally developed to synthesize data from the vast agricultural literature. One approach dealt with combining probability values of statistical tests, while the other dealt with combining indices of treatment magnitude.

The approach of combining probability values was first developed by Tippet (1931) and later refined by Fisher (1932) and by Pearson (1933). In this approach, the exact statistical probabilities from the significance test (i.e., $p$ values) are combined in order to test the overall effect (see Kerlinger, 1986, p. 101). One weakness of this approach is that it cannot give an estimate of the magnitude of the treatment effect. The second approach, combining estimates of treatment magnitude, was developed by Cochran (Cochran, 1937, 1943; Yates & Cochran, 1938). In this approach, an estimate of the mean effect of a treatment and its variability are obtained.

More recently, a series of alternative approaches have been derived from the early approaches. Bangert-Drowns (1986) classified five forms of meta-analytic methods: (1) Glassian meta-analysis (Glass, 1976; Glass, McGaw, & Smith, 1981); (2) study effect meta-analysis (Bangert-Drowns, Kulik, & Kulik, 1984; Landman & Dawes, 1982; Mansfield & Busse, 1977); (3) combined probability method (Cooper, 1979, 1982; Rosenthal, 1978); (4) approximate data pooling with tests of homogeneity (Hedges, 1982a, 1982b; Hedges & Olkin, 1985; Rosenthal & Rubin, 1982); and (5) approximate data pooling with sampling error correction (Hunter, Schmidt, & Jackson, 1983).

Before Glass introduced the concept of meta-analysis, the narrative review was the tool of choice for trying to assimilate a body of studies on a particular topic. A meta-analysis attempts to extract meaningful information out of a group of studies. However, there are differences in the degree of objectivity between a narrative reviewer and a meta-analytic reviewer.

A narrative reviewer starts by examining each study's weaknesses and strengths. Even though there are no specific rules that a narrative reviewer follows in order to establish the "quality" of a study, a popular approach is to use the categorization of Campbell and Stanley (1963), which classifies designs into preexperimental, quasi-experimental, and true experimental. Most of the time, studies are excluded from further analysis based on a subjective decision. At the same time, there is no consensus among narrative reviewers about decisions on how to weight the evidence from what they consider to be the good studies.

A meta-analytic reviewer, in contrast, follows a highly objective and public process, where a sequence of steps are clearly stated so that anyone can replicate them. All the relevant information on the different steps is included in the final report. Examples of those steps are the decisions taken about how to (a) code the variables (independent and dependent), (b) compute the effect size, (c) correct for sample size and bias, (d) apply a weighting factor, and (e) choose the appropriate statistical analysis.

The lack of consensus about methodological issues in narrative reviews is due to the fact that the process is viewed more as an *art* (i.e., where skill from the reviewer is required) than a science. An artist does not follow specified rules, but uses his or her own particular *style* (a private and subjective characteristic) to produce a piece of work. A meta-analytic reviewer, however, follows the rules of the scientific method, where objectivity and replication of methodological steps are key issues. As stated by Kerlinger (1986, p. 6), "Scientists do not accept statements as true, even though the evidence at first looks promising. They insist upon testing them. They also insist that any testing procedure be open to public inspection."

According to Halliwell and Gauvin (1982), there are three advantages of using meta-analysis as compared to narrative reviews. The first is that by the use of an objective system of coding the different study characteristics and results, the meta-analytic reviewer is less likely to incorrectly combine results of studies than is the narrative reviewer. Second, through the use of statistical tools (i.e., descriptive and inferential statistics) to summarize and analyze the information, the reviewer will have a precise overview of the pattern of results and how the different study characteristics influence the outcome measure. Finally, through an extensive literature search, and an objective coding of study characteristics and results, the reviewer can establish a practical bibliography and data bank of the topic reviewed.

Because of the relative youth of the process of meta-analysis, there is not yet a universally accepted way of conducting a meta-analysis. In the exercise and sport sciences, the methods more frequently used are the Glassian approach and the Hedges and Olkin approach, or a combination of both. Both derive the effect size (i.e., a measure of treatment magnitude) as the central unit of analysis. An effect size is a measure of the magnitude of a particular treatment, which takes into account the variability within the study from which it is calculated. As such, effect sizes can be directly compared across studies because they have been normalized. A summary of the different meta-analyses that have been conducted in the area of exercise and sport are presented in Table 5.1.

**TABLE 5.1  META-ANALYSES CONDUCTED IN THE SUBJECT AREAS OF SPORT AND EXERCISE**

| Authors | Topic | Technique used[a] | Results |
|---|---|---|---|
| Sparling (1980) | Sex differences in $\dot{V}O_2$ max | G | Removing the variability in aerobic capacity due to body size and body fatness substantially reduced magnitude of $\dot{V}O_2$ max difference between males and females. |
| Feltz & Landers (1983) | Effects of mental practice on motor skill learning and performance | G | Mental practice was more effective than no practice. Cognitive tasks had larger effects than did motor/strength tasks. |
| Kavale & Mattson (1983) | Effectiveness of perceptual-motor training | G | Perceptual-motor training is not effective for improving academic, cognitive, or perceptual-motor variables. |
| Tran, Weltman, Glass, & Mood (1983) | Effects of exercise on blood lipids and lipoproteins | G | Across all types of subjects, treatments, and research designs, the average exercising subject had reduced blood-lipid profiles. Numerous factors were found to interact with these changes. |
| Thomas & French (1985) | Gender differences in motor performance | H | Numerous motor tasks (particularly throwing) were found, which showed gender differences across age. |
| Gruber (1986) | Exercise and self-esteem development in children | G | Directed play and/or physical education programs contribute to the development of self-esteem in children. |
| Crews & Landers (1987) | Aerobic fitness and response to psychosocial stressors | H | Aerobically fit subjects had reduced psychosocial stress response compared to control subjects or baseline values. |
| Feltz, Landers, & Becker (1988) | Examined pre-post change scores to examine effects of mental practice, physical practice, and combined mental and physical practice on performance | H | Results confirmed findings from previous work, as well as extending those results to include combined physical and mental practice. More physical practice was related to greater pre-post changes in performance. |

**TABLE 5.1** (continued)

| Authors | Topic | Technique used[a] | Results |
|---|---|---|---|
| Lee & Genovese (1988) | Distribution of practice in motor learning | G | Massed practice depresses both learning and performance, when considered in terms of length of intertrial interval. |
| Oldridge, Guyatt, Fisher, & Rimm (1988) | Effect of exercise in preventing heart disease | O | Results showed a significant decrease in mortality in exercisers, compared to controls. The magnitude of benefit was correlated positively to the duration of the exercise therapy. |
| Kubitz et al. (1989) | Effects of acute exercise on sleep | G | Exercise had significant, positive effects on sleep, which were modified by methodological factors (e.g., gender, time of day). |
| Lokey & Tran (1989) | Effects of exercise on serum lipid and lipoproteins in women | G | Results showed that exercise reduced total serum cholesterol and triglyceride levels. Also, those women most at risk for heart disease responded most favorably to exercise training. |
| Whelan et al. (1989) | Effects of cognitive-behavioral interventions in athletic performance | G | Cognitive-behavioral interventions enhance athletic performance across various factors (e.g., control groups, dependent measures). |
| North et al. (1990) | Effect of exercise on depression | G | Exercise was effective in reducing depression, in psychologically normal and in psychologically abnormal subjects. Effects were found for both aerobic and anaerobic (e.g., weight training) forms of exercise. |
| Petruzzello et al. (1991) | Effect of exercise on state, trait, and psychophysiological correlates of anxiety | G | Aerobic exercise was associated with reductions in all three types of anxiety. |

[a]For technique used, G = Glassian approach, H = Hedges & Olkin approach, O = Other.

## STEPS IN A META-ANALYSIS

As outlined by Glass et al. (1981) and Thomas and French (1986), there are specific procedures to follow when conducting a meta-analysis. Such procedures should be explicitly spelled out in the written document so that other individuals can replicate the findings. This is analogous to a methods section in an experimental paper, where steps are written out in cookbook fashion so that others can replicate the study. A generic meta-analysis would include the following standard steps:

1. Identification of the problem
2. Literature search
3. Coding of moderator variables or characteristics
4. Computing of the effect size
5. Correction for bias and weighting factor
6. Statistical analysis
7. Publication

### Identification of the Problem

Areas ripe for review are often areas that have a fairly large database (i.e., at least 20 studies), but that do not, at a glance, give an immediate impression of the general findings. As a quantitative synthesis, a meta-analysis can be done in order to provide answers to specific questions (e.g., Is exercise effective in reducing depression? Does exercise modify sleep patterns?). These questions frequently, but not necessarily, have been the subject of narrative reviews that have produced conflicting findings. The meta-analysis may also be used to determine the magnitude of the effect for a particular treatment. Narrative reviews, by their nature, cannot give the interested researcher such information.

### Literature Search

The literature search should be extensive in nature. All available literature should be located by (a) using computer (and hand) searches for articles, dissertations, theses, and abstracts; (b) tracking down manuscripts in the reference lists of each obtained article; and (c) using the Social Sciences and the Science Citation Indexes to look up key articles and authors. The different sources that are used should be specified in the document. It is also possible to code for the sources of the studies used in the meta-analysis and to use them as moderator variables in the statistical analysis. Such an analysis might allow conclusions to be made regarding whether, for instance, publication status has an effect on the outcome variable (i.e., effect size).

## Coding of Moderator Variables or Characteristics

Moderator variables that could potentially modify the effect are coded either categorically or quantitatively. Such moderator variables are typically derived by examining the literature and through knowledge of questions of interest. Examples of moderator variables can include (a) subject characteristics (e.g., trained vs. untrained, male vs. female, young vs. old, physical and mental health status, percentage of body fat, maximum volume of oxygen uptake [$\dot{V}O_2$ max], age); (b) study characteristics (e.g., internal validity of the study, sample size, type of subject assignment, type of design); and (c) type of outcome measure or dependent variable (e.g., type of stress measure, type of mood state).

A major interest in many areas is to determine which mechanisms may explain why treatments have some specific effects (e.g., why exercise may reduce depression). An important aspect in coding the study characteristics is to determine a priori which types of coding characteristics could potentially have a bearing in understanding the role of those mechanisms. If such mechanisms are thought to exist, studies should be coded to allow for their examination in subsequent statistical analysis.

## Computing of the Effect Size

There are two variations on the basic computation of effect sizes. Glass (1977) computes the effect size by obtaining the difference between the mean of the experimental group and the mean of the control group and then dividing by the standard deviation of the control group. Hedges and Olkin (1985) calculate the same difference between the means but divide by the pooled standard deviation of the two groups.

## Correction for Bias and Weighting Factor

Effect sizes are positively biased in small samples. Therefore, effect sizes should be corrected for bias before further analysis is done. If this correction is not made, the mean effect size could overestimate the true effect.

Because the sample size of a particular study will influence the effect size, studies using more subjects are given more emphasis than studies with smaller Ns. To control for this effect, a weighting factor is applied to the obtained effect size. Effect sizes obtained from studies involving larger numbers of subjects are weighted more heavily than effect sizes obtained from studies with small sample sizes.

## Statistical Analysis

Standard statistical techniques (e.g., analysis of variance [ANOVA], Pearson r, regression) can be used to analyze the relationship of the different coding characteristics to the effect size (Glass, 1977). Hedges and Olkin also use specific techniques to test the effect size. First, a test of homogeneity is conducted to examine whether the group of effect sizes are estimates of the same population. If the test is not significant (i.e., the effect sizes are homogeneous), no further analysis of moderator variables is conducted. If the test is significant, it indicates that there is a reliable variability in the group of effect sizes, and a search of moderator variables is warranted. To do this, a weighted regression technique was developed (Hedges & Olkin, 1983), where the effect of the predictor variables on the effect sizes are examined (see Thomas & French, 1986, for a complete description of these procedures).

## Publication

Reporting the results of the meta-analysis in a scientific journal or book is the final step. At this point, the peer review process takes place. With a meta-analysis, peer review should be more stringent than with a single study because the results could have more influence in the scientific community, and they therefore have the potential to heavily influence (e.g., stop) future research in the area.

## EXAMPLES OF META-ANALYSIS RELATED TO PSYCHOLOGY AND EXERCISE

Examples of meta-analyses that have been conducted within exercise science are discussed in this section. Both types of analysis (i.e., Glass's approach and Hedges and Olkin's approach) have been used in exercise science, and examples of both approaches are included.

Crews and Landers (1987) followed the methodological procedures proposed by Hedges and Olkin (1985) to conduct a meta-analysis on the effects of aerobic fitness on reactivity to psychosocial stressors. The questions of interest were (a) Do aerobically fit subjects experience a reduced stress response, as compared to unfit subjects? and (b) If there is an effect, which factors moderate this effect?

The first step was to conduct a literature search that produced 34 studies, including research journals, conference abstracts, and dissertations. All studies were included in the analysis, regardless of a priori judgments of study quality. However, factors related to study quality were coded as potential moderator variables and were analyzed a posteriori. Effect sizes were computed by subtracting the mean of the unfit group from the mean of the fit group and then dividing by the pooled standard deviation. When means and standard deviations were not available, effect sizes were calculated from a $t$, $p$, or $r$ value. The effect sizes were then corrected for bias and were weighted for sample size. The 34 studies produced 92 effect sizes, based on 1449 subjects.

A series of categorical variables was used to examine the possible mediators of the effect: source (published studies, unpublished studies), exercise type (acute, chronic), gender (male, female), statistics (absence or presence of control for initial values), design (correlational, random assignment, control group, no control group), level of stressor (high, low), source of results (during stress, during recovery), and stress measures (heart rate, systolic blood pressure, diastolic blood pressure, skin response, serum or urine hormonal levels, muscle tension, psychological self-report).

A test of homogeneity of variance was conducted to determine whether the data were homogeneous. The test of homogeneity was nonsignificant, which indicated that all studies came from a common population and no further breakdown by moderating variables was required. The mean effect size of 0.48 was significantly different from zero. This means that aerobically fit subjects have a reduced response to psychosocial stress, compared to unfit subjects. This response could be due to either a reduced physiological response to stress or a faster physiological recovery. Several possible mechanisms (e.g., beta-adrenergic stimulation, hemodynamic changes, cerebral heating and serotonin levels, baroreceptor function changes, rate of insulin release, rate of endogenous opiate release) were discussed; however, because no analysis was done on the moderator variables, no specific information was available to discuss the relative merits of the proposed mechanisms.

North, McCullagh, and Tran (1990) conducted a meta-analysis examining the effects of exercise on depression, using Glass's (1977) methodology. A pilot study, using a random sample of studies, was done in order to clarify the research questions and coding sheet. A literature search was conducted using a computer search, cross-references from the bibliographies of previous studies, and the Social Sciences and the Science Citation Indexes. A coding sheet was developed that included several variables, including publication status, subject characteristics, design, and exercise treatment. The different outcome measures were transformed into effect sizes by using a standard effect-size formula [i.e., $ES = (M_1 - M_2)/SD_{pooled}$, where $ES$ = effect size and $M$ = mean]. Effect sizes were corrected for bias and weighted for sample size. A z test was done, to determine whether the mean effect size (and mean effect sizes within the different coding variables) was significantly different from zero. An ANOVA was conducted on the categorical variables, using the effect sizes as the dependent variables. When the effect was significant, post hoc analysis was conducted.

Eighty studies with 290 effect sizes were included in the meta-analysis. The overall mean effect size was –0.53, indicating that exercise groups showed decreases in depression more than did comparison groups that did not exercise. Other findings were that (a) exercise decreased depression more in subjects who were recruited from medical and psychological facilities than in subjects recruited from other sources; (b) results from published studies showed greater decreases in depression than were found in unpublished studies; (c) subjects who exercised at home showed a greater decrease in depression, compared to subjects that exercised at a medical facility or a university/college; (d) studies with medium internal validity showed a greater reduction in depression than did studies with high and low internal validity; (e) there was no difference in depression change between studies that used trait measures and studies that used state measures; (f) older subjects showed decreased depression more than did younger subjects; (g) no gender difference was found; (h) subjects receiving medical treatment decreased depression to a greater extent than subjects requiring only psychological treatment or subjects who were apparently healthy; (i) subjects who were initially depressed achieved the same amount of change in depression as did subjects who were not initially depressed; (j) the longer the exercise program, the greater the decrease in depression; (k) the greater the number of sessions, the greater the reduction in depression; (l) the number of sessions per week and the length of the exercise session did not influence depression; (m) exercise significantly decreased depression compared to no treatment or waiting-list controls; and (n) exercise plus psychotherapy was more effective in decreasing depression than exercise alone.

Several proposed mechanisms for the antidepressant effect of exercise were discussed. Among the psychological mechanisms proposed to explain the effects were the *social-interaction hypothesis* and the *time-out/distraction hypothesis*. The social-interaction hypothesis was not supported because exercise reduced depression more than so-called enjoyable activities, which tended to be group activities. The results provided mixed support for the time-out/distraction hypothesis because exercise decreased depression more than did enjoyable activities (distraction), but exercise did not differ from relaxation (time-out) in decreasing depression (see North et al., 1990, Table 13.11, p. 402).

Several physiological mechanisms were also discussed. The *cardiovascular-fitness hypothesis* states that the changes in depression are mediated by changes in cardiovascular fitness. This hypothesis was not entirely supported because changes in depression were found at 4 and 6 weeks of training, but there were no changes in cardiovascular fitness at these times. Also, anaerobic exercise decreased depression as much as or more than did aerobic exercise (see North et al., 1990, Table 13.9, p. 309, and Table 13.11, p. 402). However, there was some support for the cardiovascular-fitness hypothesis because two variables (length of exercise program and total number of exercise sessions) were significantly correlated with changes in depression. Two other possible biochemical mechanisms were discussed as possible explanations (i.e., monoamine neurotransmitters, endorphins) but could not be analyzed directly because no variable in the meta-analysis was related to these mechanisms.

Another research area that has received growing attention concerns the effect of exercise on sleep. It has been proposed (Carlson, 1981) that sleep either serves as a restitution state (e.g., tissue growth and bodily restoration), or that sleep serves adaptive purposes (e.g., keeping the organism out of danger and conserving energy). The question of interest is whether exercise helps to improve the apparent quality of sleep (e.g., long, deep, easily achieved).

Narrative reviews have been conducted (Horne, 1981; Shapiro, 1981; Shapiro & Driver, 1988; Torsvall, 1981; Trinder, Montgomery, & Paxton, 1988), but no agreement was reached in their conclusions. For example, inconsistencies in the methodology, operationalization of variables, and data analysis prevented a clear understanding of the effects of exercise on sleep. In order to have a better understanding of the area, a meta-analysis was conducted by Kubitz, Landers, Salazar, and Petruzzello (1989). A literature search of research journals, dissertation abstracts, and conference proceedings yielded 52 studies. Of those, 20 studies were not included for several reasons (e.g., no comparison group available, results reported in another study, used chronic exercise rather than acute exercise, reported no data for electroencephalograph [EEG] or sleep variables, or not enough data were available to compute the effect size). Studies were coded for potential moderating factors such as methodological variables (e.g., publication status, EEG scoring), subject variables (e.g., age, sex, fitness level), and exercise variables (e.g., type, duration, intensity of exercise).

Because 90% of the literature deals with sleep in terms of EEG measures, effect sizes were calculated for three sleep variables: (a) slow-wave sleep (i.e., sleep stages 3 and 4); (b) total sleep time; and (c) sleep onset latency (i.e., length of time to fall asleep). Effect sizes were corrected for bias, and the averaged overall effect for each sleep variable was tested for significance using the unweighted Stouffer meta-analytic z-test (Rosenthal, 1978). This indicates whether the mean effect size is different from zero. Parametric statistics (e.g., ANOVA, Tukey post hoc tests) were then used to compare between levels of the moderator variables.

Results were presented separately for each sleep variable. The mean effect size (mean = 0.19) for slow-wave sleep was significantly different from zero, which indicates that exercise increased the total amount of slow-wave sleep. This result was moderated by exercise duration, such that exercise of longer duration (60–150 minutes) produced larger increases in slow-wave sleep than exercise of shorter duration (< 60 minutes).

The mean effect size (mean = 0.33) for total sleep time was significantly different from zero, indicating that exercise produced a reliable increase in total sleep time. This effect was moderated by time of day and by gender. Exercising in the evening did not produce changes in total sleep time, but exercising during the day did produce an increase. The effect of longer sleep time was present for female, but not for male subjects.

For sleep onset latency, the mean effect size was not different from zero.

Significant moderator variables were (a) intensity of exercise and (b) whether the exercise was monitored by the researchers. Effect sizes for reported intensity (i.e., 0–50% and 50–75% of maximal oxygen consumption) were significantly different from zero but not different from each other. The mean effect size for exercise of unreported intensities was not different from zero. Overall, the results indicate that exercise produces a reliable, positive effect on sleep and that this effect is further moderated by several variables.

The relationship between exercise and anxiety has been extensively examined over the past 15 years. This research has led to many narrative reviews that have attempted to summarize the findings across the various studies. Such reviews typically include studies based on study quality and often leave out the majority of the existing literature. Many of the narrative reviews that have appeared have examined the same group of studies.

Three separate meta-analyses were conducted, to review the effects of exercise on state anxiety, trait anxiety, and psychophysiological correlates of anxiety (Petruzzello et al., 1991). Computer and hand searches of the literature yielded 104 studies that met the inclusion criteria (20 studies were excluded because insufficient information was available to calculate effect sizes). Studies were coded for subject characteristics (e.g., age, sex, mental health status), design characteristics (e.g., type of control group, subject assignment), exercise characteristics (e.g., intensity, duration, frequency), anxiety measures, and descriptive characteristics (e.g., publication status, author training). A standard formula was used to calculate effect sizes for each study $[ES = (M_{comparison} - M_{treatment})/SD_{pooled}]$. A positive effect size indicated a reduction in anxiety in the treatment group when contrasted with the comparison group.

A total of 408 effect sizes were computed based on a sample of 3048 subjects. The results substantiate the claim that exercise is associated with reductions in anxiety, but only for aerobic forms of exercise. These effects were generally independent of both subject characteristics (i.e., age and health status) and descriptive characteristics. Numerous design characteristics were different, but the differences were not uniform across the three meta-analyses.

For state anxiety, exercise was associated with reduced anxiety. However, these effects were similar to those found with other known anxiety-reducing treatments (e.g., relaxation). The trait anxiety meta-analysis revealed that random assignment resulted in larger effects than were found with intact groups. Results also indicate that training programs must exceed 10 weeks before significant changes in trait anxiety occur. For psychophysiological correlates, cardiovascular measures of anxiety (e.g., blood pressure, heart rate) yielded significantly lower effects than did other measures (e.g., electromyograph, [EMG], EEG).

The only variable that was significant across all three meta-analyses was exercise duration. Exercise of at least 21 minutes seems necessary to achieve reductions in state and trait anxiety, but there were variables confounding this relationship. Therefore, it remains to be seen what minimal duration is necessary for anxiety reduction.

The results of the meta-analyses provided an assessment of the magnitude of the effects of exercise on anxiety. In addition, the results indicate that some gaps exist in the current knowledge base, where future research efforts should be directed. At present, the largest problem in this area of research is the lack of understanding of causal mechanisms for the anxiety-reducing effect consistently seen with exercise. Because of the therapeutic value exercise offers for reducing anxiety without the dangers or costs of drug therapy or psychotherapy, it remains to be determined why exercise is associated with reduced anxiety. Numerous causal mechanisms have been proposed, but little research has been done to examine their plausibility.

While meta-analysis offers obvious advantages over the narrative review, it has not gone without its share of criticism. To present these criticisms, as well as criticisms of the narrative reviews, comparisons are made, where appropriate, between the characteristics of the two types of reviews.

## META-ANALYSIS AND THE NARRATIVE REVIEW

Criticisms of meta-analysis basically fall into two general categories. The first category includes criticisms from people with clinical backgrounds (e.g., Eysenck, 1978). To these people, the apparently complex statistical machinery of meta-analysis is (a) difficult to understand and (b) threatening to the particular perspective to which they have become accustomed (i.e., narrative reviews that selectively choose research from particular areas). Meta-analysis may cause individual researchers and their single experiments to "see themselves reduced to becoming a cog in the great statistical wheel" (Mann, 1990, p. 249). It is indeed very difficult for some researchers who have become accustomed to a methodological perspective to keep pace with new advances in methodological techniques.

The second category includes criticisms from statistically oriented researchers who accept the value of meta-analysis, but who argue about the most appropriate approach. For this reason, a number of different approaches have developed, and such development will probably continue for some time because the field is still in a state of development.

One of the major criticisms of meta-analysis concerns the fact that it combines data from studies with various degrees of quality. Mintz (1983) raised the issue of whether studies of poor quality should be included in a meta-analysis. Eysenck (1978), for example, invoked the dictum "garbage in–garbage out" to emphasize that if poor studies are put in, then poor output will be the result. On the other hand, assessments of meta-analysis (Cook & Leviton, 1980; Glass & Kliegl, 1983; Shapiro & Shapiro, 1982; Strube & Hartman, 1982) have concluded that it is preferable to retain data from studies of varying quality and then to *empirically* determine whether there are different results based on study quality. According to these authors, this would be a better approach than simply to discard the data deemed inferior in terms of the reviewer's preferred methodological criteria.

Green and Hall (1984) argue that the exclusion of studies could introduce a source of bias because the judgment of study quality may be somewhat subjective. At the same time, because a narrative reviewer is typically aware of the results of a study before making the decision of whether to include it, the reviewer might have the tendency to include studies with pleasing results. Similarly, other studies may be discarded because the results are not in agreement with the reviewer's hypotheses. Studies may also be excluded because if the apparent quality is so bad, the validity of the results are highly questionable.

Glass and Kliegl (1983) argue that a decision about whether to reject or accept studies should be based on an empirical test. An index of study quality can be obtained (i.e., coded) to test how this variable is related to other study characteristics or outcomes. If study quality is not correlated with study outcome (i.e., effect size), there is no reason not to include all the studies in the meta-analysis. Glass and his colleagues have employed regression analysis to examine the relationships between effect sizes and other study attributes. For example, a meta-analysis of the psychotherapy literature showed that an index of methodological quality accounted for only 1% of the variance in effect sizes (Glass, 1977). This implies that, within the limits imposed by the validity of the index, studies of higher and lower quality reached similar conclusions about impact (Cook & Leviton, 1980).

This strategy of coding for apparent quality has been criticized by Wilson and Rachman (1983) because of concerns about the validity of the procedure. However, it should be noted that if there are concerns about it, these concerns apply equally to the criteria that a narrative reviewer uses to exclude articles. Glass et al. (1981) have outlined specific procedures for establishing valid measures of study quality that deal with the degree of internal validity present in the study. As discussed by Cook and Campbell (1979, pp. 82–85), internal validity has primacy over other types of validity (i.e., statistical conclusion validity, construct validity, and external validity) because it deals with cause–effect relationships. The procedures outlined by Glass et al. (1981, p. 83) classify internal validity as high, medium, or low: *high* if the study used random assignment and the subject mortality was less than 15%; *medium* if the study used randomization but had differential mortality or if it was a well-designed matching study; or *low* if the matching procedures were weak or nonexistent or if mortality was severely disproportionate.

Other aspects that are related to study quality are the use of blind control, sample size, controls for cheating and recording errors, and within-subjects versus between-subjects designs (Green & Hall, 1984). Clearly, operationalizing the study quality could involve measuring several characteristics, and there is no general agreement among researchers about the different dimensions that should be taken into consideration (Gottfredson, 1978). Because of that, two strategies are possible: One is to obtain an overall index, and the other is to analyze each quality characteristic separately. A more parsimonious approach would be to choose the first option; however, the second one would give more detailed information, which could have practical implications for implementing future research.

A final point is that including all of the studies in a specific area is not a prerequisite to conduct a meta-analysis. Even though most meta-analyses follow such a practice, it is one of the decisions that has to be made during the process. The advantage of the meta-analysis is that it allows the researcher to investigate how the quality of the study affects the outcome measure.

Another criticism of meta-analysis involves the use of broad categories in averaging the effects across independent and dependent variables (Bangert-Drowns, 1986). This has been more commonly referred to as the "apples and oranges" problem. In defense of the meta-analysis, Glass et al. (1981) argue that such comparisons are exactly what meta-analysts do and should do. However, in a meta-analysis, reviewers code apples as apples and oranges as oranges; they do not just throw all the fruit into the basket, except when the interest is in the construct "fruit."

This "apples and oranges" criticism has implications at two different levels. At the level of the independent variables, the main purpose of a meta-analysis is to examine the effects of different independent variables and the interactions among them. At the level of the dependent variables, the meta-analyst should be cautious. If the interest is in an overall effect, then combining across various dependent variables would be appropriate. If, however, the interest is in the effects for related, but different, dependent variables, then the dependent variables should be analyzed separately.

For example, the meta-analysis by Petruzzello et al. (1991) examined the effects of exercise on anxiety. State anxiety, trait anxiety, and psychophysiological correlates of anxiety represented three different conceptualizations of anxiety. Because these measures were conceptually different, three different meta-analyses were conducted to examine each of these dependent variables separately. As another example, Kubitz et al. (1989), conducted three separate meta-analyses to analyze three related, but different, aspects of sleep (i.e., total sleep time, sleep onset latency, and slow-wave sleep).

A final criticism of meta-analysis is related to the use of multiple effect sizes to represent individual studies. Some critics have argued that this could result in nonindependent data points and inflated sample sizes. The obvious solution to this problem is to calculate a single effect size for each study. This, however, creates an additional problem. With a single effect size, it becomes difficult to examine potential moderator variables because the number of effect sizes in each cell of the analysis is dramatically reduced. In the Petruzzello et al. (1991) meta-analysis, one of the questions of interest involved the time course of anxiety responses following exercise. More specifically, at what point following exercise was anxiety reduction greatest, and how long did this reduction last? By calculating only a single effect size for those studies in which such an issue was directly examined, the answer to the question regarding the time course of the response could not be answered.

In attempting to solve the problem of multiple effect sizes, meta-analysts have come up with some potential solutions. There are two conditions that produce multiple effect sizes: (1) measuring the same outcome variable at different points in time (i.e., a repeated-measures condition), or (2) measuring several outcome variables (i.e., a multivariate condition). In the former case, the nonindependence of the effect sizes is taken into account when computing the repeated-measures analysis of the effect sizes.

In the case of measuring several outcome variables, three alternatives are possible. As mentioned before, one alternative is to combine the effect sizes to obtain one effect size for each study. This makes sense when the different outcomes are measuring the same construct. If the constructs being measured are different, however, this approach is not appropriate. The second approach, and perhaps the most popular, is to conduct a separate statistical analysis for each outcome measure. This approach makes sense when the correlation between the outcome measures is low (as shown by previous data or theory). The third approach is to use multivariate methods developed for meta-analytic purposes. The pioneering work was done by Hedges and Olkin (1985) and by Rosenthal and Rubin (1986). More recently, Raudenbush, Becker, and Kalaian (1988) developed a multivariate model that uses the generalized least-squares method to examine whether a treatment influences different outcomes in the same way and whether these effects are mediated by study characteristics. However, a limitation of this approach is that it requires information about the correlations among the outcome variables, and these are normally not reported.

The most glaring weakness of the narrative review seems to be its lack of quality control—namely, its unresponsiveness to the biases of the particular reviewer (Glass, 1976). For example, Morgan (1980) criticized narrative reviews of the sport personality literature as being characterized by "a tendency to include certain types of research in these reviews and exclude other types of research" (p. 53). Although subjectivity is the most severe threat to the validity of narrative reviews, these reviews have also been criticized because they may introduce bias in at least five possible ways: (1) the literature search may be so narrow that relevant studies are omitted; (2)

some of the discovered studies may be excluded on methodological grounds; (3) studies may be excluded because the theoretical constructs are considered irrelevant; (4) a large amount of information contained in primary research reports may be neglected; or (5) the reviewers may imprecisely weight their conclusions with regard to the amount of research they cover (Cook & Leviton, 1980; Cooper & Rosenthal, 1980).

When studies are excluded for any reason, it is not possible to determine whether the sample has become biased (Glass, 1977). The only practical way to examine this potential bias is to include all of the available studies—published and unpublished—related to the topic. Then an empirical test is used to determine whether different subsets of studies are associated with different effect-size magnitudes.

The narrative reviewer often uses a method referred to as a "vote count" to determine which studies support a hypothesis and which studies do not support it. This typically involves counting how often statistical tests reach conventional levels of significance (i.e., $p < .05$). While these vote-counting procedures should be considered "pre-meta-analytic," they have been criticized (Cook & Leviton, 1980; Cooper, 1990; Hedges & Olkin, 1982) for their (a) lack of statistical power, (b) susceptibility to producing wrong estimates due to publication bias, and (c) failure to assess the magnitude and direction of relationships. Light and Smith (1971) point out that while the results of a particular study may be in the hypothesized direction, if significance was not obtained, that study would be counted as support for the null hypothesis. Cronbach and Snow (1976) have also pointed out that while many studies with nonsignificant results may support the null hypothesis, it may also be rejected if most of the studies have results in the same direction. Such a conclusion would be lost, however, if studies were simply counted as supporting or not supporting a hypothesis based on $p$ values. Narrative reviewers often overlook the statistical power of the tests in question. Studies may fail to produce significance simply because sample size is too low. Light and Smith (1971) argued that estimates of effect magnitude are more useful in assessing studies because effect sizes are not as reliant on sample size as significance tests are.

Light and Smith (1971) have also pointed out that the vote-counting method is not sensitive enough for the detection of statistical interactions that can play a crucial role in theory or hypothesis testing. Inferences about theoretical constructs (e.g., anxiety, personality) often require the examination of complex patterns of data, comparing how the predicted pattern matches with the obtained pattern.

An additional advantage of meta-analysis over narrative reviews occurs in areas that have a great deal of complexity. Such complexity may be caused by either a large number of studies or a large number of variables (dependent or independent) that are of interest for the analysis (Cooper, 1979). The cognitive overload that occurs (for the narrative reviewer) because of the multiple classification of variables is magnified when there are multiple levels of the variables being investigated (Cook & Leviton, 1980).

While the discussion to this point has focused on criticisms of meta-analytic and narrative techniques for reviewing literature, the two can also be compared and contrasted on the following issues: (a) the efficiency in handling information; (b) the degree of objectivity in analyzing the data; (c) the analysis of trends and interactions present in the data; (d) the testing of hypotheses that were not tested in individual studies; and (e) the generation of new research directions (Green & Hall, 1984).

The more studies in the analysis, the more difficult it is for the narrative reviewer to handle the information. Dealing with many classifications of intervening (i.e., independent) variables and different types of outcome measures becomes increasingly difficult as more studies are included in the analysis. For a meta-analyst, however, once the study characteristics are coded and the effect sizes have been obtained, handling a few studies is as easy as handling hundreds of them.

A narrative reviewer is less likely to be objective in the analysis and selection of studies. A meta-analyst will be more objective because all of the steps in the search, selection, and analysis of the studies are described in the final report. In this way, other people can replicate the analysis or criticize any decision taken at any step.

The meta-analyst has the potential to examine the data using more complex statistical analysis than is possible for the narrative reviewer. The degree to which the effects may be mediated by intervening variables (e.g., subject characteristics, design specifications, apparent quality of the study) can be examined, and conclusions can be reached in a definitive manner (i.e., by significance tests, not so-called expert judgments). Having the ability to examine interactions in the data allows the meta-analyst to test hypotheses that could not be tested in individual studies. For example, a single study cannot provide data to examine the effect of published versus unpublished studies or the effect of study quality on the outcome variable.

Due to the more precise and objective conclusions reached (see Table 5.2 for an example), the ability to look at interactions, and the exact quantification of treatment effects, the meta-analytic review can highlight gaps in the literature and can provide a better source of insight about new research directions. Lacking such insight, narrative reviewers are often forced to digress from the topic at hand to present an often lengthy discussion of research methodology. As Green and Hall (1984) point out, the typical worn-out slogan of "more research is needed" could be changed after a meta-analysis.

One concern that does arise is that if a meta-analysis jumps to a conclusion based on a lot of poor studies, or very few studies, it will close off a subject prematurely (Mann, 1990). On the other hand, a well done meta-analysis may also lead the quantitative reviewer to state, "no more research

**TABLE 5.2   CONCLUSIONS PUT FORTH IN NARRATIVE REVIEWS AND THE CORRESPONDING FINDINGS FROM A META-ANALYTIC REVIEW**

| Meta-analytic findings | Narrative review conclusions |
|---|---|
| Exercise was associated with small but significant effects for both state ($ES$ = 0.24) and trait anxiety ($ES$ = 0.34). | Exercise reduces state anxiety but not trait anxiety. |
| Exercise of durations greater than 6 minutes is enough to produce small anxiety-reducing effects. Typical conclusions from narrative reviewers were confounded by studies that compared exercise to known anxiety-reducing treatments (e.g., relaxation) and found no differences. This was the case for 48% of the studies in the meta-analysis. When these studies were not included, durations from 6 to 20 minutes yielded anxiety reductions. | Exercise durations should exceed 20 minutes to achieve reductions in anxiety. |

*Source.* Petruzzello, Landers, Hatfield, Kubitz, & Salazar, 1991.

is needed!" For example, in reviewing the social-facilitation literature, Landers, Bauer, and Feltz (1978) suggested, based on their narrative review of a relatively small number of studies, that the effect of social facilitation may be so small as to be trivial. Nobody took this conclusion seriously, however. It was not until the meta-analysis of Bond and Titus (1983) that researchers took notice. Bond and Titus (1983) subsequently put an end to most social-facilitation research based on the conclusion that roughly less than 4% of the variance was explained by the presence of others.[1] The Bond and Titus conclusions were more accepted because they were based on the entire social facilitation literature, not just a few selected studies.

A final illustrative example highlights the differences between narrative reviews and meta-analyses. An experiment was conducted by Cooper and Rosenthal (1980) to compare the conclusions drawn from narrative reviews with the conclusions drawn from meta-analytic techniques. Subjects (i.e., reviewers) were randomly assigned to use one of the two techniques and

---

[1]The story is told of an individual who encountered another individual using a shovel to dig through a room filled with horse manure. When asked what he was doing, he replied that because the room was so full of manure, there had to be a pony in the room somewhere (adapted from Mintz, 1983). In the case of social facilitation, so much research was done with the thought that there had to be something going on, when in fact, Bond and Titus showed that there was no pony.

were given an identical set of studies to analyze. Results showed that meta-analytic reviewers estimated a larger magnitude of effect than did narrative reviewers. These results show very clearly that when the literature is apparently contradictory, narrative reviewers cannot clearly detect effects. In other words, their conclusions are more conservative because evidence that is in the right direction—but is not statistically significant—is thrown out as evidence that favors the null hypothesis. Meta-analytic reviewers, on the other hand, can precisely estimate the magnitude of the effect for each study, no matter how small. Then, through aggregation, an index of the overall effect can be tested for significance.

## FUTURE DIRECTIONS AND CONSIDERATIONS

The use of meta-analytic techniques to analyze the effects of exercise on psychological factors is relatively new. Even though it has been stated that "meta-analysis is the wave of the future. The days of the expert supposedly putting the state of the field into a review article are numbered" (Mann, 1990, p. 249), it is not likely that meta-analysis is going to replace the narrative review in the short run. An examination of Table 5.3 shows that the use of meta-analysis has increased rapidly during the past 10 years, but the rate of increase has been the same for narrative reviews.

Because meta-analysis is a statistical technique that summarizes or combines related studies (i.e., as long as they contain the necessary statistical information), any research area that has a given minimum of studies (i.e., 20) could benefit from such a quantitative summary.

One such area is the effect of exercise on cognitive functioning. While there has been a considerable amount of research to examine the effects of

**TABLE 5.3    NUMBER OF ARTICLES CLASSIFIED AS META-ANALYTIC OR NARRATIVE REVIEWS BY MEDLINE**

| Year | Meta-analysis | Narrative review |
|------|---------------|------------------|
| 1983 | 15 | 165 |
| 1984 | 14 | 185 |
| 1985 | 20 | 210 |
| 1986 | 20 | 247 |
| 1987 | 39 | 591 |
| 1988 | 74 | 809 |
| 1989 | 71 | 1006 |
| 1990 (through October) | 130 | 1584 |

*Note.* Medline is a set of computerized listings from the *Cumulated Index Medicus,* which is published by the National Library of Medicine and the U.S. Department of Health and Human Services.

exercise on the emotional aspects of human behavior (e.g., depression, anxiety, self-esteem), a smaller number of studies have been published that relate to the effects of exercise on the cognitive domain. As there are now meta-analyses conducted on those areas of emotional content (Gruber, 1986, in self-esteem; North et al., 1990, in depression; Petruzzello et al., 1991, in anxiety), it would be beneficial to have a quantitative review that examines the effect of exercise on cognitive functioning. Other areas that would benefit from a meta-analytical review include exercise and adherence, as well as exercise and selected personality traits.

As a practical guide, any area where a qualitative (i.e., narrative) review has been conducted could benefit from meta-analysis. By coding substantive and methodological features of a large and representative set of studies, a composite profile of the research literature can be obtained. This is particularly useful in appraising the current state of the art in a research domain and in guiding suggestions for future research (Shapiro & Shapiro, 1983). If the reviews have not yielded clear findings, meta-analysis can help to clarify precisely the issues that are under debate. If there is agreement in the findings of the reviews, meta-analysis provides a quantitative index for the effect's magnitude, which could be translated into practical terms or significance.

## REFERENCES

Bangert-Drowns, R. L. (1986). Review of developments in meta-analytic method. *Psychological Bulletin, 99,* 388–399.

Bangert-Drowns, R. L., Kulik, J. A., & Kulik, C. L. (1984, August). *The influence of study features on outcomes of educational research.* Paper presented at the ninety-second annual meeting of the American Psychological Association, Toronto.

Bond, C. F., & Titus, L. J. (1983). Social facilitation: A meta-analysis of 241 studies. *Psychological Bulletin, 94,* 265–292.

Campbell, D., & Stanley, J. (1963). *Experimental and quasi-experimental designs for research.* Chicago: Rand McNally.

Carlson, N. R. (1981). *Physiology of behavior* (pp. 439–469). Boston: Allyn & Bacon.

Cochran, W. G. (1937). Problems arising in the analysis of a series of similar experiments. *Journal of the Royal Statistical Society, 4,* 102–118.

Cochran, W. G. (1943). The comparison of different scales of measurement for experimental results. *Annals of Mathematical Statistics, 14,* 205–216.

Cook, T. D., & Campbell, D. T. (1979). *Quasi-experimentation: Design & analysis issues for field settings.* Boston: Houghton Mifflin.

Cook, T. D., & Leviton, L. C. (1980). Reviewing the literature: A comparison of traditional methods with meta-analysis. *Journal of Personality, 48,* 449–472.

Cooper, H. M. (1979). Statistically combining independent studies: A meta-analysis of sex differences in conformity research. *Journal of Personality and Social Psychology, 37,* 131–146.

Cooper, H. M. (1982). Scientific guidelines for conducting integrative reviews. *Review of Educational Research, 52*, 291–302.

Cooper, H. (1990). Meta-analysis and the integrative research review. In C. Hendrik & M. J. Ugart (Eds.), *Research methods in personality and social psychology.* Newbug Pond, CA: Sage.

Cooper, H. M., & Rosenthal, R. (1980). Statistical versus traditional procedures for summarizing research findings. *Psychological Bulletin, 87*, 442–449.

Crews, D. J., & Landers, D. M. (1987). A meta-analytic review of aerobic fitness and reactivity to psychosocial stressors. *Medicine and Science in Sports and Exercise, 19*, 114–120.

Cronbach, L. J., & Snow, R. E. (1976). *Attitudes and instructional methods.* New York: Irvington Publishers.

Eysenck, H. J. (1978). An exercise in mega-silliness. *American Psychologist, 33*, 517.

Feltz, D. L., & Landers, D. M. (1983). The effects of mental practice on motor skill learning and performance. *Journal of Sport Psychology, 5*, 25–27.

Feltz, D. L., Landers, D. M., & Becker, B. J. (1988). A revised meta-analysis of the mental practice literature on motor skill learning. In D. Druckman & J. Swets, *Enhancing human performance: Issues, theories, and techniques—Background papers.* Washington, DC: National Academy Press.

Fisher, R. A. (1932). *Statistical methods for research workers* (4th ed.). London: Oliver & Boyd.

Glass, G. V. (1976). Primary, secondary, and meta-analysis research. *Educational Researcher, 5*, 3–8.

Glass, G. V. (1977). Integrating findings: The meta-analysis of research. *Review of Research in Education, 5*, 351–379.

Glass, G. V., & Kliegl, R. (1983). An apology for research integration in the study of psychotherapy. *Journal of Consulting and Clinical Psychology, 51*, 28–41.

Glass, G. V., McGaw, B., & Smith, M. (1981). *Meta-analysis in social research.* Beverly Hills, CA: Sage.

Gottfredson, G. (1978). Evaluating psychological research reports. *American Psychologist, 33*, 920–934.

Green, B. F., & Hall, J. A. (1984). Quantitative methods for literature reviews. *Annual Review of Psychology, 35*, 37–53.

Gruber, J. J. (1986). Physical activity and self-esteem development in children: A meta-analysis. In G. A. Stull & H. M. Eckert (Eds.), *Effects of physical activity on children.* Champaign, IL: Human Kinetics.

Halliwell, W., & Gauvin, L. (1982). Integrating and interpreting research findings: A challenge to sport psychologists. In J. T. Partington, T. Orlick, & J. H. Salmela (Eds.), *Sport in perspective.* Ottawa, Canada: Coaching Association of Canada.

Hedges, L. V. (1982a). Estimation of effect size from a series of independent experiments. *Psychological Bulletin, 92*, 490–499.

Hedges, L. V. (1982b). Fitting categorical models to effect sizes in a series of experiments. *Journal of Educational Statistics, 7*, 119–137.

Hedges, L. V., & Olkin, I. (1982). Analyses, reanalyses, and meta-analysis. *Contemporary Education Review, 1*, 157–165.

Hedges, L. V., & Olkin, I. (1983). Regression models in research synthesis. *American Statistician, 37,* 137–140.

Hedges, L. V., & Olkin, I. (1985). *Statistical methods for meta-analysis.* New York: Academic Press.

Horne, J. A. (1981). The effects of exercise upon sleep: A critical review. *Biological Psychology, 12,* 241–290.

Hunter, J. E., Schmidt, F. L., & Jackson, G. B. (1983). *Meta-analysis: Cumulating research findings across studies.* Beverly Hills, CA: Sage.

Kavale, K., & Mattson, D. (1983). "One jumped off the balance beam": Meta-analysis of perceptual-motor training. *Journal of Learning Disabilities, 16,* 165–173.

Kerlinger, F. N. (1986). *Foundations of behavioral research.* New York: Holt, Rinehart and Winston.

Kubitz, K. A., Landers, D. M., Salazar, W., & Petruzzello, S. J. (1989). *A meta-analytic review of the effects of acute exercise on selected aspects of sleep.* Unpublished manuscript; Department of Exercise Science and Physical Education, Arizona State University.

Landers, D. M., Bauer, R. S., & Feltz, D. L. (1978). Social facilitation during the initial stages of motor learning: A re-examination of Martens's audience study. *Journal of Motor Behavior, 10,* 325–337.

Landman, J., & Dawes, R. M. (1982). Psychotherapy outcome. *American Psychologist, 37,* 504–516.

Lee, T. D., & Genovese, E. D. (1988). Distribution of practice in motor skill acquisition: Learning and performance effects reconsidered. *Research Quarterly for Exercise and Sport, 59,* 277–287.

Light, R. J., & Smith, P. V. (1971). Accumulating evidence: Procedures for resolving contradictions among different research studies. *Harvard Educational Review, 41,* 429–471.

Lokey, E. A., & Tran, Z. V. (1989). Effects of exercise training on serum lipid and lipoprotein concentrations in women: A meta-analysis. *International Journal of Sport Medicine, 10,* 424–429.

Mann, C. (1990). Meta-analysis in the breech. *Science, 249,* 476–480.

Mansfield, R. S., & Busse, T. V. (1977). Meta-analysis of research: A rejoinder to Glass. *Educational Researcher, 6,* 3.

Mintz, J. (1983). Integrating research evidence: A commentary on meta-analysis. *Journal of Counseling and Clinical Psychology, 51,* 71–75.

Morgan, W. P. (1980). The trait psychology controversy. *Research Quarterly, 51,* 50–76.

North, T. C., McCullagh, P., & Tran, Z. V. (1990). Effect of exercise on depression. *Exercise and Sport Science Reviews, 18,* 379–415.

Oldridge, N. B., Guyatt, G. H., Fisher, M. E., & Rimm, A. A. (1988). Cardiac rehabilitation after myocardial infarction: Combined experience of randomized clinical trials. *Journal of the American Medical Association, 260,* 945–950.

Pearson, K. (1933). On a method of determining whether a sample size $n$ supposed to have been drawn from a parent population having a known probability integral has probably been drawn at random. *Biometrika, 25,* 379–410.

Petruzzello, S. J., Landers, D. M., Hatfield, B. D., Kubitz, K. A., & Salazar, W. (1991). A meta-analysis on the anxiety reducing effects of acute and chronic exercise: Outcomes and mechanisms. *Sports Medicine, 11(3)*, 143–182.

Raudenbush, S. W., Becker, B. J., & Kalaian, H. (1988). Modeling multivariate effect sizes. *Psychological Bulletin, 103*, 1–10.

Rosenthal, R. (1978). Combining results of independent studies. *Psychological Bulletin, 85*, 185–193.

Rosenthal, R., & Rubin, D. B. (1982). Comparing effect sizes of independent studies. *Psychological Bulletin, 92*, 500–504.

Rosenthal, R., & Rubin, D. B. (1986). Meta-analytic procedures for combining studies with multiple effect sizes. *Psychological Bulletin, 99*, 400–406.

Shapiro, C. M. (1981). Sleep and the athlete. *British Journal of Sports Medicine, 15*, 51–55.

Shapiro, C. M., & Driver, H. S. (1988). Exercise and sleep: A review. *NATO Colloquium*. New York: Plenum.

Shapiro, D. A., & Shapiro, D. (1982). Meta-analysis of comparative therapy outcome research: A critical appraisal. *Behavioral Psychotherapy, 10*, 4–25.

Shapiro, D. A., & Shapiro, D. (1983). Comparative therapy outcome research: Methodological implications of meta-analysis. *Journal of Counseling and Clinical Psychology, 51*, 42–53.

Sparling, P. B. (1980). A meta-analysis of studies comparing maximal oxygen uptake in men and women. *Research Quarterly for Exercise and Sport, 51*, 542–552.

Strube, M. J., & Hartmann, D. P. (1982). A critical appraisal of meta-analysis. *British Journal of Clinical Psychology, 21*, 129–139.

Thomas, J. R., & French, K. E. (1985). Gender differences across age in motor performance: A meta-analysis. *Psychological Bulletin, 98*, 260–282.

Thomas, J. R., & French, K. E. (1986). The use of meta-analysis in exercise and sport: A tutorial. *Research Quarterly for Exercise and Sport, 57*, 196–204.

Tippett, L. H. C. (1931). *The methods of statistics*. London: Williams & Norgate.

Torsvall, L. (1981). Sleep after exercise: A literature review. *Journal of Sports Medicine, 21*, 218–225.

Tran, Z. V., Weltman, A., Glass, G. V., & Mood, D. P. (1983). The effects of exercise on blood lipids and lipoproteins: A meta-analysis of studies. *Medicine and Science in Sports and Exercise, 15*, 393–402.

Trinder, J., Montgomery, I., & Paxton, S. J. (1988). The effect of exercise on sleep: The negative view. *Acta Physiologica Scandinavica, 133*, 14–20.

Whelan, J. P., Meyers, A. W., & Berman, J. (1989, August). *Cognitive-behavioral interventions for athletic performance enhancement*. Paper presented at a meeting of the American Psychological Association, New Orleans.

Wilson, G. T., & Rachman, S. (1983). Meta-analysis and the evaluation of psychotherapy outcome: Limitations and liabilities. *Journal of Consulting and Clinical Psychology, 51*, 54–64.

Yates, F., & Cochran, W. G. (1938). The analysis of groups of experiments. *Journal of Agricultural Science, 28*, 556–580.

# 6

# Alternative Psychological Models and Methodologies for the Study of Exercise and Affect

**LISE GAUVIN AND LAWRENCE R. BRAWLEY**

The affective benefits of acute and chronic exercise have recently been supported by anecdotal and empirical evidence. Acute exercise provides temporary reductions in subjectively perceived anxiety and depression, as well as improved mood (North, McCullagh, & Tran, 1990; Petruzello, Landers, Hatfield, Kubitz, & Salazar, 1991), while chronic exercise is associated with improved psychophysiological reactivity to mental stress (Crews & Landers, 1987) and in some cases, alleviation of clinical depression (Martinsen, 1990; North et al., 1990) and a reduction in trait anxiety (Petruzello et al., 1991).

The study of exercise-induced affect is important for two reasons. First, a clear understanding of the efficacy and mechanisms of exercise in producing affective benefits would allow mental health and public health practitioners to appropriately prescribe exercise for therapeutic or preventive mental health purposes. Second, recent research and theorization (Sallis & Hovell, 1990) suggest that affect may play a role in people's adhering to programs of exercise. The successful adoption and prescription of exercise could result in major reductions in (a) cardiovascular morbidity and mortality, (b) mental health problems (e.g., anxiety, subclinical depression, and the treatment of clinical depression) and consequently (c) health-care costs.

Unfortunately, little is known about the actual magnitude and pervasiveness of exercise-related mood benefits, and few, if any, practical applications for mental health or exercise adherence have been drawn because the affective experience that accompanies exercise has not been thoroughly described. Little attention has been devoted to the selection of appropriate conceptual models, methodological approaches, and measurement tools that can capture the essence of what people feel during and after exercise. Rather, the mood-related conceptual models and tools used in previous research have apparently been selected on the basis of convenience and of the extent of previous use in exercise psychology rather than on the basis of a thorough examination of existing concepts and measures of mood and/or affect.

The arbitrary borrowing of definitions and measures that has been characteristic of previous research may have resulted in the unwanted inheritance of many of the problems of such measures. Before research of the type described in the preceding paragraph becomes more abundant, it is necessary to (a) identify some of the methodological and conceptual pitfalls, (b) describe several psychological models of affective experience that will provide for a clearer conceptualization of exercise and affect, and (c) describe several promising methodological approaches for the study of affect in exercise.

While there are multiple approaches to studying affect in social psychology (e.g., attitude–affect, affect associated with attributions, affect associated with various kinds of interpersonal relations), the approach designed to describe the nature of affective experience from a social- and/or personality-psychology perspective is favored in this chapter. It is our position that if any progress is to be made in understanding affect as an antecedent or a consequence of exercise, earlier research pitfalls must be avoided and multidimensional approaches to the study of exercise and affect must be entertained. The remainder of this chapter provides evidence for this suggestion.

## METHODOLOGICAL AND CONCEPTUAL SHORTCOMINGS

The understanding of exercise-related affect has been pursued in training studies or in response to an acute bout of physical exercise through the administration of standardized paper and pencil questionnaires such as the Profile of Mood States (POMS; McNair, Lorr, & Droppleman, 1971), the Multiple Affect Adjective Check List (MAACL; Zuckerman & Lubin, 1965), the State–Trait Anxiety Inventory (STAI; Spielberger, Gorsuch, & Lushene, 1970), and the Activation–Deactivation Adjective Checklist (AD-ACL; Thayer, 1986). Each of these questionnaires includes a series of adjectives designed to tap some aspect of emotional, cognitive, and/or physiological functioning. The subject is required to rate subjective feelings over a given period of time.

The use of this approach has allowed researchers to substantiate the existence of exercise-related emotional fluctuations. However, the data may be contaminated by ceiling effects, floor effects, expectancy effects, large between-subject variability and problems of conceptual and operational definitions of affect. These problems pose difficulties in data interpretation, as illustrated next.

### Ceiling and Floor Effects

Ceiling effects and floor effects occur when subjects' scores on dependent measures are at the extreme of the theoretical range of a given measurement scale. The results of a study (Gauvin & Szabo, 1992) designed to examine the time course of exercise-related mood shifts resulting from a 20-minute bout of moderate-intensity (65% of maximal oxygen uptake) cycling illustrate this problem. In this study, regular exercisers and sporadic exercisers of both sexes from a university student population filled out the POMS before exercise, and then at 2, 30, and 120 minutes after the exercise and at a time in the day when the subjects felt most relaxed.

As can be seen from Figure 6.1, the mean vigor scores[1] are all above a $T$-score[2] of 50, while the mean tension scores are all well below a $T$-score

---

[1]The POMS provides subscale scores on 6 different aspects of mood—namely, tension, depression, anger, fatigue, vigor, and confusion. For the purposes of the illustration, *vigor* refers to the extent to which the subject feels full of pep and energy, while *tension* refers to the extent to which the subject feels anxious and stressed.

[2]A $T$-score transformation produces a normal distribution with a mean of 50 and a standard deviation of 10. In the case of the POMS, Lorr et al. (1971) present tables for transformation of raw scores into $T$-scores that are based on norms for a college student population.

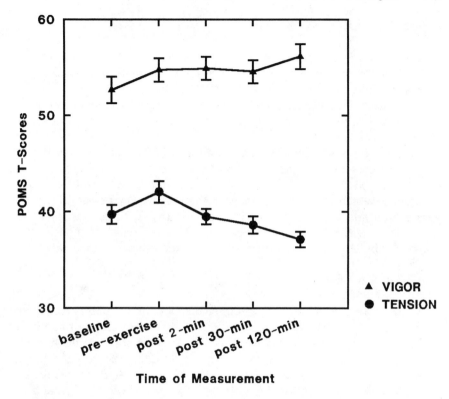

**Figure 6.1.**    Data from Gauvin and Szabo (1992) illustrating ceiling and floor effects in the exercise and affect literature.

of 45.[3] In the case of the vigor scores, there may be a ceiling effect, while in the case of the tension scores, there may be a floor effect. College students may not feel more invigorated following exercise if they were already slightly above the average to begin with. Similarly, decreases in tension would not be expected to be very large if the subject were very low on tension at the outset. Thus, level of prior mood state seems to be an important consideration in research where a change in mood is expected to be induced by presentation of an exercise stimulus.

---

[3]There were no significant main effects for life-style or gender for both the vigor and the tension scores. There was a significant main effect of time for the tension scores, indicating that tension significantly decreased from baseline and preexercise to postexercise. No time main effects were observed for vigor.

### Between-Subject Variability

Another issue that has received little attention is between-subject variability in mood. In the study of mood-related phenomena, mood is assumed to be a variable, transient state, subject to influence from a variety of factors. Despite this fact, very little attention has been devoted to how to control for homogeneity of prior mood state and to control for other mood-influencing factors in exercise research.

To illustrate this point, the data relating to POMS tension scores from Gauvin and Szabo (1992) are illustrated in the form of box plots[4] in Figure 6.2. As can be seen, the "whiskers" on each box plot reveal very large variability, which was not evident with the standard error bars. There are even many outlying scores (shown by the asterisks). Thus, there is a need to find some way to account for large individual differences in mood, which may contribute to abnormal distributions in the typically small samples.

### Subject and Experimenter Expectancy Effects

*Expectancy effects* refer to unintentional behavior on the part of the experimenter or the subject, which increase the likelihood of certain hypotheses being confirmed (Rosenthal & Rosnow, 1984). In the study of the affective benefits of exercise, it is difficult to defend the idea that subjects and experimenters are blind to the hypotheses under investigation. Fitness clubs and public health organizations disseminate messages across Canada and the United States about the beneficial effects of exercise on well-being. Subjects obviously enter the testing session with a clear vision of what might result from exercising. Through repeated administration of questionnaires, it is easy for subjects to convey their expectancies and to present themselves in a socially desirable way. Furthermore, experimenters are often physically active people, whose knowledge and personal experience of physical activity would lead them to believe in the affective beneficence of exercise. They may unknowingly lead subjects to believe that they are in a better mood by behaving or speaking in a way that directs compliant volunteers to respond in a hypothesized direction. Few, if any, studies have developed safeguards against the problem of expectancies.

---

[4]A *box plot* is a graphic display of a batch of numbers which presents a clearer picture of the structure of the batch of data points (Emerson & Strenio, 1983). Box plots are considered to be a visual analogue to the analysis of variance (ANOVA). The line within the box represents the median, the box represents the fourth spread (location of data points in the lower fourth and upper fourth), the whiskers indicate the location of $3/2$ of the inter fourth spread, and the asterisks represent outlying scores.

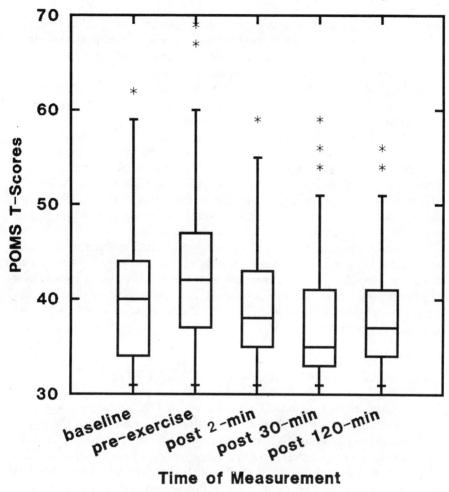

Figure 6.2.    Box-plotgraph of the tension data from Gauvin and Szabo (1992).

## Conceptual and Operational Definitions of Mood/Affect

A *conceptual definition* outlines the meaning of a variable in abstract terms, while an *operational definition* describes how a concept is measured in any concrete situation (Rosenthal & Rosnow, 1984). Few studies on exercise and mood have included conceptual and operational definitions of *affect*, and even fewer studies have been designed to test theoretical hypotheses (Petruzello et al., 1991). As a consequence, only very global statements about the affective beneficence of exercise can be made.

Further, the absence of a reliable conceptual definition and the lack of a conceptual model or theoretical framework leads to an obvious research problem. There is no explicit linking among conceptual definition, theoretical model, and operational definition of affect. As a consequence, measurement suffers. The result for the literature is what we currently observe: inconsistent descriptions of affect that make it difficult to draw between-study comparisons and to achieve even the most basic level of research—namely, description. The lack of precise and consistent definitions of affect are further compounded when attempting to answer the more complex questions of when, under what conditions, and why affect changes due to exercise. That is, affect becomes difficult to manipulate or control in laboratory or field contexts, because we are not precise in what we are measuring or controlling. Although these are generic problems to the social/behavioral sciences that are well recognized, exercise scientists and psychologists alike have often ignored them in the study of affect.

Previous research is wanting, from both conceptual and methodological standpoints. Conceptually, researchers have not employed theories and models of affect. Empirically, very little attention has been given to how best to measure and study affect in exercise. A discussion of alternative psychological models and methodologies for the study of exercise-induced affect therefore is warranted.

## PSYCHOLOGICAL CONCEPTUALIZATIONS OF AFFECT

Not surprisingly, researchers have experienced difficulty in defining the concepts of emotion/affect/mood. This difficulty is reflected in the range, number, and focus of models that are currently available in the literature, as well as the ongoing search for a definition of the terms *affect, mood,* and *emotion.* The description of affective experience in social psychology has been approached in one of two ways (Vallerand, 1984). One group of authors, referred to as categorical theorists (e.g., Ekman, 1982; Frijda, 1987; Izard, 1977), have tried to identify a small number of basic emotions (e.g., anger, fear) and then proceeded to develop models for understanding each emotion. A second group of researchers has attempted to describe the dimensions along which all emotional experience may vary. This latter approach seems better suited to the understanding of exercise and affect because the models stemming from it are intended to be broad, encompassing conceptualizations of affective experience. Because the affective experience that accompanies exercise has not been thoroughly described, a model of affect that has a wider breadth is more likely to capture the essence of exercise-induced affect than a model that, at the outset, limits the focus of investigation to specific emotions. Selected models stemming from the application of this second approach are therefore reviewed next.

## Dimensions of Affective Experience

One of the most frequently employed approaches in the description of affective experience has been to have subjects rate a list of words that are used in mood inventories, either in terms of similarity or as a function of semantic differential scales. Multidimensional scaling techniques or factor analysis have then been applied to the data. Variations in both statistical techniques and data interpretation have led researchers to propose different conceptual models and measurement strategies.

**The Circumplex Model of Affect.**   Russell's (1978, 1980) circumplex model of affect suggests that affective experience can be represented in two-dimensional space. The two essential dimensions along which emotional experience fluctuates are *hedonic tone,* anchored by pleasure–displeasure, and *activation,* anchored by arousal–sleepiness.

Russell, Weiss, and Mendelsohn (1989) have developed a one-item measurement tool, called the "Affect Grid," to allow for rapid assessment of people's affective states. The Affect Grid consists of a 9 x 9 matrix where the horizontal axis represents variations in unpleasant–pleasant feelings, while the vertical axis represents changes in sentiments of sleepiness–arousal. The subject is required to rate her or his current affective state by placing an "X" in the appropriate cell within the matrix. Scores provide an indication of the location of the subject's affective state within a two-dimensional space defined by hedonic tone and activation. Psychometric data support the test's validity and to some extent its reliability. The affect grid is fairly simple to use once the subject has been acquainted with the use of the 9 x 9 grid. It was designed for ongoing measurement of mood and presents two advantages: (1) It requires a very short period of time to answer, and (2) it is less heavily dependent on a subject's understanding of the meaning associated with various words typically used in mood inventories.

Further, one of the important contributions of Russell's work has been to highlight the preponderance of the hedonic tone and activation dimensions. In fact, empirical evidence suggests that a major portion of the variance (45%) in affective experience can be accounted for by these two dimensions of affect.

Russell's (1978, 1980) circumplex model of affect has been virtually ignored by researchers in exercise psychology, although Hardy and Rejeski (1989), Rejeski, Best, Griffith, and Kenney (1987) and Kenney, Rejeski, and Messier (1987) have produced descriptive evidence that indirectly pertains to the circumplex model.

Specifically, Hardy and Rejeski (1989) had sedentary subjects exercise for 30 minutes at 30%, 60%, and 90% of their maximal capacity, and then data on their rated perceived exertion (RPE) and the Feeling Scale (FS) were collected. The FS is an 11-point bipolar scale ranging from –5 to +5, which measures how bad–good a person feels while exercising and provides a measure of the hedonic tone dimension. They found that increasing exercise intensities were accompanied by decreases in FS scores and increases in RPE. It might therefore be concluded that exercise of increasing intensity provides affective decrements. However, as mentioned by Hardy and Rejeski (1989), the correlations between FS and RPE were only moderate, explaining between 10.8% to 30.2% of the variance. Likewise, recovery data on the FS were not collected, thus precluding any conclusions about what happens after exercise.

In a study designed to examine the reactions to exercise stress in males differing on sex-role orientation, Rejeski et al. (1987) had college students cycle for 6 minutes at 85% of their $\dot{V}O_2$ max and then to exhaustion at 110% of $\dot{V}O_2$ max. They found that masculine males and androgenous males reported higher levels of hedonic tone, as measured through the FS, than the feminine males. This finding emerged even though the heart rates of subjects differing in sex-role orientation were not significantly different.

Finally, Kenney et al. (1987) examined the effects of a distress-management training program on the psychological responses of novice female runners to high-intensity exercise. Half the subjects participated in a 5-week distress-management training program, which consisted of information about exercise and distress management, an introduction to coping behaviors, and a practice of coping behaviors. All subjects participated in a 5-week training period and then were required to run for 15 minutes at 75% of their $\dot{V}O_2$ max and then to run to exhaustion at 85% of their $\dot{V}O_2$ max. FS and RPE data were collected every minute during the lower-intensity exercise and again when subjects indicated that they had reached exhaustion in the higher intensity portion of the exercise stimulus. Results indicated that subjects who received the distress-management training reported lower RPEs and higher scores on the FS during the latter part of the low-intensity exercise than the control subjects. The experimental subjects also reported higher FS scores just prior to exhaustion than the control subjects.

These three studies, along with extant literature, point to the dynamic nature of affect during and following exercise, as well as to the importance of individual differences and coping skills for determining affective outcomes. The onset of exercise, especially higher-intensity exercise, may be associated with decrements along the hedonic-tone dimension (pleasure–displeasure), while the removal of the exercise stimulus may produce increases in hedonic tone. Likewise, between-group differences may exist as a function of individual differences and coping skills. Future research should therefore focus on describing when changes in hedonic tone and self-perceptions of activation occur throughout exercise stimuli of varying intensities, as well as during the recovery period from exercise. The identification of relevant individual-difference variables is also needed. In studies of acute exercise, data should be collected at least at the following times: prior to exercise, once physiological steady state has been achieved, periodically during the exercise stimulus, and every 5 to 10 minutes during recovery from exercise. In studies of the effects of chronic exercise, these patterns of change in hedonic tone and activation should be examined prior to any physical training and then periodically throughout the training and maintenance phases of exercise. Such time-course data could reveal whether the effects of acute exercise on affect are related to any possible effects of chronic exercise on mood.

Furthermore, the description of exercise-induced mood changes according to the circumplex model of affect appears to be relevant for two reasons. First, the aforementioned data indicate that there may be movement along the hedonic tone dimension both during and following exercise. Likewise, exercise produces significant changes in activation. The circumplex model of affect thus seems particularly well suited to the study of exercise and mood because exercise may induce changes in both dimensions of the model. Second, as mentioned by Russell (1980), the dimensions of hedonic tone and activation appear to account for about 45% of the variance in affective experience. Therefore, the importance of these dimensions cannot be ignored.

Given the availability of the Affect Grid and its relation to the circumplex model, it is worth commenting on its potential use in exercise research. Russell et al. (1989) have suggested that the Affect Grid is convenient and easy to use while people are performing selected tasks. Many exercise psychology researchers have successfully had subjects rate their mood using a simple unidimensional rating scale during exercise. The viability of using a two-dimensional matrix such as the Affect Grid requires testing because it may be too difficult to visually focus on while performing exercise, especially at high intensities. Given the necessity to measure affect at different points prior to, during, and following the exercise stimulus, the complexity of the Affect Grid may render it impractical. A method involving two successive ratings on bipolar scales may prove to be preferable. However, a concurrent validity study is required, to examine which of the two measurement strategies is more reliable and more practical for ongoing measurement of affect during exercise.

**The Two-Factor Structure of Affect.** The two-factor model of affect (Watson, Clark, & Tellegen, 1988; Watson & Tellegen, 1985; Zevon & Tellegen, 1982) was yielded from factor-analytic and multidimensional-scaling studies similar to those conducted by Russell (1978, 1980). The distinguishing characteristic of this model hinges on a methodological feature. Russell's (1980) dimensional structure emerges when employing unrotated factor structures, while Watson and Tellegen's (1985) structure emerges when factor structures are varimax rotated. Methods of rotation are typically used to increase the interpretability of a solution (Tabachnick & Fidell, 1989). On the basis of the rotated solution, Watson and Tellegen (1985) contend that the two fundamental dimensions of affect are positive and negative affect. The positive affect (PA) dimension reflects the extent to which a person feels enthusiastic, active, and alert. A person low on PA would experience depression, lethargy, and fatigue. The negative affect (NA) component reflects the extent to which a person experiences aversive mood states, such as anger, contempt, disgust, guilt, fear, and nervousness. A person low on NA would experience calmness and serenity.

Watson, Clark, and Tellegen (1988) have developed a brief paper-and-pencil questionnaire to measure PA and NA, called the "Positive Affect Negative Affect Schedule" (PANAS). The PANAS requires about 2 minutes to fill out and consists of 20 emotion-related words. The subject rates his or her mood or feelings on a scale from 1 (not at all) to 6 (extremely). The time frame of the PANAS can also be modified by including instructions to rate feelings at the present moment, today, during the past few days, the past week, the past few weeks, the past year, and in general. Psychometric data support its validity and reliability.

Watson and Tellegen's (1985) model of affect has been used in only three published studies (Clark & Watson, 1988; McIntyre, Watson, & Cunningham, 1990; Watson, 1988) and one pilot study (Ainsworth, Hardy, Depue, & Leon, 1990), to understand the relationship between exercise and affect. On the basis of extant literature (North et al., 1990; Petruzello et al., 1991; Salazar et al., Chapter 5, this volume), it might be expected that exercise would be related to decreased NA because previous literature suggests that exercise alleviates state anxiety (i.e., one of the constituent aversive states of NA). Likewise, exercise should be linked to higher PA because previous reviews suggest that exercise and depression (i.e., low PA) are negatively related.

In fact, the data relevant to Watson and Tellegen's (1985) model indicate that exercise may be more strongly related to PA than to NA. For example, Clark and Watson (1988) recruited Japanese university students to fill out daily mood questionnaires and to record daily activities over a period of 3 months. A 57-item mood inventory designed to tap PA and NA was translated and adapted for use with this population. They found that PA was highly correlated with social events and particularly physically active social events (e.g., hiking, skiing, cycling). NA was not associated with physical activity.

In another study, Watson (1988) collected daily mood ratings from college students over a period of 6–8 weeks. A 24-item mood inventory measuring PA and NA was employed. Subjects indicated how much sleep and stress they had experienced during the day, as well as whether they had exercised. Within-subject correlations, as well as between-subject correlations, were computed. Within-subject correlations indicated that exercise was weakly but consistently correlated to PA but not to NA. Between-subject analyses indicated that frequency of exercise was positively correlated with daily PA and negatively correlated with daily NA.

In their work, McIntyre et al. (1990) studied the PA and NA of college students as a function of different daily activities. Over a 1-week period, subjects filled out the PANAS 4 times: baseline, after social interaction, after exercise, and before an academic exam. Results indicated that PA was higher than baseline following social interaction and exercise, and that NA was higher than baseline before the exam. No other differences were significant.

Finally, Ainsworth et al. (1990) randomly assigned male and female volunteers to a 12-week brisk-walking condition or a 12-week flexibility-exercise condition. Subjects filled out the PANAS twice a day, in the morning and the evening, for a 16-week period. Results indicated very few effects of exercise, although PA tended to be higher in the evening and tended (although not significantly) to increase in the walking treatment group. The flexibility-exercise group demonstrated decreasing NA over time.

Taken together, these four studies are noteworthy for several reasons. First, they all included repeated measurements of mood over an extended period of time. This approach is certainly more conducive to increasing our understanding of the role of acute and chronic exercise in modulating affective life than one-shot pre–post designs.

Second, the results suggest that acute exercise (e.g., hiking, skiing, exercise) is related to PA but not always to NA. As mentioned previously, a perusal of existing literature reviews might have pointed to a relationship between exercise and NA, as well as between exercise and PA. However, little is known about the extent to which paper-and-pencil measures of affect used in previous research (e.g., POMS, STAI, MAACL) equate with the two-factor structure of affect proposed by Watson and Tellegen (1985). Furthermore, in the three published studies described herein, neither acute nor chronic exercise was experimentally manipulated. The effects of properly controlled acute exercise bouts, sustained and intense exercise training, or exercise deprivation have not been thoroughly examined. Therefore, firm conclusions cannot be made.

It is noteworthy to mention that the two-factor structure of affect has gained widespread recognition in the field of psychology as one of the most widely used and elegant models of affective experience. Describing exercise-induced affect according to this model would therefore offer greater possibility of generalization, as long as researchers simultaneously avoid the research pitfalls mentioned earlier.

**The Frequency, Intensity, and Variability of Affect.**  Recent work by another group of researchers (Diener & Emmons, 1985; Diener, Larsen, Levine, & Emmons, 1985; Larsen, 1987) is also based on the two-pronged distinction between PA and NA. These researchers share with Watson and Tellegen (1985) the view that PA and NA are separate and fundamental dimensions of emotional experience. However, their addition to the study of affect has been to describe other aspects of PA and NA—namely, frequency, intensity, and variability over time. *Frequency* refers to how often the individual experiences PA or NA over time; *intensity* designates the typical strength of the person's affective reactions; and the *variability* refers to the frequency of mood shifts in a person over time. Measurement of these three characteristics of mood can be obtained through the use of the Experience Sampling Method (ESM—Hormuth, 1986; Stone & Neale, 1982), which involves repeated measurements of a number of mood dimensions at random times during the day, over an extended period of time. That is, subjects are required to fill out a mood rating scale that includes nine mood adjectives (happy, satisfied, joyful, fun, unhappy, depressed, angry/hostile, frustrated, worried/anxious) every time the pager ("beeper") they are carrying around sounds off. A six-point rating scale ranging from "Not at all" to "Extremely much" is used. Composite mood scores are then obtained for the frequency and intensity of positive and negative affect over time. The time-series data provide indicators of mood variability and can be analyzed through spectral analysis[5] (Larsen, 1987).

An example of a recent study using this methodology was conducted by Gauvin and Fei (1992). In order to test the hypothesis that an increase in fitness can enhance mood over time, they randomly assigned 32 sedentary Chinese to either a treatment or an attention control group. The treatment group participated in an 8-week session of triweekly, 1-hour exercise periods, which included a 20- to 30-minute aerobic stimulus. The attention control group participated in an 8-week session of social dance periods of the same length and frequency as the exercise session. During the aerobic stimulus of each session the experimental subjects' heart rate reached an average of 155.25 beats per minute (bpm), while the heart rate of the attention control subjects reached an average of only 106.80 bpm. The experimental subjects were therefore working at a significantly higher workload than the attention control subjects. Experience sampling data on moods were collected for 3 weeks prior to and beginning the treatment, during 3 weeks at the midpoint of treatment, and for 3 weeks at the end of and following the treatment.

---

[5]*Spectral analysis* is a statistical technique, which decomposes time-series data into sine–cosine waves of various frequencies and amplitude (Larsen, 1987). Amounts of variance explained by different types of sine–cosine waves can be obtained. The researcher is thus able to determine whether variations in the data are explained by frequent and repeated mood shifts, by slow and progressive mood changes, or by moderate-speed mood changes.

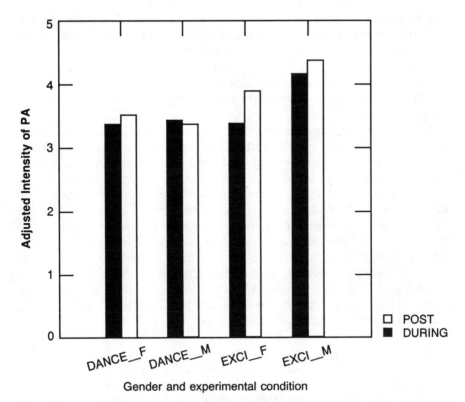

**Figure 6.3.** Intensity of positive affect at different times in training in males and females in the exercise treatment and social-dance control groups (Gauvin & Fei, 1992). Data are residuals adjusted for pretraining differences.

At the beginning of the study, all subjects—control and experimental alike—had a high frequency of PA (i.e., their daily PA always outweighed their daily NA). Thus no effect on frequency of PA could be observed. However, as shown in Figure 6.3, results indicated that in the exercise treatment group the intensity of PA significantly increased throughout the testing period.[6] Thus, exercise did not increase the frequency of PA in a person's life but rendered daily PA more intense, at least as indicated at the time points across the time course of the study. Such a finding emphasizes the limitation of only using pre–post designs and a unidimensional approach to describing exercise-related affect (e.g., frequency), which has been

---

[6]The results were analyzed using a 2 x 2 x 3 (Condition x Sex x Time: During–Post) analysis of covariance, using pretraining scores as a covariate because groups initially differed on intensity of positive affect despite random assignment.

characteristic of previous research. Previous interpretations might have concluded a null effect or a ceiling effect if the only affect characteristic described was frequency. By using the ESM and the conceptual distinction between frequency and intensity of affect, misleading interpretations are more likely to be avoided and the aspects of affect that do change over time due to exercise can be described. These findings obviously await further replication and extension.

Recently, Gauvin and Szabo (in press) studied the mood changes and psychosomatic symptoms associated with exercise deprivation. College students who reported exercising at least three times a week and who were highly committed to exercise participated in an ESM procedure wherein they filled out mood and symptom questionnaires four times a day for 35 days. The experimental group refrained from exercising between Days 15 and 21, while the control group maintained their normal level of physical activity. Results indicated that PA and NA were not affected by the manipulation, although subjects in the experimental group reported almost twice as many physical symptoms (e.g., headaches, chest pains, stomach pains, tense or sore muscles) between days 15 and 28, in comparison to the control group. These data suggest that exercise may be related to factors other than affect, such as reported physical well-being.

Although the ESM approach and the distinctions among frequency, intensity, and variability[7] of PA and NA provide greater opportunity (because multiple measures are used) to demonstrate the effect of exercise on affect, if indeed a true impact is made, the conclusion drawn from these two studies is one of only partial support for the link between exercise and affect. However, the fact that this impact occurs in different manifestations (e.g., intensity of PA in the Gauvin and Fei study and frequency of reports of physical symptoms in the Gauvin and Szabo study) speaks to the potential advantage of using the ESM multiple-measure approach in future exercise studies.

Furthermore, use of the ESM approach and the distinctions among frequency, intensity, and variability of PA and NA is suited to allowing investigators to determine whether chronic exercise significantly modifies subjects' typical pattern of mood. Likewise, it can be determined whether changes elicited by acute exercise are large or small in comparison to typical patterns of mood change within a given subject. Finally, the question of whether affective responses to acute exercise change from one phase of training to another could also be examined in order to acquire a sense of the relation between the acute and the chronic effects of exercise.

---

[7]While analyses of the variability of these data have not yet been completed, they too could reveal interesting perspectives.

**The Potency Dimension.** Many researchers view two-dimensional models to be incomplete. Even Russell (1978) indicates that other dimensions of affective experience probably exist. Phenomenological reports about affect in exercise (e.g., Ravizza, 1984; Sachs, 1984) also indicate that exercise-induced affect apparently includes more dimensions than hedonic tone and activation or broad dimensions of PA and NA. One way to validate these anecdotal claims is to examine other dimensions of affective experience.

The third most frequently mentioned dimension of affective experience is potency. *High potency* refers to sentiments of personal empowerment, whereas *low potency* refers to sentiments of powerlessness. This affective dimension was identified by several researchers (McKinnon & Keating, 1989; Morgan & Heise, 1988), who have collected new data on words used in mood inventories and reexamined their underlying dimensional structure. Instead of requiring subjects to provide judgments of similarity, each word and the emotion it represented was evaluated in terms of three semantic differential scales: Good–Nice vs. Bad–Awful, Fast–Lively–Young vs. Slow–Old–Quiet, and Big–Powerful vs. Small–Powerless, representing the dimensions of hedonic tone, activation, and potency.

Results of these studies revealed a three-dimensional structure including several important nuances. The first dimension emerging from the data was hedonic tone: Affective experience ranges from positive to negative. The second and third dimensions revealed were the activation (e.g., high vs. low intensity) and potency (e.g., powerful vs. powerless) dimensions. The interesting distinctions were that positive emotions could be discriminated by the activation dimension alone, while negative emotions required both the activation and the potency dimensions for discrimination. Positive emotions were all rated high on potency, in contrast to the variation observed in negative emotions. Some negative emotions were rated as being as potent as the positive emotions (e.g., anger), while others were rated as being low on potency (e.g., sadness). In other words, when people experience any form of PA, they tend to feel powerful. However, when NA is experienced, people can feel either powerful or powerless.

Although the potency dimension of affective experience has not been examined in exercise-psychology research, research on self-efficacy cognitions during exercise suggests that cognitions related to powerfulness (i.e., being confident one can successfully perform the behavior) can moderate or mediate affective consequences of exercise. McAuley and Courneya (1992) found that affective reactions to acute exercise were higher on the hedonic tone dimension (as measured by the FS) among subjects who displayed high self-efficacy, while affective reactions to exercise were more negative in subjects who reported low self-efficacy. Consequently, affective reactions to exercise may differ among individuals as a function of potency-related cognitions. The extent to which thoughts about potency and feelings of potency are related could therefore be examined.

Furthermore, one of the mechanisms through which exercise has been hypothesized to improve mood is described as the "mastery hypothesis" (Morgan & O'Connor, 1989; Petruzello et al., 1991). The *mastery hypothesis* suggests that through exercising, people conquer challenges that provide feelings of competence. This is to say that participating in exercise would induce increased feelings of potency coupled with changes in self-efficacy cognitions. One way to test the viability of the mastery hypothesis would therefore be to examine whether, for differing levels of self-efficacy, the subject's emotional state increases along the potency dimension as the exercise unfolds or as exercise training progresses and whether hedonic tone, activation, PA, or NA covary with potency. Experimental manipulations designed to vary self-efficacy and to enhance feelings of potency would help to ascertain the viability of these hypotheses. Development of an appropriate measurement technology for gauging potency-related affect is also required.

**Cognitive Appraisal Dimensions.** Above and beyond the dimensions of hedonic tone, activation, and potency, Smith and Ellsworth (1985) have proposed and documented that affective experience is differentiated along other dimensions of cognitive appraisal. College students rated 15 different emotional experiences (e.g., happiness, sadness, fear, anger, boredom, challenge, interest, hope, frustration, contempt, disgust, surprise, pride, shame, and guilt) as a function of 8 dimensions of cognitive appraisal (e.g, pleasantness, attentional activity, control, certainty, goal-path obstacle, legitimacy, responsibility, and anticipated effort). Results revealed that emotional experience varied along six of these dimensions.

The first dimension was the pleasantness dimension; affective experiences range from positive to negative. For instance, happiness and pride were rated as positive, while fear and anger were rated as unpleasant. The second dimension was anticipated effort; affective experiences differ in the extent of effort a person expects to have to exert effort. For example, challenge was viewed as requiring high effort, while happiness required low effort. The third dimension was certainty; affective experiences differ in the extent to which future occurrences are predictable or unpredictable. For example, surprise and hope were viewed as unpredictable, whereas boredom and sadness were seen as predictable. The fourth dimension was attentional activity; affective experiences differ in the extent to which subjects focus their attention on or off the current events. Subjects indicated that when experiencing positive emotions, they paid attention to events unfolding but that when they experienced boredom, they tried to focus their attention on something else. The fifth dimension was self versus other responsibility/control; affective experiences differ in the extent to which people attribute causes of events to themselves or to others. Guilt, pride and shame were associated with self-responsibility/control, whereas surprise is associated with other responsibility. The sixth and final dimension was situational control. Affective experiences were differentiated depending on whether subjects felt a person was responsible or whether a situational factor was responsible. In anger experiences, subjects rated people to be responsible for events, whereas in sadness, subjects rated people to be the victims of circumstance.

Cognitive appraisal dimensions of affect have not been examined directly in exercise, although several hypotheses can be formulated about their influence. For example, if attentional focus does indeed result in different affective experiences, then its measurement is paramount in the study of affect. Data on associative and dissociative techniques while performing marathons (Schomer, 1986) point to the fact that subjects may vary in their attentional focus while exercising. Some subjects focus inwardly on bodily sensations, through association, while others focus externally on visual or auditory sensations or other thoughts, through dissociation. The dissociative strategies tend to be related to higher performance while the associative strategies tend to be related to lower performance and to be viewed as less enjoyable, especially at high workloads (Gill & Strom, 1985).

Several authors have suggested that information-processing factors may explain some of the effects of exercise on mood (Petruzzello et al., 1991; Rejeski, Hardy, & Shaw, 1991). For example, physiological changes associated with acute exercise may be interpreted by some subjects as anxiety, and thus, removal of exercise would result in alleviation of subjectively perceived anxiety. Unfortunately, the affective consequences of using different foci of attention while exercising have not been formally examined, even though techniques such as exercising to music have been unsuccessfully employed to dissipate some of the less-pleasurable sensations associated with exercise (Steptoe & Cox, 1988). Future research could examine this issue.

Another mechanism that has been suggested to contribute to the affective beneficence of exercise is the distraction hypothesis (Morgan & O'Connor, 1989; Petruzzello et al., 1991). The *distraction hypothesis* suggests that when people exercise, they take a break from their concerns and therefore experience changed moods. Presumably, this would mean that subjects are focusing their attention on the exercise per se or on the environmental stimuli, as opposed to their daily concerns. Although exercise has been compared to other forms of distraction, the issue of what people focus on or think about during exercise has never been examined empirically or manipulated experimentally. By having subjects focus alternatively on their daily concerns or on the sensations and perceptions arising from the exercise experience, this question may be addressed.

These examples illustrate that other dimensions of affective experience might also pertain to exercise. Thus, future research should contain measures or otherwise control for these factors. In sum, the affect literature, which stems from a broad and encompassing approach to affect, offers a wealth of models and methodologies that have relevance for the study of exercise and mood. Useful alternative conceptualizations of affect that could be tested in the future include Russell's (1980) circumplex model of affect, Watson and Tellegen's (1985) two-dimensional model of affect, and the characteristics of frequency, intensity, and variability of PA and NA, as well as other dimensions of affect. Likewise, the ESM, the PANAS, the Affect Grid, the FS, and scales designed to measure other dimensions of affective experience await further validation for the study of exercise and affect. As may have become apparent, one more major issue in the study of exercise and affect requires examination—namely, the link between affect and other psychological parameters that occur during and following exercise.

## A Taxonomy of Emotion Words

Clore, Ortony, and Foss (1987; Ortony, Clore, & Foss, 1987) have approached the study of emotion through an examination of people's perceptions of the affective connotations of emotion words. Specifically, these researchers established a list of 535 emotion words that were used in the affect literature and classified them conceptually into one of eight categories. Their basic contention was that all words used in the emotion literature do not necessarily refer to affect but may designate cognitive states, behavioral intentions, or somatic states.

The first two categories defined by Clore et al. (1987; Ortony et al., 1987) regroup words that refer to external conditions, as opposed to intrapersonal conditions. These are subjective evaluations (e.g., attractive) and objective descriptors (e.g., unprotected). The words referring to internal conditions were divided into nonmental and mental categories. The nonmental categorized words referred to physical and bodily states (e.g., drowsy). The mental categorized states were further subdivided into affective states (e.g., happy), affective–behavioral conditions (e.g., cheerful), affective–cognitive conditions (e.g., encouraged), behavioral–cognitive conditions (e.g., careful), and cognitive conditions (e.g., certain).

Subsequently, these 535 words were presented in varying semantic contexts to subjects who were asked to rate whether they felt that each word referred to their idea of an emotion. The researchers hypothesized that any word that actually referred to affect would be rated as such, whether it was presented in the "I am _____" or the "I feel _____" forms (e.g., "I am anxious" and "I feel anxious" both refer to emotions). Words referring to subjective evaluations or to cognitive states would not always be rated as affect-laden in the "I am _____" and "I feel _____" forms (e.g., "I feel attractive" and "I am attractive"; the first may refer to an emotion, while the second may refer to an objective evaluation). Thus, an empirically derived taxonomy of emotional words was produced distinguishing words into cognitive, affective, physical and bodily, and external categories.

It should be noted that many of the words used in previous work in developing exercise mood questionnaires and in ascertaining the dimensions underlying emotion do not refer to affect but to bodily states or cognitive conditions, as defined by Clore et al. (1987) and Ortony et al. (1987). To illustrate this point, we analyzed the emotion words used in the FS, the MAACL, the POMS, the AD-ACL, the STAI, the PANAS, and the ESM questionnaire. Table 6.1 presents a tabulation of the number of emotion words in each questionnaire, which falls into the theoretically defined categories of Ortony et al. (1987). Table 6.2 presents tabulations of the number of emotion words in each questionnaire, as a function of the empirically derived categories of Clore et al. (1987).

As can be seen from Table 6.1, only about half of the items on the MAACL, the POMS, the AD-ACL, the STAI, and the PANAS include affect-laden words (e.g., affective, affective–cognitive and affective–behavioral words), as defined by Ortony et al. (1987). The ESM questionnaire appears to include the highest proportion of affect words—72.7%. Table 6.2 reveals a similar pattern. Once the words in each questionnaire are categorized into the empirically derived categories, approximately 50% or fewer of the items are categorized as affective according to the Clore et al. (1987) taxonomy. In contrast, 90% of the items on the ESM questionnaire have an affective connotation.

These findings raise the methodological issue that many of the questionnaires used in previous exercise research may not provide adequate operational measures of affect. That is, they measure selected portions of affective experience, along with cognitive conditions, subjective evaluations, or bodily states. While it is true that laypersons use colloquial expressions, and possibly not affect-laden terms, to express their emotions, it is also true that in research, an attempt must be made to employ only those affect words that are unambiguous and that generalize as emotions. Future research and measurement attempts should employ those words that are truly face-valid and classified as affect-laden. Clear distinctions as to the psychological meaning associated with each word should be made, so that subjects can use these words to respond. Thus, the classifications of Ortony et al. (1987) and Clore et al. (1987) may be useful in describing and creating a conceptual and operational definition of *affect*, which is suitable for exercise research.

Finally, it is not untenable that changes in bodily function due to exercise are associated with changes both in affect and in information processing of related somatic experiences and thoughtful appraisals. The process of conceptually defining and building a model of exercise-induced affect, with

**TABLE 6.1  PROPORTION OF ITEMS IN EACH SCALE FALLING INTO ORTONY ET AL.'S (1987) THEORETICAL CLASSIFICATION OF EMOTION WORDS**

| Category | Questionnaire | | | | | | |
|---|---|---|---|---|---|---|---|
| | FS | MAACL | POMS[a] | AD-ACL | STAI[a] | PANAS | ESM |
| Physical & bodily state | — | — | 5 (7.6%) | 4 (20.0%) | 4 (17.4%) | 1 (5.0%) | — |
| Affective condition | — | 38 (28.8%) | 23 (34.8%) | 3 (15.0%) | 12 (52.2%) | 9 (45.0%) | 8 (72.7%) |
| Affective–behavioral condition | — | 11 (8.3%) | 3 (4.5%) | 1 (5.0%) | — | — | — |
| Affective–cognitive condition | — | 13 (9.8%) | 4 (6.1%) | — | 3 (13.0%) | 2 (10.0%) | 2 (18.2%) |
| Behavioral–cognitive condition | — | 15 (11.4%) | 6 (9.1%) | 3 (15.0%) | — | — | — |
| Cognitive condition | — | 5 (3.8%) | 6 (9.1%) | — | 1 (4.3%) | 4 (20.0%) | — |
| Subjective evaluation | 2 (100%) | 7 (5.3%) | 1 (1.5%) | — | 1 (4.3%) | 1 (5.0%) | — |
| Objective descriptor | — | 5 (3.8%) | 1 (1.5%) | 1 (5.0%) | — | — | — |
| Not in list | — | 38 (28.8%) | 17 (25.8%) | 8 (40.0%) | 2 (8.7%) | 3 (15.0%) | 1 (9.1%) |
| Total | 2 (100%) | 132 (100%) | 66 (100%) | 20 (100%) | 23 (100%) | 20 (100%) | 11 (100%) |

[a]The POMS and the STAI actually include 65 and 20 items, respectively. Ortony et al.'s (1987) classification associates a psychological and physical meaning with the words *relaxed* and *comfortable*. The item *relaxed* is included in both the POMS and the STAI and therefore was classified twice. Likewise one of the items in the STAI includes two emotion words—namely feeling "over-excited or rattled." Two items on the ESM include two emotion words—namely "angry/hostile" and "worried/anxious." They, too, were classified as two separate items.

**TABLE 6.2  PROPORTION OF ITEMS IN EACH SCALE FALLING INTO CLORE ET AL.'S (1987) EMPIRICAL CLASSIFICATION OF EMOTION WORDS**

| Category | Questionnaire | | | | | | |
|---|---|---|---|---|---|---|---|
| | FS | MAACL | POMS[a] | AD-ACL | STAI[a] | PANAS | ESM |
| Cognitive condition | — | 19 (14.4%) | 9 (13.6%) | 3 (15.0%) | 4 (17.4%) | 4 (20.0%) | — |
| Affective condition | — | 50 (37.9%) | 29 (22.0%) | 3 (15.0%) | 11 (47.8%) | 11 (55.0%) | 10 (90.9%) |
| Physical & bodily state | — | 2 (1.5%) | 6 (4.5%) | 3 (15.0%) | 2 (8.7%) | 1 (5.0%) | — |
| External condition | 2 (100%) | 23 (17.4%) | 5 (3.8%) | 3 (15.0%) | 4 (17.4%) | 1 (5.0%) | — |
| Not in list | — | 38 (25.8%) | 17 (25.8%) | 8 (40.0%) | 2 (8.7%) | 3 (15.0%) | 1 (9.0%) |
| Total | 2 (100%) | 132 (100%) | 66 (100%) | 20 (100%) | 23 (100%) | 20 (100%) | 11 (100%) |

[a]The POMS and the STAI actually include 65 and 20 items, respectively. Ortony et al.'s (1987) classification associates a psychological and physical meaning with the words *relaxed* and *comfortable*. The item *relaxed* is included in both the POMS and the STAI and therefore was classified twice. Likewise, one of the items in the STAI includes two emotion words—namely feeling "over-excited or rattled." Two items on the ESM include two emotion words, namely "angry/hostile" and "worried/anxious." They, too, were classified as two separate items.

methods such as a taxonomy, should disentangle what portions of the phenomenology of exercise refer to affect, to self-perception of bodily function and exertion (i.e., related somatic experiences), and to cognitions (i.e., thoughtful appraisals). This will help in the process of conceptually defining affect and building a model.

## SUMMARY AND CONCLUSION

The understanding of exercise-induced affect will require a significant departure from previously used methods and approaches. Future research on the effects of acute exercise should include measures of the different dimensions of affective experience, cognitive appraisal dimensions of affect, RPE, and self-perceptions of physiological activation. The intent would be to clarify conceptual and operational definitions of affect. If this is done, then it is more likely that research can focus on the more ambitious project of disentangling the time-course of changes in each one of these parameters, as well as comparing the magnitude of changes in exercise-induced affect to the subject's typical pattern of mood change. This disentangling will require controlling prior mood state and expectancy effects. Researchers must also experimentally manipulate (a) exercise intensity and duration (to provide insight into the dose–response issue), (b) focus of attention, (c) efficacy information, and (d) anticipated effort as mediator or moderator variables influencing exercise-induced affect. Such investigations may yield a more comprehensive description of the phenomenology of acute exercise than presently exists.

Suggesting how research should progress toward the understanding of the effects of chronic exercise is more problematic. The discussion in this chapter highlights the value of measuring positive and negative affect, through methods such as the ESM, and of attempting to clarify the relation between acute and chronic exercise effects. In this regard, it does seem imperative to collect data at all training phases and to decipher both when major changes in affect occur and the speed of such changes.

While most of the suggestions advocated will ultimately produce descriptive information that may lead to conceptual and operational definitions, future research demands a more thorough foundation. Once a substantive description of the phenomenology of acute exercise and a better grasp of the affective consequences of chronic exercise have been acquired, then the more challenging issues regarding the mechanisms underlying affective changes due to exercise and the relation between mental health and exercise adherence can be approached adequately. The specific issues outlined in this chapter emphasize a few of the many steps necessary to achieve these goals.

## REFERENCES

Ainsworth, B. E., Hardy, C. J., Depue, R. A., & Leon, A. S. (1990, September). *Comparison of the effects of moderate aerobic exercise and flexibility exercise on mood.* Paper presented at the annual conference of the Association for the Advancement of Applied Sport Psychology, San Antonio, TX.

Clark, L. A., & Watson, D. (1988). Mood and the mundane: Relations between daily life events and self-reported mood. *Journal of Personality and Social Psychology, 54,* 296–308.

Clore, G. L., & Ortony, A. (1991). What more is there to emotion concepts than prototypes? *Journal of Personality and Social Psychology, 60,* 48–50.

Clore, G. L., Ortony, A., & Foss, M. A. (1987). The psychological foundations of the affective lexicon. *Journal of Personality and Social Psychology, 53,* 751–766.

Crews, D. J., & Landers, D. M. (1987). A meta-analytic review of aerobic fitness and reactivity to psychosocial stressors. *Medicine and Science in Sports and Exercise, 19,* S114–S120.

Diener, E. (1984). Subjective well-being. *Psychological Bulletin, 95,* 542–575.

Diener, E., & Emmons, R. E. (1985). The independence of positive and negative affect. *Journal of Personality and Social Psychology, 47,* 1105–1117.

Diener, E., Larsen, R. J., Levine, S., & Emmons, R. A. (1985). Frequency and intensity: The two dimensions underlying positive and negative affect. *Journal of Personality and Social Psychology, 48,* 1253–1265.

Ekman, P. (Ed.) (1982). *Emotions in the human face* (2nd ed.). New York: Cambridge University Press.

Emerson, J. D., & Strenio, J. (1983). Boxplots and batch comparison. In D. C. Hoaglin, F. Mosteller, & J. W. Tukey (Eds.), *Understanding robust and exploratory data analysis* (pp. 58–96). New York: Wiley.

Frijda, N. H. (1987). *The emotions.* New York: Cambridge University Press.

Gauvin, L., & Fei, X.-W. (1992). *The effects of chronic exercise on the frequency and intensity of mood in Chinese males and females.* Manuscript in preparation.

Gauvin, L., & Szabo, A. (1992). *Effects of acute exercise on mood: Toward an understanding of their significance, time-course and mediating variables.* Manuscript submitted for publication.

Gauvin, L., & Szabo, A. (in press). Application of the Experience Sampling Method to the study of the effects of exercise withdrawal on well-being. *Journal of Sport and Exercise Psychology.* Manuscript submitted for publication.

Gill, D. L., & Strom, E. H. (1985). The effect of attentional focus on performance of an endurance task. *International Journal of Sport Psychology, 16,* 217–223.

Hardy, C. J., & Rejeski, W. J. (1989). Not what, but how one feels: The measurement of affect during exercise. *Journal of Sport and Exercise Psychology, 11,* 304–317.

Hormuth, S. E. (1986). The sampling of experiences in situ. *Journal of Personality, 54,* 262–293.

Izard, C. E. (1977). *Human emotions.* New York: Plenum.

Kenney, E. A., Rejeski, W. J., & Messier, S. P. (1987). Managing exercise distress: The effect of broad spectrum intervention on affect, RPE, and running efficiency. *Canadian Journal of Sport Sciences, 12,* 97–105.

Larsen, R. J. (1987). The stability of mood variability: A spectral analytic approach to daily mood assessment. *Journal of Personality and Social Psychology, 52,* 1195–1204.

Martinsen, E. W. (1990). Benefits of exercise for the treatment of depression. *Sports Medicine, 9,* 380–389.

McAuley, E., & Courneya, K. S. (1992). Self efficacy relationships with affective and exertion responses to exercise. *Journal of Applied Social Psychology, 22,* 312–326.

McIntyre, C. W., Watson, D., & Cunningham, A. C. (1990). The effects of social interaction, exercise, and test stress on positive and negative affect. *Bulletin of the Psychonomic Society, 28,* 141–143.

McKinnon, N. J., & Keating, L. J. (1989). The structure of emotions: Canada–United States comparisons. *Social Psychology Quarterly, 52,* 70–83.

McNair, D. M., Lorr, M., & Droppleman, L. F. (1971). *Manual for the profile of mood states.* San Diego, CA: Educational and Industrial Testing Service.

Morgan, R. L., & Heise, D. (1988). Structure of emotions. *Social Psychology Quarterly, 51,* 19–31.

Morgan, W. P., & O'Connor, P. (1989). Psychological models. In R. K. Dishman (Ed.), *Exercise adherence: Its impact on public health* (pp. 91–121). Champaign, IL: Human Kinetics.

North, C. T., McCullagh, P., & Tran, W. (1990). Effect of exercise on depression. *Exercise and Sport Science Reviews, 19,* 379–415.

Ortony, A., Clore, G. L., & Foss, M. A. (1987). The referential structure of the affective lexicon. *Cognitive Science, 11,* 361–384.

Petruzzello, S. J., Landers, D. M., Hatfield, B. D., Kubitz, K. A., & Salazar, W. (1991). Effects of exercise on anxiety and mood: A meta-analysis. *Sports Medicine, 11,* 143–182.

Ravizza, K. (1984). Qualities of the peak experience in sport. In J. M. Silva & R. S. Weinberg (Eds.), *Psychological foundations in sport* (pp. 452–461). Champaign, IL: Human Kinetics.

Rejeski, W. J., Hardy, C. J., & Shaw, J. (1991). Psychometric confounds of assessing state anxiety in conjunction with acute bouts of vigorous exercise. *Journal of Sport and Exercise Psychology, 13,* 65–74.

Rejeski, W. J., Best, D. L., Griffith, P., & Kenney, E. (1987). Sex-role orientation and the responses of men to exercise stress. *Research Quarterly for Exercise and Sport, 58,* 260–264.

Rosenthal, R., & Rosnow, R. L. (1984). *Essentials of behavioral research: Methods and data analysis.* New York: McGraw-Hill.

Russell, J. A. (1978). Evidence of convergent validity on the dimensions of affect. *Journal of Personality and Social Psychology, 36,* 1152–1168.

Russell, J. A. (1980). A circumplex model of affect. *Journal of Personality and Social Psychology, 39,* 1161–1178.

Russell, J. A. (1991). In defense of a prototype approach to emotion concepts. *Journal of Personality and Social Psychology, 60,* 37–47.

Russell, J. A., Weiss, A., & Mendelsohn, G. A. (1989). Affect grid: A single-item scale of pleasure and arousal. *Journal of Personality and Social Psychology, 57,* 491–502.

Sachs, M. L. (1984). The runner's high. In M. L. Sachs & G. W. Buffone (Eds.), *Running as therapy: An integrated approach* (pp. 273–287). Lincoln, NE: University of Nebraska Press.

Sallis, J. F., & Hovell, M. F. (1990). Determinants of exercise behavior. *Exercise and Sport Science Reviews, 18,* 307–330.

Schomer, H. H. (1986). Mental strategies and perception of effort of marathon runners. *International Journal of Sport Psychology, 17,* 41–50.

Smith, C. A., & Ellsworth, P. C. (1985). Patterns of cognitive appraisal in emotion. *Journal of Personality and Social Psychology, 48,* 813–838.

Spielberger, C. D., Gorsuch, R. L., & Lushene, R. (1970). *State–Trait Anxiety Inventory manual.* Palo Alto, CA: Consulting Psychologists Press.

Steptoe, A., & Cox, S. (1988). Acute effects of aerobic exercise on mood. *Health Psychology, 7,* 329–340.

Stone, A. A., & Neale, J. M. (1982). Development of a methodology for assessing daily experiences. In A. Baum & J. Singer (Eds.), *Advances in environmental psychology: Environment and health* (Vol. 4, pp. 49–83). New York: Erlbaum.

Tabachnick, B. G., & Fidell, L. S. (1989). *Using multivariate statistics.* New York: Harper & Row.

Thayer, R. E. (1986). Activation–deactivation adjective check list: Current overview and structural analysis. *Psychological Reports, 58,* 607–614.

Vallerand, R. J. (1984). Emotion in sport: Definitional, historical and social psychological perspectives. In W. F. Straub & J. M. Williams (Eds.), *Cognitive sport psychology* (pp. 65–78). New York: Sport Science Associates.

Watson, D. (1988). Intraindividual and interindividual analyses of positive and negative affect: Their relation to health complaints, perceived stress, and daily activities. *Journal of Personality and Social Psychology, 54,* 1020–1030.

Watson, D., Clark, L. A., & Tellegen, A. (1988). Development and validation of brief measures of positive and negative affect: The PANAS scales. *Journal of Personality and Social Psychology, 54,* 1063–1070.

Watson, D., & Tellegen, A. (1985). Toward a consensual structure of mood. *Psychological Bulletin, 98,* 219–235.

Zevon, M. A., & Tellegen, A. (1982). The structure of mood change: An idiographic/nomothetic analysis. *Journal of Personality and Social Psychology, 43,* 111–122.

Zuckerman, M., & Lubin, B. (1965). *Manual for the Multiple Affect Adjective Check List.* San Diego, CA: Educational and Industrial Testing Service.

# 7

# Sympathetic Response to Acute Psychosocial Stressors in Humans: Linkage to Physical Exercise and Training

**FRANÇOIS PÉRONNET AND ATTILA SZABO**

## THE SYMPATHETIC SYSTEM: A BRIEF OVERVIEW

The autonomic or "involuntary" system has two anatomically and functionally distinct components: (1) the sympathetic system, and (2) the parasympathetic nervous system. Together, these two systems regulate several physiological processes and are highly responsive to situations that disturb internal physiological equilibrium (for a more detailed description, the reader is referred to Burn [1975] or Guyton [1986]). The sympathetic division of the autonomic system comprises both a nervous component—namely, the sympathetic nervous system—and an endocrine component, which is represented by the circulating plasma catecholamines. These molecules arise in part from the sympathetic nerve fibers (mainly norepinephrine) and in part from the adrenal medulla (epinephrine and norepinephrine).

## The Sympathetic Nervous System

The sympathetic nervous system is composed of a large number of nerve fibers. These fibers originate from the thoracic-lumbar region of the spinal cord and connect within the ganglion of the sympathetic chain. From here, postganglionic, mainly noradrenergic, fibers branch to various organs and tissues. The most extensive distribution of sympathetic fibers is to the smooth muscles of blood vessels, including arterioles and venules, throughout the body. Certain tissues receive direct sympathetic innervation not only to their vessels but also to the tissue cells themselves. These include the iris; lachrymal, salivary, and sweat glands; smooth muscles in the bronchioles; the mucosa of the lungs; the heart; the gastrointestinal tract; the liver; the pancreas; the genital organs, and the urinary bladder; hair-raising muscles; and adipose tissue. This complex system of communication is designed to quickly send specific messages from the neurovegetative centers to the peripheral organs. The main features of this system are its *quickness* and its *specificity*, in that transmission along the nerve fibers is very fast, and different messages can be sent to different organs or tissues at the same time. As a general rule, only part of the sympathetic nervous system is activated upon stimulation at any time, in a coordinated manner, in order to regulate the functions of the organs involved in the response to a particular homeostatic challenge. Therefore, the often-used terminology of "sympathetic activity" may result in erroneous interpretations, which may imply a general activation of the whole system when reference is made only to a part of the system.

The majority of sympathetic fibers release norepinephrine, while a smaller fraction of them release acetylcholine as their neurotransmitter. Indeed, some tissues, such as the smooth muscles of the arterioles in the skeletal muscle tissue, receive both noradrenergic and cholinergic innervation. Furthermore, besides norepinephrine and acetylcholine, both types of sympathetic fibers may also release smaller amounts of other substances (known as cotransmitters), such as epinephrine, dopamine, and various peptides, the functions of which are not clearly understood at present.

## Plasma Catecholamines

Some tissues do not receive sympathetic innervation and thus are excluded from sympathetic nervous control. Among them is one tissue of particular importance in the present context: skeletal muscle tissue. Muscle cells are not innervated by sympathetic fibers. Most sympathetic fibers branching toward the muscles innervate the smooth muscles of the blood vessels. While these fibers are of primary importance in the regulation of muscle blood flow, they are unable to control the metabolic or contractile activity of the muscle cells themselves. Muscles, like other tissues with sparse or no sympathetic innervation, rely on the endocrine component of the sympathetic system, which is represented by plasma catecholamines. Circulating catecholamines are distributed via the blood vessels to every organ and tissue in the body in equal (arterial) concentration. The circulating catecholamines include both epinephrine and norepinephrine. Epinephrine is secreted by the adrenal medulla, which also secretes significant amounts of norepinephrine into the circulation.

The proportion of epinephrine versus norepinephrine released from the adrenal medulla varies across species. In humans, the adrenal medulla contains and releases about 85% epinephrine (Goldstein, 1987). Accordingly, the adrenal medulla is only a minor source for circulating norepinephrine in humans. Most of the circulating norepinephrine arises from sympathetic nerve endings. Indeed, a portion of the norepinephrine released as a neurotransmitter from the sympathetic nerve terminals escapes the synaptic junctions and enters circulation.

## Norepinephrine: Neurotransmitter and Hormone

The nervous component of the sympathetic system could also act as an endocrine component. Norepinephrine is released from sympathetic nerve terminals in order to transmit messages at synaptic junctions: Its primary purpose is to act as a neurotransmitter at local levels. However, noradrenergic fibers in the sympathetic nervous system do not form synapses identical to those in other nervous tissues. Instead, they form special synapses, termed "synapse en passant," within the interstitial fluid of the tissue. These special synapses are made up of long and dense networks of fibers that are equipped with special structures, known as "varicosities."

Norepinephrine is stored in specialized vesicles within the varicosities. When a depolarization travels along the fiber, norepinephrine is released from every varicosity and floods the interstitial fluid, in which it can reach its receptor sites. Due to this special organization and functioning, norepinephrine may be considered a "local hormone" released over a comparatively large area, in comparison to synaptic junctions encountered in other parts of the nervous system. Consequently, a fiber or varicosity cannot be considered as having tight control over a fixed number of cells, but rather as having a loose control over a small volume of surrounding tissue. In addition, when norepinephrine is released from the varicosities and diffuses in the interstitial fluid, its action is terminated mainly by uptake and reincorporation within the sympathetic fiber. Because the catecholamine uptake mechanism is very efficient, norepinephrine is quickly removed from the interstitial fluid, taken up, and stored again within the storage vesicles for later use.

In order to better understand the physiology of the sympathetic system, the sympathetic fibers should be viewed not only as the source of, but also as a site of clearance for norepinephrine, as well as a site of clearance for epinephrine. They act as vacuums for the epinephrine and norepinephrine molecules that venture into their vicinity. As such, sympathetic fibers protect the tissue against the effects of both locally released and circulating catecholamines.

The physiological evidence for this role is exemplified by the phenomenon of presynaptic hypersensitivity. This phenomenon is readily observable when sympathetic nerve endings are destroyed or the uptake mechanism is blocked—for example, by cocaine. In both cases, the absence of catecholamine uptake into the nerve endings leads to a marked hypersensitivity to catecholamines in the affected tissues. Thus, the phenomenon of presynaptic hypersensitivity illustrates that the catecholamine uptake mechanism plays an important role in the regulation and fine tuning of the control exerted by the sympathetic system. However, as mentioned earlier, a portion of the norepinephrine locally released from the sympathetic fibers escapes uptake at the nerve endings, diffuses into circulation, and can act on distant target cells. Therefore, any portion of the sympathetic nervous system also can be considered to be an endocrine organ, able to exert not only local control, but also a systemic control over a wide range of physiological functions.

## Adrenergic Receptors

Although epinephrine and norepinephrine are two related molecules, they perform distinct physiological functions. Their specific action depends on the extent of sympathetic innervation, on the epinephrine/norepinephrine ratio in circulation, and on the type of receptors present in the tissue. With no or minimal sympathetic innervation, the concentration of catecholamines in the interstitial fluid for a given arterial concentration is likely to be high, while in tissues having dense sympathetic innervation, plasma catecholamines are likely to exert only weak effects because of the powerful uptake mechanism. In addition, these effects will vary with the nature of the circulating catecholamines and the type of adrenergic receptors.

Two major types ($\alpha$ and $\beta$) of adrenergic receptors with various subtypes have been identified. The affinity of epinephrine and norepinephrine for the various receptors is different. Epinephrine is more potent on $\alpha$ and $\beta_2$

adrenergic receptors. Located on the smooth muscle, $\alpha_1$ (postsynaptic) receptors control vasoconstriction in the arterioles and venules. Situated on nerve terminals and having affinity for both epinephrine and norepinephrine, $\alpha_2$ (presynaptic) receptors reduce the release of norepinephrine. The $ß_2$ receptors have virtually no affinity for norepinephrine. Postsynaptic $ß_2$ receptors control vasodilation in the skeletal muscle, while presynaptic $ß_2$ receptors, which are present on the nerve terminals, enhance the release of norepinephrine. Norepinephrine is more potent than epinephrine on the $ß_1$ receptors, which are found, for example, in the heart and adipocytes.

It should be emphasized that adrenergic receptors are not static structures but are proteins or a combination of proteins that exhibit substantial plasticity. Depending on the activity of the tissues, the action of various hormones, and the concentration of plasma catecholamines, adrenergic receptors can be either activated or inactivated. *Upregulation* is the process of activation of adrenergic receptors, resulting from cell externalization and/or de novo synthesis of receptors. *Downregulation* refers to the process of inactivation of adrenergic receptors, resulting from internalization of the receptors, sequestration within a compartment of the cell, or breakdown of the protein molecules. As a consequence of up- and downregulation, the number of receptors on the cell surface, along with cell sensitivity to epinephrine and norepinephrine, are constantly changing.

## The Measures of "Sympathetic Activity"

Sympathetic responses to various stimuli may be assessed via direct and/or indirect indices. Direct indices are mainly represented by plasma (e.g., Hjemdahl, Freyschuss, Juhlin-Dannfelt, & Linde, 1984) and urinary (e.g., Frankenhaeuser, 1975) catecholamines, plasma catecholamine turnover (e.g., Kjær, Christensen, Sonne, Richter, & Galbo, 1985), and recordings of sympathetic electrical nerve activity (e.g., Delius, Hagbarth, Hongell, & Wallin, 1972). Plasma dopamine-ß-hydroxylase (the enzyme that converts dopamine into norepinephrine) activity (Péronnet, Nadeau, de Champlain, & Chartrand, 1982) and plasma chromogranin (a protein specific to the storage vesicles) concentration have also been used in the assessment of sympathetic activity (Dimsdale & Ziegler, 1991). Indirect indices are often used because they may reflect the degree of participation of the sympathetic system in the regulation of various physiological functions. These indices, among others, include cardiovascular measures such as preejection period, electrocardiographic (ECG) T-wave amplitude, total peripheral resistance, local resistance, blood pressure, heart rate, cardiac output, and skin conductance level. Still another way to assess sympathetic function in a particular tissue is by examining the adrenergic receptor attributes, such as density or sensitivity, in that particular tissue.

The accuracy with which the aforementioned indices reflect sympathetic activity in a particular tissue is debatable. Because the adrenal medulla is the major source of circulating epinephrine, changes in plasma epinephrine concentration reflect fairly well the changes in adrenal medullary activity. Thus, plasma epinephrine concentration may be considered as a reliable and direct measure of adrenal medullary activity. In contrast, circulating norepinephrine may have multiple, differing sites of origin, and its plasma concentration is dependent on numerous factors, including local sympathetic nerve activity, uptake, adrenal medullary activity, and local blood flow. Only about 20% of the released norepinephrine escapes the synaptic junctions and diffuses into the circulation (Hoeldtke, Cilmi, Reichard, Boden, & Owen, 1983). Consequently, important increases in local sympathetic nerve activity may be accompanied by only minimal changes in plasma norepinephrine levels (Seals, Victor, & Mark, 1988; Victor, Leimbach, Seals, Wallin, & Mark, 1987).

In addition, although increases in plasma norepinephrine levels reflect large changes in sympathetic nerve activity, they do not reveal the source of norepinephrine or its target tissue(s), if any. Furthermore, it is unknown how much or how intense sympathetic nerve activity is needed to detect changes in plasma norepinephrine levels. Localized sympathetic nerve activity may result in significant physiological changes in a particular tissue without simultaneous changes in whole plasma norepinephrine levels. Therefore, plasma norepinephrine is not a precise index of sympathetic activity. The same situation applies to urinary catecholamines. While urinary epinephrine marks changes in adrenal medullary activity, only a small fraction of norepinephrine ends up in urine (Frankenhaeuser, 1975).

The most accurate reflection of sympathetic nerve activity is direct electrical recording (Seals, Victor, & Mark, 1988; Victor et al., 1987). However, electrical activity of sympathetic nerves can only be recorded on a limited number of peripheral nerves, which provide only an incomplete picture about the activation of the sympathetic system. They are merely measures of local regional sympathetic activity. As for indirect indices of sympathetic activity, these may reflect a decrease or an increase in sympathetic activity, but they display a composite action and thus may reflect the activity (or activities) of another regulatory system(s) as well.

Finally, changes in adrenergic receptor characteristics may also reveal the degree of control exerted by the sympathetic system in a particular tissue. In humans, changes in adrenergic receptors are often measured on lymphocytes or blood platelets because of convenient accessibility. However, it remains unclear how representative these are of other receptors in other organs.

## SYMPATHETIC RESPONSE TO PSYCHOSOCIAL STRESSORS

As early as the beginning of this century, Cannon established a pioneering linkage between the adrenal gland and heightened emotional states.

Following a series of experiments with cats who secreted significant amounts of "adrenin" when frightened by barking dogs (Cannon & de la Paz, 1911), Cannon introduced the "fight-or-flight" concept that he associated with an internal "emergency system" responsive to a number of different challenges.

## The Significance of the Somatic Response to Psychosocial Stress

The autonomic system is responsive to psychosocial stress via both the sympathetic and the parasympathetic division. These autonomic responses to psychosocial stress, while in themselves complex, are only a part of a larger and substantially more complex general somatic response. This larger response includes neuromuscular, neuroendocrine, cardiovascular, and metabolic components. The significance of the somatic response to acute psychosocial stress may be incorporated into three inferred "theories," which describe the physiological changes taking place as: (1) nonspecific, (2) vestigial, and (3) adapted or borrowed.

The first of these theories, under its most extreme and simplistic forms, suggests that the somatic response to psychosocial stress is the same for all stressors (i.e., nonspecific) and is generalized to the entire organism. Only the degree of activation will vary with the intensity of the stimulus. In addition, the somatic response is considered useless (unadapted) or even detrimental (inappropriate) for adequate coping. Although some situations of very intense psychosocial stress do exist, such as a direct physical threat, when the somatic response does appear generalized, inappropriate, and nonspecific, in most cases of mild challenges, the somatic response (a) varies not only in degree but also in its nature, (b) is not necessarily generalized, and (c) may have some value in coping with the situation. Describing the somatic response to psychosocial stress as nonspecific, generalized, and inappropriate may only indicate a lack of understanding.

The second theory suggests that the somatic response to psychosocial stress is a vestigial legacy of our evolutionary past. These responses have had adaptive values for the survival of our ancestors and were developed at that time through the process of natural selection. For some reason, they were retained although they do not appear to serve any purpose anymore. Two examples of these vestigial responses are the hair-raising reactions in the case of extreme fear and the sweating of the palms of the hands and the soles of the feet experienced by some individuals in response to even mild psychosocial stress. Hair-raising (which results from the contraction of hair-raising muscles innervated by sympathetic fibers) has an adaptive value for some mammals because it results in an increase in the apparent size of the animal, which can be a deterrent for a predator or a competitor. Due to the limited development of hair in our species, this purpose has been lost, although the function has been preserved. Similarly, sweating of the palms of the hands and of the sole of the feet could have been of value for a distant ancestor who climbed trees using both "hands" and "feet" (as contemporary monkeys still do) by securing its grips on the branches. (It is not uncommon for workers to spit into the palms of their hands to secure their grip on a shovel.)

The somatic response to psychosocial stress can include vestigial components without any obvious purpose for contemporary man. Some of these vestigial components have no adaptive value in normal day-to-day life in parts of the civilized world, in which physical threats and fights are not common. However, in the physical and social world of our ancestors and of a large number of our contemporary societies, physical threats by predators or competitors from the same species were and still are common. The responses to these threats, which have evolved by natural selection, include several strategies, such as flight, fight, fainting, frightening, signalization (i.e., to warn of impending danger and to ask for help), and hiding. Most of these responses are somatic in nature and involve a certain amount of physical activity and accordingly an adaptation of circulation and metabolism to sustain the energy demand of the exercising muscles (the exception is fainting, but again, a special somatic response is developed, due to a reduction of heart rate through an increased vagal tone). Accordingly, somatic responses to psychosocial stress have an adaptive value in the natural situation in which our species has evolved and in which we still live, to a large extent.

In the very artificial setting of a laboratory, the somatic response to a psychosocial stressor, such as an arithmetic task, serves little purpose. It does, however, take place in this unnatural situation because natural selection has not selected any specific response, and therefore the organism "borrows" the response pattern available to cope with a physical threat. Such borrowing is not unusual in situations for which no adapted organized response pattern is available to the organism. For example, in a severe pathological condition such as heart failure, the borrowed endocrine and cardiovascular response is the response to dehydration. This is due to the fact that the reduction in cardiac output and in renal blood flow is apparently "misinterpreted" as a sign of dehydration. In the case of psychological stressors, it is difficult to identify the signals that are misinterpreted and that therefore trigger the organized response pattern adapted to cope with a physical threat, but this response definitely occurs.

## General Overview of Psychosocial Stressors

The most extensively studied psychosocial stressors are contrived laboratory tasks, while real-life stressors have not been studied to a large extent. Both laboratory and real-life stressors can be grouped into two categories: active and passive coping stressors. *Active coping stressors* involve tasks or situations for which the outcome is subject dependent—that is, an active response leading to the end result is under the subject's control. An example of an active laboratory stressor is mental counting, and an example of an active real-life stressor is parachute jumping. In both situations, measurable performance from the subject's part is required. Passive stressors are tasks or situations for which the outcome cannot be modified by the subject because control over the situation is not possible. Exposure to unavoidable pain or to noise in the laboratory and to real-life flight emergency both exemplify passive coping stressors.

One of the most extensively employed active laboratory stressors is the Stroop color-word task (Stroop, 1935). This task involves the visual presentation of color words, such as *blue*, printed in conflicting colors, for example, red. The subject's task is to ignore the word *blue* and to correctly name the color of the print (in this case, red). There are a number of modified versions of the Stroop task. One of them—introduced by Frankenhaeuser, Mellis, Rissler, Bjorkvall, and Patkai (1968)—includes the simultaneous auditory and visual presentation of color words both of which have to be ignored and only the color of visual stimulus (color word) should be named.

Another popular laboratory active coping stressor is mental arithmetic. This is a form of challenge in which the subject is required to perform basic mathematic operations mentally for a predetermined length of time. Video games of a competitive nature are often used in studies on Type A behavior because they are believed to elicit strong physiological reactions in Type A individuals. Reaction time tasks are of two types: (1) performance reaction time task, when the subject is expected to accomplish something as fast as possible in order to receive a reinforcement (points, coins, etc.) and (2) avoidance reaction-time task, when the subject has to quickly respond to a signal in order to avoid an unpleasant event (electric shocks, loud noise bursts, harassment, etc.). These stressors bear a strong structural similarity to video games. Other forms of somewhat less common active laboratory stressors are reading while exposed to delayed auditory feedback, memory tasks, quizzes, and Raven's progressive matrices, which is a mental challenge in which a geometric pattern that corresponds to a progressive geometric schema has to be selected from a number of alternatives, within a limited time interval (Raven, 1965).

Passive laboratory stressors involve circumstances in which the subject has no control over the situation. These may include exposure to films that elicit various emotional reactions (Levi, 1965). For example, films on accidents (Hull, Young, & Ziegler, 1984), surgery, or erotic scenes (Cantor, Zillman, & Day, 1978; Obrist et al., 1978); imagery of stressful events, such as combat experience (Pitman, Orr, Forgue, Altman, & de Jong, 1990); exposure to unpleasant auditory sounds (Dienstbier, LaGuardia, Barnes, Tharp, & Schmidt, 1987) or to a fearful stimulus (Bandura, Taylor, Williams, Mefford, & Barchas, 1985), with no avoidance possibility.

Real-life stressors, besides being classified as active or passive, may be further characterized as acute or chronic stressors. The sympathetic response mechanism to acute and to chronic stress may be significantly different. The active real-life stressors examined, among others, include public speech (Bassett, Marshall, & Spillane, 1987; Dimsdale & Moss, 1980), public defense of a Ph.D. thesis (Johansson, Collins, & Collins, 1983), rappelling (Brooke & Long, 1987), and competition stress in elite athletes (Hoch, Werle, & Weicker, 1988), stress in pilots (Krahenbuhl et al., 1980), in parachute jumpers (Fenz & Jones, 1974), in race-car drivers (Taggart & Carruthers, 1971) and combat stress in soldiers (Austin et al., 1967; Roman, Older, & Jones, 1967). The passive real-life stressors studied, among others, include dental procedures (Taggart, Hedworth-Whitty, Carruthers, & Gordon, 1976), in-flight emergencies (Krahenbuhl, Harris, Malchow, & Stern, 1985), and loss of employment—which is a chronic type of stressor (Baum, Fleming, & Reddy, 1986).

## Sympathetic Response to Laboratory Stressors

Empirical evidence indicates that laboratory psychosocial stressors elicit measurable sympathetic responses in humans. For example, increased sympathetic responses to Stroop color-word task administered under different conditions have been consistently reported (Table 7.1), using urinary and plasma catecholamine levels and nerve activity as indices of sympathetic activity. Frankenhaeuser et al. (1968) showed a significant increase from 3.3 to 5.4 ng/minute in urinary epinephrine excretion, in response to a modified version of the Stroop test, while urine norepinephrine levels remained unchanged. In line with urinary catecholamines, plasma epinephrine concentration may increase about 50–100% or even more, while plasma venous norepinephrine concentration may rise only about 0–20% in response to the Stroop test.

The lack of significant increases in venous norepinephrine concentration, however, does not imply an absence of response from the sympathetic system. Hjemdahl et al. (1984) reported an increase from 1.53 to 2.13 nanomoles (nM) in arterial plasma norepinephrine concentration in response to the Stroop test, while antecubital venous plasma norepinephrine concentration did not change significantly (Figure 7.1). This finding not only indicates that arterial norepinephrine concentration may be a better index of sympathetic response to stress than venous plasma norepinephrine levels but also demonstrates that there is significant nervous sympathetic response to psychosocial stress accompanying adrenal medullary response. The nervous sympathetic response was confirmed by studies that have revealed an elevation in sympathetic electrical nerve activity in response to psychosocial stressors. For example, Freyschuss et al. (1990) showed that muscle sympathetic-nerve activity recorded from the right peroneal nerve increased in response to the Stroop task, along with arterial plasma epinephrine and norepinephrine concentration and indirect (cardiovascular) indices of sympathetic activity.

Consistent and strong sympathetic responses to mental arithmetic (al-

**TABLE 7.1 EXAMPLES OF SYMPATHETIC RESPONSES TO THE STROOP COLOR WORD TASK**

| Source | Subjects | Sympathetic measures | Sympathetic response | Time of sampling |
|---|---|---|---|---|
| Frankenhaeuser, Mellis, Rissler, Bsorkvall, & Patkai (1968) | 25 ♂ | Urinary EPI, NE | 64% ↑ EPI NE (no change) | End of 6 x 4 min |
| Freyschuss, Hjemdahl, Juhlin-Dannfelt, & Linde (1988) | 30 ♂ | A & V EPI, NE | 120% ↑ EPI(A) 40% ↑ NE(A) | 3 min 3 min |
| Freyschuss, Fagius, Wallin, Bohlin, Perski, & Hjemdahl (1990) | 10 ♂ | A & V EPI, NE, & MSNA | 59% ↑ EPI(A), 82% ↑ EPI(V), 23% ↑ NE(A), 25% ↑ NE(V) MSNA ↑ > ↓ | 3 min 3 min 3 min 3 min continuous |
| Hjemdahl, Freyschuss, Juhlin-Dannfelt, & Linde (1984) | 12 ♂ | Plasma (A) & (V) EPI, NE | 118% ↑ EPI(A), 54% ↑ EPI(V), 39% ↑ NE(A), NE (no change) | 3 min 10 min 3 min |
| Hull, Young, & Ziegler (1984) | 35 ♂ & 20 ♀ | Plasma (V) EPI, NE | 58% ↑ EPI, 16% ↑ NE | 5 min 5 min |

| Study | N / Sex | Measure | Results | Time |
|---|---|---|---|---|
| Seraganian, Hanley, Hollander, Roskies, Smilga, Martin, Collu, & Oseasohn (1985) | 32 ♂ | Plasma (V) EPI, NE | (% ?) ↑ EPI, 25 pg/ml ↑ EPI, (% ?) ↑ NE, 3 pg/ml ↑ NE | 3 min, 3 min |
| Sinyor, Schwartz, Péronnet, Brisson, & Seraganian (1983) | 30 ♂ | Plasma (V) EPI, NE | ? ↑ EPI, ? ↑ NE | 1 min & 3 min, 1 min & 3 min |
| Sinyor, Péronnet, Brisson, & Seraganian (1988) | 6 ♂ | Plasma (V) EPI, NE | ? ↑ EPI, ? ↑ NE | 1 min & 3 min, 1 min & 3 min |
| Sothman, Horn, Hart, & Gustafson (1987) | 19 ♂ | Plasma (V) EPI, NE | [a]56%/17% ↑ EPI, 68%/71% ↑ EPI, 0.9%/8% ↑ NE, −4.4%/39% ↑ NE | 6 min, 12 min, 6 min, 12 min |
| Tidgren & Hjemdahl (1989) | 12 ♂ | Plasma (A), & renal (V) DA, EPI, NE | 54% ↑ DA(V), 197% ↑ EPI(A), 146% ↑ EPI(V), 78% ↑ NE(A), 171% ↑ NE(V) | 10 min, 3 min, 10 min, 3 min, 3 min |

*Note.* ↑ = increase; ♂ = males; ♀ = females; (% ?) = percentage unknown; ? = unknown; A = arterial; EPI = epinephrine; MSNA = muscle sympathetic nerve activity; NE = norepinephrine; V = venous; min = minute(s).
[a] Reported separately for fit/unfit subjects.

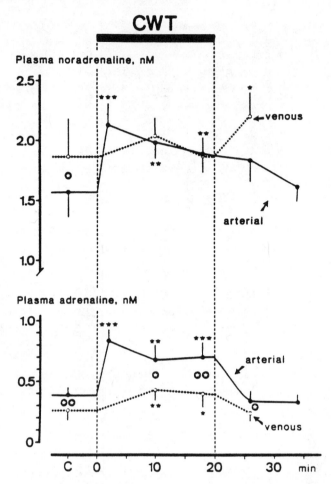

**Figure 7.1.** Arterial and antecubital venous plasma norepinephrine and epineph-rine concentrations in connection with the Stroop color-word task (CWT). Mean values ± standard error from 10–12 paired observations are given. Black asterisks indicate significant changes from prestress values (*p < .05, **p < .01, ***p < .001) and white circles the significance between arterial and venous concentrations (same significance level code). Reprinted with permission from Hjemdahl et al. (1984). *Acta Physiologica Scandinavica, 527* (page 27, Figure 2).

though different forms with different length of exposure were utilized) have also been reported (e.g., Anderson, Wallin, & Mark, 1987; Blumenthal et al., 1990; LeBlanc, Côté, Jobin, & Labrie, 1979; Matsukawa et al., 1991; Seraganian et al., 1985; Sinyor, Péronnet, Brisson, & Seraganian, 1983; Stoney, Matthews, McDonald, & Johnson, 1988; Ward et al., 1983). These responses often exceed those observed in response to the Stroop test (Table

7.2). Plasma epinephrine levels may increase almost 75% after the first minute and as much as double after the second minute into the task (see LeBlanc et al., 1979). Sympathetic nerve activity has been shown to increase in leg muscles, but not in forearm muscle (Anderson, Wallin, & Mark, 1987). In contrast, Matsukawa et al. (1991) showed that leg-muscle sympathetic nerve activity decreased 34% in healthy males and increased 7% in borderline hypertensives during mental arithmetic. Associated with these changes in fiber electrical activity, norepinephrine levels may show variable changes, but mostly increases in response to mental arithmetic.

One reason why mental arithmetic may produce a highly variable pattern of sympathetic and/or cardiovascular response is because it exists in a variety of forms and/or versions. It may be presented via auditory or visual media, can be of high, low, or medium intensity, may require continuous or intermittent answers or may be computerized, with built-in control for subject's mathematical ability (Turner et al., 1986). Furthermore, it may require verbal, written, or motoric (e.g., joystick selection) answers. Although very popular, verbal responses may be inappropriate because vocalization of numbers alone, without accompanying mental calculation, also can produce significant increases in heart rate (Brown, Szabo, & Seraganian, 1988).

Other laboratory stressors, such as reaction-time tasks (Allen & Crowell, 1989; de Geus, van Doornen, de Visser, & Orlebeke, 1990; Gasic, Grünberger, Korn, Oberhummer, & Zapatoczky, 1985; Glass, 1983; Morell, 1989; Sherwood, Allen, Obrist, & Langer, 1986; van Doornen & de Geus, 1989), Raven's progressive matrices (Seraganian et al., 1985; Steptoe, Moses, & Edwards, 1990a; Steptoe, Moses, Matthews, & Edwards, 1990b), quizzes (Seraganian, Roskies, Hanley, Oseasohn, & Collu, 1987; Seraganian et al., 1985; Sinyor et al., 1983), and video games (Cléroux, Péronnet, & de Champlain, 1985; Glass, 1983; Goldstein, Eisenhofer, Sax, Keiser, & Kopin, 1987; Tischenkel et al., 1989) requiring active coping also produce elevated sympathetic reactivity. For example, Goldstein et al. (1987) have studied plasma norepinephrine dynamics during psychosocial stress (a video game), following infusion of radioactive norepinephrine. Antecubital venous plasma norepinephrine levels did not change, but arterial levels increased 20%, along with total body spillover (rate of appearance of norepinephrine in arterial blood).

Transition from active to passive types of stressors is accompanied by a transition in psychophysiological response as well. Bandura et al. (1985) studied this transitional response from active to passive coping in phobic subjects. Spider-phobic females were presented with increasingly threatening interactive situations with a large Wolf spider. As long as subjects thought that they were in control, or able to cope with the situation, plasma epinephrine and norepinephrine levels remained low. Moderate levels of control, comprising a certain degree of uncertainty, resulted in elevated

**TABLE 7.2   EXAMPLES OF SYMPATHETIC RESPONSES TO MENTAL ARITHMETIC**

| Source | Subjects | Sympathetic measures | Sympathetic response | Time of sampling |
|---|---|---|---|---|
| Anderson, Wallin, & Mark (1987) | 6 ♂ | Leg & arm MSNA | ↑ Leg MSNA, arm MSNA (no change) | continuous |
| Blumenthal, Fredrikson, Kuhn, Ulmer, Walsh-Riddle, & Appelbaum (1990) | 37 ♂ | Plasma (V) EPI, NE | [a]80 – 180% ↑ EPI, 14 – 39% ↑ NE | continuous for 15 min – mean value employed |
| LeBlanc, Côté, Jobin, & Labrie (1987) | 12 ♂ | Plasma (V) EPI, NE | [a]74% & 157% ↑ EPI, 9% & 22% ↑ NE | 1 min & 2 min 1 min & 2 min |
| Matsukawa, Gotoh, Uneda, Miyajima, Shionoiri, Tochikubo, & Ishii (1991) | 20 ♂ | Plasma (V) EPI, NE MSNA | 69%[b] 88%[c] ↑ EPI, 9%[b] 13%[c] ↑ NE, −34%[b] 7%[c] ↑ MSNA | 2 min 2 min continuous |
| Seraganian, Haley, Hollander, Roskies, Smilga, Martin, Collu, & Oseasohn (1985) | 32 ♂ | Plasma (V) EPI, NE | (% ?) ↑ EPI, 56 pg/ml ↑ EPI, (% ?) ↑ NE 61 pg/ml | 3 min 3 min |

| Study | N | Measure | Results | Timing |
|---|---|---|---|---|
| Sinyor, Schwartz, Péronnet, Brisson, & Seraganian (1983) | 30 ♂ | Plasma (V) EPI, NE | [a,d]122%/100% ↑ EPI, 1 min; 89%/26% ↑ NE | 1 min |
| Sinyor, Péronnet, Brisson, & Seraganian (1988) | 6 ♂ | Plasma (V) EPI, NE | ↑*140%/129% ↑ EPI, 1 min; 37%/10% ↑ NE | 1 min |
| Stoney, Matthews, McDonald, & Johnson (1988) | 19 ♀ & 20 ♂ | Plasma (V) EPI, NE | 14% ↑ EPI (♂), 10% ↑ EPI (♀), 8% ↑ NE (♂), –3% ↑ NE (♀) | continuous continuous continuous continuous |
| Ward, Mefford, Parker, Chesney, Taylor, Keegan, & Barchas (1983) | 8 ♂ | Plasma (V) EPI, NE | 191% ↑ EPI, 24% ↑ NE | continuous continuous |

*Note.* (% ?) = percentage unknown; ↑ = increase; ♂ = males; ♀ = females, EPI = epinephrine; MSNA = muscle sympathetic nerve activity; NE = norepinephrine; V = venous; min - minute(s).

[a] Approximate values.
[b] Normotensives.
[c] Borderline hypertensives.
[d] Presented separately for fit/unfit subjects.
[e] Presented separately for before/after exercise training condition.

plasma epinephrine and norepinephrine levels. Finally, when subjects perceived themselves as completely unable to cope with the situation, a sharp drop in the concentration of both catecholamines occurred. This study demonstrated that active and passive type stressors elicit different patterns of sympathetic responses. Extremely stressful situations may even result in fainting, which is also an example of passive coping. However, there are no systematic laboratory studies on psychosocial-stress situations eliciting fainting.

Levi (1965) has shown that passive coping in the laboratory elicits significant increases in urinary catecholamines. Subjects viewing various motion pictures showed significant increases in urinary epinephrine levels following both pleasant amusing and unpleasant aggression-provoking scenes. An anxiety-provoking (horror) film elicited as much as a 41% increase in urinary epinephrine, as well as a 34% increase in urinary norepinephrine excretion. However, Hull, Young, and Ziegler (1984) found no significant changes in plasma catecholamine levels and cardiovascular measures in response to a passive coping stressor (scenes of industrial accidents).

In general, the knowledge about the psychophysiological response to passive coping stressors is limited. One reason for this is the ethical restriction from exposing human subjects to high-potency stressors. Passive stressors in real-life situations, such as the loss of a loved one, the loss of employment, or the like, are not only more powerful, but also can be characterized as chronic stressors, in comparison to artificially created acute stressors employed under laboratory settings. Laboratory stressors are generally of low intensity and often may be less stressful to the subject than the overall context of being tested.

### Sympathetic Response to Real-Life Stressors

Although sympathetic responses to real-life stressors are difficult to study, several experiments have examined this issue. As manifested in Table 7.3, these stressors apparently elicit larger plasma catecholamine responses than laboratory stressors in general. It is also evident that real-life stressors that require active coping (e.g., Dimsdale & Moss, 1980; Hoch, Werle, & Weicker, 1988; Johansson, Collins, & Collins, 1983; Taggart & Carruthers, 1971) may produce greater sympathetic responses than those that require passive coping (e.g., Krahenbuhl et al., 1985; Taggart et al., 1976). However, discrepancies in the sympathetic response to identical life stressors are not uncommon. Dimsdale and Moss (1980) reported significant increases in plasma epinephrine, but less pronounced increases in plasma norepinephrine levels in response to public speaking. Conversely, Taggart, Carruthers, and Somerville (1973) found no changes in plasma epinephrine, but reported significant changes in plasma norepinephrine levels in response to the same type of stress. It was suggested that differences in the

**TABLE 7.3  EXAMPLES OF SYMPATHETIC RESPONSES TO SOME REAL-LIFE STRESSORS**

| Source | Subjects | Sympathetic measures | Sympathetic response | Type of stressor |
|---|---|---|---|---|
| Bassett, Marshall, & Spillane (1987) | 22 ♂ & 7 ♀ | Urine DA, EPI, NE | [a]14% ↑ DA, 56% ↑ EPI, 25% ↑ NE | Public speech |
| Brooke & Long (1987) | 18 ♂ | Plasma (V) EPI, NE | 48%/30%[b] ↑ EPI, 21%/3% ↑ NE | Rappelling |
| Dimsdale & Moss (1980) | 9 ♂ | Plasma (V) EPI, NE | 124% ↑ EPI, 58% ↑ NE | Public speech |
| Hoch, Werle, & Weicker (1988) | 10 ♂ | Plasma (V) EPI, NE | [a]224%/480%[c] ↑ EPI, 38%/180% ↑ NE | Championship contest |
| Johansson, Collins, & Collins (1983) | 1 ♂ & 1 ♀ | Urine EPI, NE | [a]160%/193%[3] ↑ EPI, ? ↑ NE | Ph.D. defense |
| Krahenbuhl, Marett, & King (1977) | 10 ♂ | Urine EPI, NE | 19–823% ↑ EPI, 50–436% ↑ NE | Various tasks in training of pilots |
| Krahenbuhl, Marett, & Reid (1978) | 20 ♂ | Urine EPI, NE | 615% ↑ EPI, 42% ↑ NE | Pilot training |

**TABLE 7.3** (continued)

| Source | Subjects | Sympathetic measures | Sympathetic response | Type of stressor |
|---|---|---|---|---|
| Krahenbuhl, Harris, Malchow, & Stern (1985) | 40 ♂ | Urine DA, EPI, NE | 11% ↓ DA, 61% ↑ EPI, 34% ↑ NE | Flight emergency |
| Taggart & Carruthers (1971) | 16 ♂ | Plasma (V) EPI, NE | 189% ↑ EPI, 181% ↑ NE | Racing driving |
| Taggart, Carruthers, & Somerville (1973) | 21 ♂ & 2 ♀ | Plasma (V) EPI, NE | EPI (no change) ? ↑ NE | Public speech |
| Taggart, Hedworth-Whitty, Carruthers, & Gordon (1976) | 21 ♀ | Plasma (V) EPI, NE | [a]76% ↑ EPI, 9% ↑ NE | Dental procedure |

*Note.* ? = unknown; ♂ = males; ♀ = females; ↑ = increase; DA = dopamine; EPI = epinephrine; P = plasma; NE = norepinephrine; V = venous; U = urine.

[a] Approximate values.

[b] Reported separately for fit/unfit subjects.

[c] Increases from baseline (taken 1 day in advance) to pre/post contest values.

[d] Reported separately for the two subjects.

methods used, such as the time of sampling, between the two studies may have accounted for these discrepancies (Dimsdale & Moss, 1980). However, other factors, such as the components of the speech, as well as audience and auditorium characteristics, all may alter the degree of the perceived challenge and hence the somatic response profiles.

## Methodological Limitations in Stress Research

The first methodological barrier is represented by the fluctuation of biological measures. Most physiological variables can be classified as either *controlling variables* (e.g., plasma catecholamines), or as *controlled variables* (e.g., heart rate). The former show consistent fluctuations regardless of homeostatic state, while the latter are more stable in a state of equilibrium. In stress situations, changes in both variables are measured in relation to a baseline value. However, within-subject variability in baseline measures from one week to another, both in controlling (Péronnet et al., 1986b) and in controlled variables (Szabo & Gauvin, 1992), have been demonstrated. There is a general consensus that baseline values should not be taken on the day of testing because of anticipatory effects that may influence baseline recordings (e.g., Brooke & Long, 1987). Instability in baseline measures, however, calls against such reasoning. Some sort of pre- and/or posttreatment resting measure appears to be more valid because changes from that value may reflect treatment effect, but comparison to a previous value may be erroneous. Both Péronnet et al. (1986b) and Szabo and Gauvin (1992) have shown that group data are reproducible over time even if individual measures may highly fluctuate. If groups are large enough, this may partially solve the problem, but if groups are small, changes in individual baseline values may alter the magnitude of change induced by the treatment.

Another methodological problem arises from the adoption of stressors. Perhaps the greatest problem in stress research is still the characterization of stress. The type of stress may influence the sympathetic response of the organism. A generalized activation of the sympathetic system may occur in response to extreme life-threatening situations (Goldstein, 1987), but this can be examined only in real-life situations. Most scientific accounts, however, originate from laboratory studies that use fairly mild challenges (due to ethical constraints on research with human subjects). Laboratory stressors are artificial and may elicit somatic responses that may not necessarily mirror the organism's response in a real-life stress situation.

As previously mentioned, two types of stressors—active and passive—can be differentiated on the basis of controllability. Using the animal kingdom as an example, Folkow and Neil (1971) differentiated between a "defense reaction" and a "playing dead" reaction. The former, a form of fight-or-flight response, may be associated with heightened physiological responsiveness or active coping, while the latter may be associated with lowered physiological reactions or passive coping. It appears that active and passive stressors elicit different types of responses in different individuals representing a continuum on the sympathetic–parasympathetic axis. Consequently, comparisons between studies that use active versus passive stressors may lead to erroneous conclusions.

Repeated exposure to a stressor removes the novelty effect, which is often the most stressful aspect of a particular challenge. This results in lowered physiological response to the stressor, due to habituation (Szabo & Gauvin, 1992). If not controlled for, lowered physiological responses as a consequence of habituation may be erroneously interpreted as treatment effects. As covered in many experimental psychology textbooks, one possible control measure in such situations is to habituate the subjects to the challenge prior to the administration of the treatment.

Subject selection is also critical in stress research. Random assignment into treatment and control groups may present unwanted restrictions on subjects, while self-selection may lead to changes due to expectations rather than the treatment per se. On one hand, we should consider the fact that although a treatment may be thought to be beneficial, such as exercise, if it is a burden on the person to whom it is prescribed, it may be more detrimental than beneficial. On the other hand, the psychological changes associated with self-selection, including expectancy, may be an integral part of the benefits. Perhaps the merits and demerits of self-selection versus random assignment should be weighed empirically, one against the other.

## SYMPATHETIC RESPONSE TO EXERCISE AND TRAINING

### From Rest to Exercise

Sympathetic activity increases above resting values during dynamic exercise. This increase can be manifested through a 0.1- to 50-fold augmentation in plasma norepinephrine and epinephrine levels, which increase exponentially with increasing work intensities (Vendsalu, 1960). The rise in plasma catecholamines is a function of relative (% of maximum volume of oxygen uptake, $\dot{V}O_2$ max), not absolute, workload. A 2-fold increase in plasma epinephrine and a 3-fold increase in plasma norepinephrine concentration may be observed at 80% $\dot{V}O_2$ max during graded running (Galbo, 1983). A very short intense bout of exercise lasting about 2 minutes may also produce significant increases in plasma catecholamine concentration and urinary catecholamine excretion. The plasma concentration of the two catecholamines—norepinephrine and epinephrine—do not behave identically during exercise, in that norepinephrine concentration increases earlier and at relatively lower intensity levels than does epinephrine (Galbo, 1983, 1986). Plasma norepinephrine levels rise immediately at the onset of an exercise and then stabilize at a certain point, with little or no further increase from that point on. However, plasma epinephrine levels show a slow but continuous increase as exercise duration is prolonged (Figure 7.2).

An increase in plasma norepinephrine levels during exercise is presumably due to increased sympathetic nerve activity. There is a strong positive correlation ($r$ = +0.80) between muscle sympathetic-nerve activity and plasma norepinephrine from rest to exercise during arm cycling (Seals, Victor, & Mark, 1988). However, the magnitude of increase in muscle sympathetic-nerve activity is much higher than the increase in plasma norepinephrine concentration when percentage changes from resting baseline values are related (Seals, Victor, & Mark, 1988). An increase in plasma epinephrine and norepinephrine concentration from rest to exercise may occur in two ways: increased secretion or decreased clearance rate. While both may play an important role, changes in plasma epinephrine levels cannot be fully explained in terms of decreased clearance (Kjær, 1989). Although there is a tendency toward decreased clearance with increasing relative workloads, Kjær et al. (1985) have shown that no more than approximately a 20% change in clearance rate of plasma epinephrine takes place during exercise. This finding indicates that changes in plasma epinephrine concentration during exercise are primarily a consequence of increased epinephrine release into the circulation from the adrenal medulla. Higher plasma norepinephrine levels from rest to exercise also appear to be due to increased norepinephrine release into plasma.

While evidence in humans is limited, Péronnet et al. (1988) have shown that the skeletal-muscle vascular bed is the main contributor to increased plasma norepinephrine levels from rest to exercise in dogs. This does not necessarily imply increased sympathetic activity, but it may be a reflection of increased perfusion of skeletal muscles, which could favor norepinephrine washout from the interstitial fluid. Furthermore, Péronnet et al. (1988) also demonstrated that clearance rate was not significantly reduced from rest to exercise. Consequently, it appears that increases in both plasma epinephrine and norepinephrine levels from rest to exercise are due to increased release rather than reduced clearance rate.

**Factors Influencing Sympathetic Response to Exercise.** The characteristics of sympathetic responses to exercise are influenced by many factors (Galbo, 1983). Altitude and oxygen availability could alter plasma catecholamine responses to exercise, with higher altitudes or lower oxygen availability producing higher increases in plasma catecholamine levels. Extreme temperatures also may trigger higher plasma catecholamine concentrations during exercise. After sodium depletion or dehydration during prolonged exercise, plasma catecholamine levels may be higher. Finally, the availability of metabolic fuels, such as glucose, may largely and in inverse proportion influence plasma catecholamine levels (Galbo, 1983). Therefore, it is essential to exert some sort of control over these variables in studies involving both exercise and plasma catecholamines concurrently.

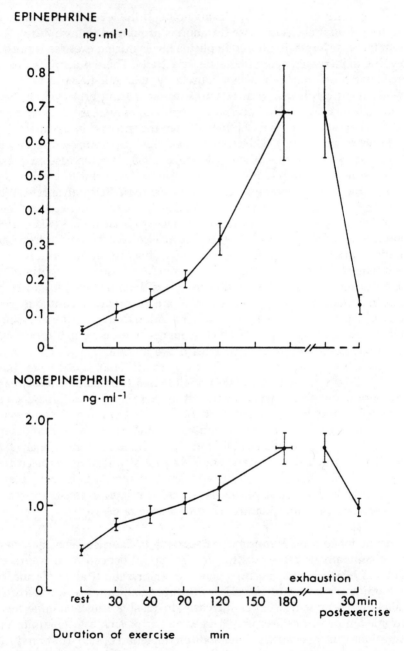

**EPINEPHRINE**

ng · ml⁻¹

**NOREPINEPHRINE**

ng · ml⁻¹

Duration of exercise    min

**Figure 7.2.**   Mean concentrations of epinephrine and norepinephrine (± standard error, $n = 7$) in a forearm vein during prolonged running at 60% $\dot{V}O_2$ max. Reprinted with permission from Galbo, H. (1983). *Hormonal and Metabolic Adaptation to Exercise,* Georg Thieme Verlag: Stuttgart (page 7, Figure 4).

Another appreciable difficulty that researchers encounter in studies with humans is the selection of a representative sample. Frequently, there is great variability in the age and sex ratio of the subjects. Variability in such factors, which are critical in sympathetic response to exercise, further amplifies the inherent variability due to individual differences in physiological studies. There is evidence that plasma catecholamine levels increase with age (Fleg, Tzankoff, & Lakatta, 1985; Hagberg et al., 1988; Lehmann & Keul, 1986; Mazzeo & Grantham, 1989). During graded maximal treadmill exercise, plasma norepinephrine and epinephrine are higher in older than in younger subjects, while at submaximal workloads, only plasma norepinephrine appears to vary across age groups (Fleg, Tzankoff, & Lakatta, 1985). Graded cycling triggers higher plasma norepinephrine and plasma epinephrine concentrations in older subjects, pointing to an age-dependent change in plasma catecholamine levels in response to exercise. Decreased receptor sensitivity or increased catecholamine clearance rate with age may be partly responsible for such findings (Lehmann & Keul, 1986).

Gender is another critical factor. While both sexes exhibit similar degrees of plasma catecholamine increases in response to exercise at identical heart rates and hence similar relative workloads, women show noticeable variation in plasma catecholamine levels during various phases of the menstrual cycle (Sutton et al., 1980). Furthermore, there is evidence that at identical absolute workloads, women demonstrate significantly higher sympathetic activity than men, probably due to smaller muscle/workload ratios (Lehmann, Berg, & Keul, 1986). Therefore studies employing both sexes and using exercise as one of the variables may have to (a) control for the menstrual-cycle phase and (b) relate to relative exercise workload when plasma catecholamines are one of the dependent variables.

One of the major problems when repeated sampling is performed is the unreliability of individual plasma catecholamine levels at rest and during exercise (Péronnet et al., 1986b). This may be due to the rapid and large fluctuations in plasma catecholamines over time. Although group data may be reproducible (Péronnet et al., 1986b), if small samples are used, high individual variability may mask true treatment differences. Unfortunately, in psychophysiological experiments using invasive blood-sampling technique, there is a tendency to employ relatively small samples, either because of the cost of individual biochemical assays along with monetary compensation to the subjects, or because of the amount of work and time involved in the gathering and analysis of such data. If, however, large enough sample sizes are used, the random within-subject variability may cancel out across the groups, and comparison may be attempted.

## At Rest, Following Exercise

Physiological indices of recovery from exercise to resting levels can be measured in terms of time. In most instances, plasma catecholamines return to resting levels within minutes following a bout of acute exercise. For example, 30 minutes after compete exhaustion, almost total recovery in norepinephrine levels are readily observable, while epinephrine remains about 40% above resting levels (Galbo, 1983). Thus, while the increase in epinephrine levels is retarded in response to exercise, so is recovery in comparison to norepinephrine levels. However, Péronnet, Massicotte, Paquet, Brisson, and de Champlain (1989) observed a 50% decrease in epinephrine levels (compared to reference baseline values) 1 hour following an acute bout of exercise. This may be attributed to changes in forearm blood flow during the recovery period following exercise and/or may represent a reduction in the activity of the adrenal medulla (Péronnet et al., 1989). Finally, plasma catecholamines may rise for a short period of time following exercise. This has been shown following exercise in the upright position and was attributed to postexercise hypotension (Watson et al., 1980), which can be avoided by having the subjects lie down as soon as the exercise is interrupted.

## At Rest, After Training

Training apparently does not modify the activity of the sympathetic system at rest. A number of investigators have independently reported that resting plasma norepinephrine levels remained unchanged after a training program (Cléroux, Péronnet, & de Champlain, 1985; Lehmann, Dickhuth, Schmid, Porzig, & Keul, 1984; Péronnet et al., 1981; Svedenhag, 1985; Svedenhag, Wallin, Sundlöf, & Henrikksson, 1984). Furthermore, no changes in muscle sympathetic nerve activity at rest were observed following training (Svedenhag, 1985). However, resting plasma epinephrine concentrations in some instances were found to be slightly higher in trained subjects (Kjær et al., 1985; Svedenhag, Henriksson, & Juhlin-Dannfelt, 1984), while in other cases, no changes were reported (Lehmann et al., 1984; Winder, Hagberg, Hickson, Ehsani, & McLane, 1978). After carefully weighing the data, Svedenhag (1985) concluded that resting plasma-epinephrine concentrations remain unchanged following training.

## During Exercise, After Training

Sympathetic activity during exercise is modified following training, as revealed by plasma norepinephrine measurements. After only 1 week of intensive aerobic training, a major reduction in norepinephrine response to a given absolute workload can be seen (Winder et al., 1978). Thus, higher workload is needed to elicit similar norepinephrine response to those of pretraining values, suggesting that plasma norepinephrine dynamics during exercise are a function of the relative rather than the absolute work intensity. This is confirmed by Péronnet et al. (1981), who have shown that norepinephrine response remains constant in relation to relative workload. Similar to plasma norepinephrine concentrations, increases in plasma epinephrine levels during exercise appear to be a function of relative workload, and thus the training state; however, no consistent findings are reported in the literature (Svedenhag, 1985).

It is worth mentioning here the control mechanisms that are thought to regulate the sympathetic response to exercise (for a complete review, the reader is referred to Rowell, 1980, 1986). Experimental evidence in humans and animals suggests that in response to short-duration exercise, neurovegetative centers in the hypothalamus and the limbic system, which regulate the degree and the pattern of activation of the sympathetic system—including the adrenal medulla—are themselves under the control of information coming from the following sources: (1) motor or premotor areas (intercentral control) that initiate and control motor activity, and (2) active muscle tissues and joints (reflex control). Information originating from the motor and premotor areas in the brain first triggers an initial sympathetic response at the onset of exercise or even a few seconds before the exercise is actually started.

This feed-forward control of neurovegetative centers is only able to trigger and sustain a crude sympathetic adjustment to the exercise performed. However, reflex feedback originating from working muscles and joints provides information on the metabolic state of the muscle cells and on tensions in the connective tissue to the neurovegetative centers, and it then precisely adjusts the degree and pattern of sympathetic activation, in order that cardiovascular adjustments can match the metabolic demand of the working muscles. The reduction in sympathetic (and cardiovascular) response to a given absolute workload, following training, is believed to be mainly a direct consequence of the improvement in the ability of each muscle cell to perform work and in the ability of the cardiovascular system to supply blood flow and hence oxygen to the working muscles. Accordingly, for a given absolute workload, the amount of muscle fibers recruited and therefore the central motor command are reduced following training. Consequently, the feed-forward control mechanism from the motor and premotor centers to the neurovegetative centers, and the sympathetic response that parallels the central motor command, are reduced.

The reflex control of the neurovegetative centers is also reduced because of (a) the improvement in the ability of the cardiovascular system to supply blood and oxygen to the working muscles, and (b) the ability of each muscle cell to perform work in aerobic conditions; both of these result in less disturbance in the interstitial fluid of the muscle. On the other hand, for a given relative workload (e.g., 75% $\dot{V}O_2$ max), which obviously is also a higher absolute workload after training, two processes are similar to those observed before training for the same relative workload: (1) the central motor command and the parallel sympathetic response triggered by the feed-forward mechanism, and (2) the metabolic disturbances and the sympathetic response triggered by the reflex control mechanism. Accordingly, the sympathetic and cardiovascular responses are similar to those observed before training. It should be recognized that here we use a circular argument; the two different absolute workloads that induce the same sympathetic and the same cardiovascular response are, by definition, the same relative workload before and after training.

According to this current interpretation of the control mechanisms of the sympathetic response to exercise, there are only minor effects, if any, of exercise training on the sympathetic system per se. The key element is that exercise training does not modify the structure or the functioning of the sympathetic system, nor does it change the control mechanism that regulates its response to exercise. In other words, it is not the change in sympathetic activity that modifies work capacity, but rather, the changes in work capacity that alter the sympathetic response to a given absolute workload.

## EXERCISE TRAINING AND SYMPATHETIC RESPONSE TO PSYCHOSOCIAL STRESS

A number of studies have actually compared sympathetic response during stress to sympathetic response during exercise (Dimsdale & Moss, 1980; Fibiger & Singer, 1984; Hoch, Werle, & Weicker, 1988). The outcome of these studies point in the same direction, suggesting that sympathetic response to stress and to exercise are clearly distinct. Dimsdale and Moss (1980) observed a 2-fold increase in plasma epinephrine levels during public speaking, compared to a threefold increase in norepinephrine levels after a short-duration stepping exercise. These findings suggest that while the sympathetic nervous system is highly implicated in physical exercise of short duration, the adrenal gland is highly involved in the psychological stress response. Hoch, Werle, and Weicker (1988) provide support for this difference by revealing higher plasma epinephrine levels in a championship contest (i.e., psychological stress due to emotional strain of the high-level competition), in contrast to higher plasma norepinephrine concentrations found in a training fight in elite fencers. While the studies by Dimsdale and Moss (1980) and Hoch, Werle, and Weicker (1988) adopted a real-life stress situation, Fibiger and Singer (1984) also found higher plasma epinephrine levels in response to psychosocial stress and higher plasma norepinephrine levels in response to exercise under laboratory conditions. These observations substantiate that there is no one single sympathetic activity or sympathetic response; rather, there are a number of sympathetic responses to different stimuli or challenges. The challenge of psychosocial stress and the challenge of exercise are different, and so are the sympathetic responses to them. This, in turn, further substantiates that similarities in sympathetic response to psychosocial stress and physical exercise are only superficial.

## Sympathetic Response to Psychosocial Stress During Exercise

As outlined earlier, during both mental stress and physical exercise, there is an increase in sympathetic activity. If the two types of challenges are superimposed, an additional response, as revealed by cardiovascular indices, may be observed (Myrtek & Spital, 1986; Roth, Bachtler, & Fillingim, 1990). Thus, the magnitude of the cardiovascular response to mental stress and exercise is greater than the magnitude of the response to either challenge alone. These additional responses were observed after 3 minutes at 25 watts (Myrtek & Spital, 1986) and following 10 minutes at 50 watts (Roth et al., 1990) of light to moderate cycling exercise.

While cardiovascular (indirect) indices point toward synergistic response patterns, it is not clear whether direct sympathetic indices would confirm these results and indicate that mental challenge may elicit additional responses during exercise. This issue can be addressed only indirectly. For example, Hoch, Werle, and Weicker (1988) studied sympathetic response of top German national-level fencers in a training session (simulated competition) and during competition. Venous plasma catecholamines were assayed 1 day before the fight, 1 minute after announcement of the opponent, and immediately after the fight, in both training and championship competition. Norepinephrine levels significantly increased from rest to pre- and posttraining session and from pre- to postcompetition but were significantly lower after competition than after the training session (Figure 7.3a). Plasma epinephrine levels increased from rest to pre- and posttraining fights and from rest to pre- and postcompetition fights, as well as from pre- to postfight in both conditions (Figure 7.3b). Furthermore, epinephrine levels were significantly higher following the championship competition than after simulated (training) competition. These data elegantly demonstrate that venous plasma norepinephrine concentration is lower, while epinephrine concentration is higher in situations where emotional stress is added to physical activity performance. While no additional increases in plasma norepinephrine levels can be observed when emotional stress is encountered during exercise, a significant additional response of plasma epinephrine appears prominent. We are unaware of similar experiments performed under laboratory conditions.

Two studies have looked at personality parameters—namely, anxiety and affective states—during exercise. The first (Péronnet et al., 1986a), using male students with high and low trait anxiety, examined plasma epinephrine and norepinephrine response to mild and moderate short-duration exercise. The findings revealed no differences between high and low trait-anxiety groups in resting plasma catecholamines and during mild (40% $\dot{V}O_2$

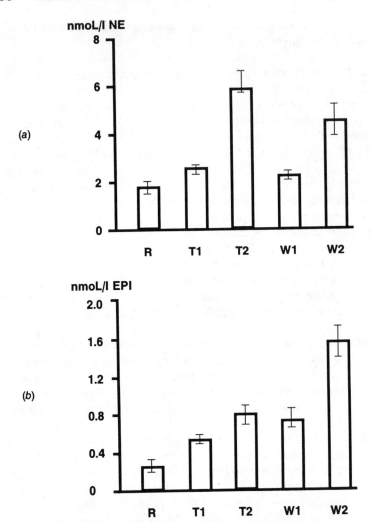

**Figure 7.3.** **(a)** Plasma norepinephrine (NE) values (mean value ± standard error of the mean) at rest ($n = 10$), during training ($n = 10$), and during competition ($n = 9$). R = resting value 1 day before the fight; T1,W1 = 1 minute after the announcement of the opponent (T = Training, W = Competition); T2,W2 = immediately after the fight. A significant increase was registered from R to T1, R to T2, T1 to T2, and W1 to W2, and a significant decrease is shown from T2 to W2 ($p < .05$).

**(b)** Plasma epinephrine (EPI) values in training and competition. A significant increase was found from R to T1, R to T2, R to W1, R to W2, T1 to T2, W1 to W2, and T2 to W2 ($p < .05$). Reprinted with permission from Hoch et al. (1988), *International Journal of Sports Medicine, 9,* Supplement (page S142, Figures 2A & 2B).

max) bicycle exercise. Plasma epinephrine levels were not different in the two groups in any situation. However, at moderate exercising levels (60% of the individual $\dot{V}O_2$ max), plasma norepinephrine levels in high trait-anxiety males were twice as high (2510 vs. 1243 pg/mL) as in low trait-anxiety subjects, while no changes were observed in heart rate (175 bpm in high trait anxiety vs. 174 in low trait anxiety). State–trait anxiety inventory data gathered immediately following the evaluations were significantly different for the two groups. Another study, by Hardy, McMurray, and Roberts (1989), evaluated psychophysiological reactivity in Type A/B male and female students during mild- (40% $\dot{V}O_2$ max), moderate- (60% $\dot{V}O_2$ max), and high-intensity (80% $\dot{V}O_2$ max) bicycle ergometer exercise. Their findings, resembling those of Péronnet et al. (1986a), revealed no differences in plasma catecholamines at mild and moderate levels of exercise but revealed greater norepinephrine response to high-intensity exercise in Type A subjects (2317 picograms [pg]/mL in Type A's vs. 1689 pg/mL in Type B's). Furthermore, as did Péronnet et al. (1986a), these authors found no difference in heart rate (i.e., 160 bpm in Type A's vs. 164 bpm in Type B's) at the workload where plasma norepinephrine distinguished the two groups. The Type A's in this study also showed greater negative affect during high-intensity cycling but more positive affect during mild and moderate intensities, in comparison to Type B's. Thus, the two studies (Hardy, McMurray, & Roberts, 1989; Péronnet et al., 1986a) that have examined stress-related personality factors point in the same direction, indicating that personality factors associated with heightened emotional states (Dembroski, MacDougall, & Shields, 1977; Manuck & Garland, 1979; Sothman, Horn, Hart, & Gustafson, 1987) are also associated with higher plasma norepinephrine levels during moderate- and high-intensity exercise levels.

## Psychosocial Stress Response Following an Acute Bout of Exercise

Sympathetic response to psychosocial stress following an acute bout of exercise has received little attention. Péronnet et al. (1989) evaluated the stress response in young trained males on two occasions: approximately 90 minutes after either a 2-hour mild to moderate (50% $\dot{V}O_2$ max) bicycle-exercise condition or a 2-hour film-watching (neutral content) condition. After the 2-hour exercise condition, subjects demonstrated significantly lower plasma epinephrine response to the Stroop color word task than after the control condition (0.21 vs. 0.41 nmol/L). However, another study, which used an identical paradigm except that the exercise duration lasted 30 minutes instead of 2 hours (Szabo et al., 1990), failed to demonstrate any differences in plasma catecholamine responses to mental arithmetic and to the Stroop color word task between control and exercise conditions. These findings point to the possibility that duration may be a critical determinant when the effects of acute exercise on sympathetic reactivity to psychosocial stress are studied.

Changes in indirect indices of sympathetic activity, including lower blood pressure, following an acute bout of exercise have been reported in both normotensive and hypertensive subjects (Bennett, Wilcox, & McDonald, 1984; Fitzgerald, 1981; Floras et al., 1989; Hannum & Kasch, 1981; Kaufman, Hughson, & Schaman, 1987; Paulev, Jordal, Kristensen, & Ladefoged, 1984; Wilcox, Bennett, Brown, & McDonald, 1982). When reactivity to psychosocial stress was examined in conjunction with exercise, neither Péronnet et al. (1989) nor Szabo et al. (1990) were able to demonstrate reduced blood-pressure response to psychosocial stress following 120-minute and 30-minute cycling tasks, respectively, in normotensive subjects. However, Rajeski, Gregg, Thompson, and Berry (1991) found diminished mean arterial pressure response to the Stroop task in trained cyclists following both light (50% $\dot{V}O_2$ max for 30 minutes) and heavy (80% $\dot{V}O_2$ max for 60 minutes) cycling exercise. The heavy exercise appeared to be more effective in reducing mean arterial pressure than the light exercise. The authors found no differences in heart rate response to the stressor across conditions.

Indeed, heart rate response to psychosocial stress appears to be unaffected by an acute bout of exercise. Fifteen minutes of bicycling at 40, 55, or 70% $\dot{V}O_2$ max did not alter heart-rate response to mental arithmetic (McGowan, Robertson, & Epstein, 1985). Similarly, cycling for 2 hours at 50% $\dot{V}O_2$ max (Péronnet et al., 1989), for 30 minutes at 60% $\dot{V}O_2$ max (Szabo et al., 1990), for 20 minutes at 60% $\dot{V}O_2$ max (Russell, Epstein, & Erickson, 1983), or for 15 minutes at 70% $\dot{V}O_2$ max (Duda, Sedlock, Melby, & Thaman, 1988) failed to modify heart-rate response to Stroop color word task and/or mental arithmetic. These data indicate that neither duration nor intensity of ergometer cycling can be related to lower heart-rate response to these types of psychosocial stressors after exercise. It is noteworthy that paralleling these negative findings, the impact of an acute bout of exercise on psychological states is also controversial (see Tuson & Sinyor, Chapter 4, this volume).

### Stress Response Following Chronic Exercise

**Summary of Cross-Sectional Studies.** A few cross-sectional studies have examined whether fitness level is associated with sympathetic reactivity to psychosocial stress. These studies have selected highly fit and relatively unfit subjects and compared their sympathetic and/or cardiovascular responses to active and/or passive coping stressors. Except for one, investigations that compared plasma epinephrine response to psychosocial stress between the two fitness groups (Table 7.4) failed to reveal any significant differences (Claytor, Cox, Howley, Lawler, & Lawler, 1988; Hull, Young, &

Ziegler, 1984; Sinyor et al., 1983; Sothman et al., 1987). The only study that reported a difference attempted to create a real-life stress situation by using rappelling (Brooke & Long, 1987). Faster recovery for plasma epinephrine levels in fit than in unfit males was found (5, 15, 30 minutes: 84, 55, 50 vs. 98, 63, 54 pg/mL), while there were no major differences in plasma norepinephrine levels (755, 604, 471 vs. 813, 520, 419 pg/mL). It should be pointed out, however, that Brooke and Long (1987) used an active stressor that was highly dependent on physical fitness level. For example, although both groups were inexperienced and not different in perceived efficacy in mastering the rappelling task, highly fit subjects may have had initially higher self-confidence in their ability to accomplish a task that strongly depended on physical ability, as compared to relatively unfit subjects. This, in turn, may have resulted in less fear associated with rappelling and lower emotional arousal in response to the stressor in highly fit versus relatively unfit subjects. Highly fit and relatively unfit people show no differences in plasma norepinephrine response to psychosocial stress (Brooke & Long, 1987; Claytor et al., 1988; Hull, Young, & Ziegler, 1984).

Plasma norepinephrine levels may be lower in fit subjects as the length of exposure to the psychosocial stress increases, however (Sothman et al., 1987). Furthermore, fit subjects may show an earlier peak plasma norepinephrine response to mental challenge than their unfit counterparts following the onset of exposure (Sinyor et al., 1983). The meaning of such findings is not clearly understood, but it may be associated with the concept of "toughness" (see Dienstbier, 1991). Finally, studies using indirect indices, mostly cardiovascular measures, also report mixed findings on fitness associated psychosocial stress response (e.g., Garber, Siconolfi, & Carleton, 1985; Hollander & Seraganian, 1984; Holmes & Roth, 1985; Light, Obrist, James, & Strogatz, 1987; Nixon, Robertson, & Epstein, 1986; Plante & Karpowitz, 1987; Shulhan, Scher, & Furedy, 1986; van Doornen & de Geus, 1989). In the case of studies that report different cardiovascular response to psychosocial stress between highly fit and relatively unfit individuals, it is not clear to what degree the differences in cardiovascular responses could be attributed to stress reactivity itself. It is possible that mere differences in the cardiovascular physiology (brought about by exercise training) between differing fitness groups may account for the differences observed in psychosocial-stress situations.

**Summary of Longitudinal Studies.**    The presumption that aerobic exercise benefits physiological response to stress has two foundations. The first is the oversimplistic similarity in sympathetic and cardiovascular response to stress and exercise, whereas the second is the dramatic improvement in cardiovascular functions brought about by aerobic training, within a relatively short period of time (Nadel, 1985). Studies examining the effects of exercise training on sympathetic response to mental challenge have usually

**TABLE 7.4  CATECHOLAMINE RESPONSE TO STRESS AS A FUNCTION OF FITNESS**

| Source | Subjects | Catecholamine measured | Type measured | Findings of stressor |
|---|---|---|---|---|
| Brooke & Long (1987) | High & low fit ♂ | Plasma (V) EPI, NE | Rappelling | EPI—positive NE—negative |
| Claytor, Cox, Howley, Lawler, & Lawler (1988) | High & low fit ♂ | Plasma (V) EPI, NE | Reaction-time tasks | EPI—negative NE—negative |
| Hull, Young, & Ziegler (1984) | High & low fit ♂ & ♀[a] | Plasma (V) EPI, NE | Passive & active, psychological & physical | EPI—negative NE—positive (on physical stress only) |
| Sinyor, Schwartz, Péronnet, Brisson, & Seraganian (1983) | High & low fit ♂ | Plasma (V) EPI, NE | Arithmetic, Stroop, & quiz | EPI—negative NE—positive |
| Sothman, Horn, Hart, & Gustafson (1987) | High & low fit ♂ | Plasma (V) EPI, NE | Stroop & anagrams | EPI—negative NE—positive |

*Note.* ♂ = males; ♀ = females; EPI = epinephrine; NE = norepinephrine; V = venous; negative = no differences between fitness groups; positive = differences between fitness groups.
[a]Employed subjects in different fitness categories.

employed a short-duration aerobic training program lasting from 7 to about 20 weeks (Cléroux, Péronnet, and de Champlain, 1985; de Geus et al., 1990; Dienstbier et al., 1987; Holmes & McGilley, 1987; Sinyor et al., 1988).

Two of these studies used indirect indices of sympathetic activity (de Geus et al., 1990; Holmes & McGilley, 1987), another two also measured plasma epinephrine and norepinephrine concentrations (Cléroux, Péronnet, & de Champlain et al., 1985; Sinyor et al., 1988), and a fifth assessed urinary catecholamine excretion in response to psychosocial stress (Dienstbier et al., 1987) before and after training. Two of these studies had no control groups (Cléroux, Péronnet, & de Champlain et al., 1985; Sinyor et al., 1988), and one of them (Cléroux, Péronnet, & de Champlain et al., 1985) used labile hypertensive subjects. Although testing an identical hypothesis—that is, the effects of aerobic training on sympathetic or cardiovascular response to psychosocial stress—a great variability emerged in the designs, as well in the findings of these studies. Inconsistencies in subject attributes, types of stressors used, sympathetic/cardiovascular measures, and training characteristics make comparison difficult.

Two of the studies found no difference in reactivity to psychosocial stress following the aerobic training program (de Geus et al., 1990; Sinyor et al., 1988). Holmes and McGilley (1987) found lower heart rate response (approximately 90 bpm vs. 102 bpm in relatively unfit subjects) to stress after training, while Cléroux, Péronnet, and de Champlain (1985) revealed lower systolic blood-pressure response (approximately 5 mm Hg) to psychosocial stress after moderate training in labile hypertensive subjects. However, Cléroux, Péronnet, and de Champlain (1985) found no differences in plasma norepinephrine and epinephrine levels after training in response to a challenging video game stressor.

In contrast, Dienstbier et al. (1987) reported increased urinary catecholamine levels in response to a passive-coping laboratory stressor after a semester-long training program. Increased urinary catecholamine excretion in response to psychosocial stress following exercise training is difficult to interpret. Dienstbier et al. (1987) suggest that training could increase "the ability to excrete catecholamines." In fact, this has been reported in response to exercise: For a given absolute workload, urinary catecholamine excretion was increased following training (Taylor, Schoeman, Esfandiary, & Russell, 1971). However, this is likely to be due to a lower reduction in renal blood flow in response to exercise following training (Taylor et al., 1971). Renal vasoconstriction due to increased sympathetic activity in response to mental stress has been reported in humans (Tidgren & Hjemdahl, 1989). The increased urinary catecholamine excretion reported by Dienstbier et al. (1987) can thus be suggestive of a *reduction* in the response of the renal sympathetic fibers following training.

Some studies have compared the influence of aerobic training on sympathetic/cardiovascular response to psychosocial stress, in relation to other forms of training and/or interventions. A general pattern of inconsistency has emerged from these experiments as well. For example, three studies showed no difference between aerobic and anaerobic training groups when their posttraining stress-response profile was assessed (Seraganian et al., 1987; Sinyor et al., 1986; Steptoe et al., 1990b). Furthermore, indirect sympathetic indices revealed no changes in response to psychosocial stress following training in any of the groups. Three other studies have reported lower cardiovascular response to stress after training in the aerobic, but not in the anaerobic group (Blumenthal et al., 1988; Blumenthal et al., 1990; Sherwood, Light, and Blumenthal, 1989). Blumenthal et al. (1990) point out that these findings might be due to aerobic-training-induced adaptation in the cardiovascular system rather than to a change in cardiovascular response to stress. Blumenthal et al. (1990) also reported a posttraining reduction in plasma epinephrine response to psychosocial stress. Holmes and Roth (1988) showed lower cardiovascular response during stress, but not during recovery, in an aerobic training group, as compared to a relaxation training group, following an 11-week experimental period. In contrast, Keller and Seraganian (1984) showed faster heart rate and electrodermal response during recovery, but not during psychosocial stress, in aerobic-training, compared to meditation-training or music-appreciation groups, after a 10-week training program.

Examination of these longitudinal studies suggests that there are no clearly identifiable changes in sympathetic response to psychosocial stress after physical exercise training as revealed by direct sympathetic indices, such as circulating catecholamines (Table 7.5). The two studies that showed lower blood-pressure response to stress after training (Cléroux, Péronnet, & de Champlain, 1985; Sherwood, Light, & Blumenthal, 1989) used labile or borderline hypertensives, indicating that changes in this population following aerobic exercise training may take place. No comparable findings using normotensive subjects have been reported. The studies that reported lower reactivity to psychosocial stress following aerobic training (Blumenthal et al., 1990; Holmes & Roth, 1988) may have found overall changes in cardiovascular parameters rather than in reactivity per se. While it may be argued that the duration of the training programs employed may have been insufficient to induce changes in sympathetic response, the changes observed with labile or borderline hypertensives invalidate this speculation.

A thoughtful analysis of the results of the longitudinal studies substantiates the fact that the mechanisms that govern sympathetic responses to physical exercise and psychosocial stress, respectively, are different. Therefore, no parallel changes in sympathetic response to stress and physical exercise can be expected. This is not to rule out the possibility that some changes in sympathetic response to psychosocial stress may occur after training, but simply to redraw attention to the fact that if changes do occur, they may not be the result of training-induced changes in sympathetic response.

**TABLE 7.5   THE EFFECTS OF EXERCISE TRAINING ON CATECHOLAMINE RESPONSE TO STRESS**

| Source | Subjects | Catecholamine measured | Type of measured | Type of training | Findings stressor |
|---|---|---|---|---|---|
| Blumenthal, Fredrikson, Kuhn, Ulmer, Walsh-Riddle, & Applebaum (1990) | 37 ♂ | Plasma (V) EPI, NE | Aerobic & anaerobic (12 weeks) | Mental arithmetic | EPI/aerobic positive NE—negative |
| Cléroux, Péronnet, & deChamplain (1985) | 8 ♂ | Plasma (V) EPI, NE | Aerobic (20 weeks) | Video game | EPI & NE—negative |
| Dienstbier, LaGuardia, Barnes, Tharp, & Schmidt (1987) (Study 1) | 35 ♂ | Urine EPI, NE | Aerobic (one semester | Passive coping (unpleasant | EPI—NE positive (increase) |
| Dienstbier, LaGuardia, Barnes, Tharp, & Schmidt (1987) (Study 2) | 42 ♂ & ♀ | Urine CAs (EPI + NE combined) | Aerobic (one semester | Passive coping (unpleasant | CAs—positive (increase) |
| Dienstbier, LaGuardia, Barnes, Tharp, & Schmidt (1987) (Study 3) | 39 ♀ | Urine CAs (EPI + NE combined) | Aerobic (one semester long) | Stroop & arithmetic | CAs—negative |
| Seraganian, Hanley, Hollander, Roskies, Smilga, Martin, Collu, & Oseasohn (1985) | 32 ♂ | Plasma (V) EPI, NE | Aerobic, anaerobic & stress management (10 weeks) | Six active coping laboratory stressors | No changes reported |
| Sinyor, Péronnet, Brisson, & Seraganian (1988) | 6 ♂ | Plasma (V) EPI, NE | Aerobic (10 weeks) | Arithmetic & Stroop | EPI & NE—negative |

*Note.* ♂ = males; ♀ = females; CAs = catecholamines; EPI = epinephrine; NE = norepinephrine; V = venous; negative = no training effects; positive = changes in catecholaminergic response to stress after training.

## CONCLUDING REMARKS

Following an extensive review of the literature, we are unable to confirm that physical exercise training results in modification of sympathetic response to psychosocial stress. Although some studies have reported lower sympathetic response to various stressors, these findings are generally inconsistent and may not be directly related to modified sympathetic response. While methodological limitations and/or experimental flaws may have contributed to the emergence of heterogeneous findings across studies, these alone could not totally mask a general trend of modified sympathetic response to psychosocial stress, if there were any.

Because sympathetic response to an absolute workload during exercise is modified after physical training, the hypothesis that sympathetic response to psychosocial stress also could be modified by exercise training has emerged. However, as discussed earlier in this chapter, the control mechanisms governing the sympathetic response to physical exercise and to psychosocial stress are different and hence changes in one cannot be directly linked to changes in the other.

One general trend emerging from empirical data that supports the existence of different sympathetic control mechanisms involved in exercise and psychosocial stress is the distinct epinephrine/norepinephrine ratio during exercise and psychosocial stress (van Doornen, de Geus, & Orlebeke, 1988). However, the difference in the sympathetic control mechanism is only one factor that argues against the simplistic analogy between sympathetic response to exercise and the response to psychosocial stress. The other argument against this analogy is that sympathetic response to physical exercise itself is not modified following exercise training. Although sympathetic response to an absolute workload is different following exercise training, the sympathetic response to a relative workload remains unchanged (Péronnet et al., 1981). The observed change in sympathetic response to an absolute workload during exercise following training can be attributed to changes in work capacity rather than to changes in sympathetic control mechanisms.

Consequently, the assumption that sympathetic response to exercise is changed following training is somewhat erroneous because what is changed indeed is the ability of the muscle to perform work and the ability of the cardiovascular system to supply blood and oxygen to the working muscle. This phenomenon results in different signals through the feedforward and feedback mechanisms' control of the sympathetic centers, and thus, sympathetic response appears to be different following exercise training. Taken together, these facts—as well as the lack of clear empirical evidence—suggest that no direct linkage between sympathetic response to physical exercise training and response to psychosocial stress can be established.

Assessing sympathetic response in a stress situation by measuring plasma catecholamines reveals little or no information about the origin, action, and destination of the response. Higher catecholamine levels in response to a particular situation do not imply more than seeing a higher heart-rate response to the same situation. Therefore, it is unclear whether increases or decreases can be paralleled with deterioration or improvement of sympathetic response. It is often believed that lower sympathetic response represents some sort of improvement. However, we should ask the question whether lower catecholamine levels or lower heart rates are necessarily mirroring a better coping mechanism with stress? The application of a treatment (such as an exercise training program) is often accompanied by the expectancy that lower physiological values in response to a particular stressor will be observed following the intervention. If such an observation becomes evident, then there is indeed a general tendency to interpret the findings as a sign of improvement. However, it is also suggested that increased catecholamine secretion may be associated with better performance and emotional stability (Dienstbier, 1991). Thus, it may be inappropriate to interpret changes in sympathetic indices before a deeper understanding of their role within an overall mechanism is achieved. At present, we believe that this mechanism is not clearly known and that it is unclear whether lower versus higher sympathetic responses to psychosocial stressors are more "desirable" for better coping.

## REFERENCES

Allen, M. T., & Crowell, M. D. (1989). Patterns of autonomic response during laboratory stressors. *Psychophysiology, 26,* 603–614.

Anderson, E. A., Wallin, B. G., & Mark, A. L. (1987). Dissociation of sympathetic nerve activity in arm and leg muscle during mental stress. *Hypertension Dallas 9* (Suppl. 3), 114–119.

Austin, F. H., Gallagher, T. J., Brictson, C. A., Polis, B. D., Furry, D. E., & Lewis, C. E. (1967). Aeromedical monitoring of naval aviators during aircraft combat operation. *Aerospace Medicine, 38,* 593–596.

Bandura, A., Taylor, C. B., Williams, S. L., Mefford, I. N., & Barchas, J. D. (1985). Catecholamine secretion as a function of perceived coping self-efficacy. *Journal of Consulting and Clinical Psychology, 53,* 406–414.

Bassett, J. R., Marshall, P. M., & Spillane, R. (1987). The physiological measurement of acute stress (public speaking) in bank employees. *International Journal of Psychophysiology, 5,* 265–273.

Baum, A., Fleming, R., & Reddy, D. M. (1986). Unemployment stress: Loss of control, reactance and learned helplessness. *Social Science and Medicine, 22,* 509–516.

Bennett, T., Wilcox, R. G., & McDonald, I. A. (1984). Post-exercise reduction of blood pressure in hypertensive men is not due to acute impairment of baroreflex function. *Clinical Science, 67,* 97–103.

Blumenthal, J. A., Emery, C. F., Walsh, M. A., Cox, D. R., Kuhn, C. M., Williams, R. B., & Williams, R. S. (1988). Exercise training in healthy type A middle-aged men: Effects on behavioral and cardiovascular responses. *Psychosomatic Medicine, 50,* 418–433.

Blumenthal, J. A., Fredrikson, M., Kuhn, C. M., Ulmer, R. L., Walsh-Riddle, M., & Appelbaum, M. (1990). Aerobic exercise reduces levels of cardiovascular and sympathoadrenal responses to mental stress in subjects without prior evidence of myocardial ischemia. *American Journal of Cardiology, 65,* 93–98.

Brooke, S. T., & Long, B. C. (1987). Efficiency of coping with a real-life stressor: A multimodal comparison of aerobic fitness. *Psychophysiology, 24,* 173–180.

Brown, T. G, Szabo, A., & Seraganian, P. (1988). Physical versus psychological determinants of heart rate reactivity to mental arithmetic. *Psychophysiology, 25,* 532–537.

Burn, J. H. (1975). *The autonomic nervous system* (5th ed.). Oxford: Blackwell Scientific Publications.

Cannon, W. B., & de la Paz, D. (1911). Emotional stimulation of adrenal secretion. *American Journal of Physiology, 27,* 64–70.

Cantor, J. R., Zillman, D., & Day, K. D. (1978). Relationship between cardiorespiratory fitness and physiological responses to films. *Perceptual and Motor Skills, 46,* 1123–1130.

Claytor, R. P., Cox, R. H., Howley, E. T., Lawler, K. A., & Lawler, J. A. (1988). Aerobic power and cardiovascular response to stress. *Journal of Applied Physiology, 65,* 1416–1423.

Cléroux, J., Péronnet, F., & de Champlain, J. (1985). Sympathetic indices during psychological and physical stimuli before and after training. *Physiology & Behavior, 35,* 271–275.

de Geus, E. J. C., van Doornen, L. J. P., de Visser, D. C., & Orlebeke, J. F. (1990). Existing and training induced differences in aerobic fitness: Their relationship to physiological response patterns during different types of stress. *Psychophysiology, 27,* 457–478.

Delius, W., Hagbarth, K. E., Hongell, A., & Wallin, B. G. (1972). Manoeuvres affecting sympathetic outflow in human muscle nerves. *Acta Physiologica Scandinavica, 84,* 82–94.

Dembroski, T. M., MacDougall, J. M., & Shields, J. L. (1977). Physiologic reactions to social challenge in persons evidencing the type A coronary-prone behavior pattern. *Journal of Human Stress, 3,* 2–10.

Dienstbier, R. A. (1991). Behavioral correlates of sympathoadrenal reactivity: The toughness model. *Medicine and Science in Sports and Exercise, 23,* 846–852.

Dienstbier, R. A., LaGuardia, R. L., Barnes, M., Tharp, G., & Schmidt, R. (1987). Catecholamine training effects from exercise programs: A bridge to exercise-temperament relationships. *Motivation and Emotion, 11,* 297–318.

Dimsdale, J. E., & Moss, J. (1980). Plasma catecholamines in stress and exercise. *Journal of American Medical Association (JAMA), 25,* 340–342.

Dimsdale, J. E., & Ziegler, M. G. (1991). What do plasma and urinary measures of catecholamines tell us about human response to stressors? *Circulation, 83*(Suppl. 2), 36–42.

Duda, J. L., Sedlock, D. A., Melby, C. L., & Thaman, C. (1988). The effects of physical activity level and acute exercise on heart rate and subjective response to a psychological stressor. *International Journal of Sport Psychology, 19,* 119–133.

Fenz, W. D., & Jones, G. B. (1974). Cardiac conditioning in a reaction time task and heart rate control during real life stress. *Journal of Psychosomatic Research, 18,* 199–203.

Fibiger, W., & Singer, G. (1984). Physiological changes during physical and psychological stress. *Australian Journal of Psychology, 36,* 317–326.

Fitzgerald, W. (1981). Labile hypertension and jogging: New diagnostic tool or spurious discovery? *British Medical Journal, 282,* 542–544.

Fleg, J. L., Tzankoff, S. P., & Lakatta, E. G. (1985). Age-related augmentation of plasma catecholamines during dynamic exercise in healthy males. *Journal of Applied Physiology, 59,* 1033–1039.

Floras, J. S., Sinkey, C. A., Aylward, P. E., Seals, D. R., Thoren, P. N., & Mark, A. L. (1989). Postexercise hypotension and sympathoinhibition in borderline hypertensive men. *Hypertension, 14,* 28–35.

Folkow, B., & Neil, E. (1971). *Circulation.* New York: Oxford University Press.

Frankenhaeuser, M. (1975). Experimental approaches to the study of catecholamines and emotion. In L. Levi (Ed.), *Emotions: Their parameters and measurement* (pp. 209–234). New York: Raven Press.

Frankenhaeuser, M., Mellis, I., Rissler, A., Bjorkvall, C., & Patkai, P. (1968). Catecholamine excretion as related to cognitive and emotional reaction patterns. *Psychosomatic Medicine, 30,* 109–120.

Freyschuss, U., Fagius, J., Wallin, B. G., Bohlin, G., Perski, A., & Hjemdahl, P. (1990). Cardiovascular and sympathoadrenal responses to mental stress: A study of sensory intake and rejection reactions. *Acta Physiologica Scandinavica, 139,* 173–183.

Freyschuss, U., Hjemdahl, P., Juhlin-Dannfelt, A., & Linde, B. (1988). Cardiovascular and sympathoadrenal responses to mental stress: Influence of ß-blockade. *American Journal of Physiology, 255,* H1443–H1451.

Galbo, H. (1983). *Hormonal and metabolic adaptation to exercise.* Stuttgart, Germany: Georg Thieme Verlag.

Galbo, H. (1986). Autonomic neuroendocrine responses to exercise. *Scandinavian Journal of Sports Sciences, 8,* 3–17.

Garber, C. E., Siconolfi, S. F., & Carleton, R. A. (1985). Circulatory reactivity to mental stress in trained and untrained women. *Medicine and Science in Sports and Exercise, 17,* 281.

Gasic, S., Grünberger, J., Korn, A., Oberhummer, I., & Zapatoczky, H. G. (1985). Biochemical, physical and psychological findings in patients suffering from cardiac neurosis. *Neuropsychobiology, 13,* 12–16.

Glass, D. C. (1983). Behavioral, cardiovascular and neuroendocrine responses to psychological stressors. *International Review of Applied Psychology, 32,* 137–151.

Goldstein, D. S. (1987). Stress-induced activation of the sympathetic nervous system. *Baillière's Clinical Endocrinology and Metabolism, 1,* 253–277.

Goldstein, D. S., Eisenhofer, G., Sax, F. L., Keiser, H. R., & Kopin, I. J. (1987). Plasma norepinephrine pharmacokinetics during mental challenge. *Psychosomatic Medicine, 49,* 591–605.

Guyton, A. C. (1986). The autonomic nervous system. In *Textbook of medical physiology* (7th ed.). Philadelphia: Saunders.

Hagberg, J. M., Seals, D. R., Yerg, J. E., Gavin, J., Gingerich, R., Premachandra, B., & Holloszy, J. O. (1988). Metabolic responses to exercise in young and older athletes and sedentary men. *Journal of Applied Physiology, 65,* 900–908.

Hannum, S. M., & Kasch, F. W. (1981). Acute postexercise blood pressure response of hypertensive and normotensive men. *Scandinavian Journal of Sports Sciences, 3,* 11–15.

Hardy, C. J., McMurray, R. G., & Roberts, S. (1989). A/B types and psychophysiological responses to exercise stress. *Journal of Sport and Exercise Psychology, 11,* 141–151.

Hjemdahl, P., Freyschuss, U., Juhlin-Dannfelt, A., & Linde, B. (1984). Differentiated sympathetic activation during mental stress evoked by the Stroop test. *Acta Physiologica Scandinavica, 527*(Suppl.), 25–29.

Hoch, F., Werle, E., & Weicker, H. (1988). Sympathoadrenergic regulation in elite fencers in training and competition. *International Journal of Sports Medicine, 9,* 141–145.

Hoeldtke, R. D., Cilmi, K. M., Reichard, G. A., Jr., Boden, G., & Owen, O. E. (1983). Assessment of norepinephrine secretion and production. *Journal of Laboratory and Clinical Medicine, 101,* 772–782.

Hollander, B. J., & Seraganian, P. (1984). Aerobic fitness and psychophysiological reactivity. *Canadian Journal of Behavioral Sciences, 16,* 525–529.

Holmes, D. S., & McGilley, B. M. (1987). Influence of a brief aerobic training program on heart rate and subjective response to a psychologic stressor. *Psychosomatic Medicine, 49,* 366–374.

Holmes, D. S., & Roth, D. L. (1985). Association of aerobic fitness with pulse rate and subjective responses to psychological stress. *Psychophysiology, 22,* 525–529.

Holmes, D. S., & Roth, D. L. (1988). Effects of aerobic training and relaxation training on cardiovascular activity during psychological stress. *Journal of Psychosomatic Research, 32,* 469–474.

Hull, E. M., Young, S. H., & Ziegler, M. G. (1984). Aerobic fitness affects cardiovascular and catecholamine responses to stressors. *Psychophysiology, 21,* 353–360.

Johansson, G., Collins, A., & Collins, V. P. (1983). Male and female psychoneuroendocrine response to examination stress: A case report. *Motivation and Emotion, 7,* 1–9.

Kaufman, F. L., Hughson, R. L., & Schaman, J. P. (1987). Effect of exercise on recovery blood pressure in normotensive and hypertensive subjects. *Medicine and Science in Sports and Exercise, 19,* 17–20.

Keller, S., & Seraganian, P. (1984). Physical fitness level and autonomic reactivity to psychosocial stress. *Journal of Psychosomatic Research, 28,* 279–287.

Kjær, M. (1989). Epinephrine and some other hormonal responses to exercise in man: With special reference to physical training. *International Journal of Sports Medicine, 10,* 2–15.

Kjær, M., Christensen, N. J., Sonne, B., Richter, E. A., Galbo, H. (1985). Effect of exercise on epinephrine turnover in trained and untrained male subjects. *Journal of Applied Physiology, 59,* 1061–1067.

Krahenbuhl, G. S., Constable, S. H., Darst, P. W., Marett, J. R., Reid, G. B., & Reuther, L. C. (1980). Catecholamine excretion in A-10 pilots. *Aviation, Space and Environmental Medicine, 51,* 661–664.

Krahenbuhl, G. S., Harris, J., Malchow, R. D., & Stern, J. R. (1985). Biogenic amine/metabolite response during in-flight emergencies. *Aviation, Space, and Environmental Medicine, 56,* 576–580.

Krahenbuhl, G. S., Marett, J. R., & King, N. W. (1977). Catecholamine excretion in T-37 flight training. *Aviation, Space and Environmental Medicine, 48,* 405–408.

Krahenbuhl, G. S., Marett, J. R., & Reid, G. B. (1978). Task-specific simulator pretraining and in-flight stress of student pilots. *Aviation, Space and Environmental Medicine, 49,* 1107–1110.

LeBlanc, J., Côté, J., Jobin, M., & Labrie, A. (1979). Plasma catecholamines and cardiovascular responses to cold and mental activity. *Journal of Applied Physiology, 47,* 1207–1211.

Lehmann, M., Berg, A., & Keul, J. (1986). Sex-related differences in free plasma catecholamines in individuals of similar performance ability during graded ergometric exercise. *European Journal of Applied Physiology, 55,* 54–58.

Lehmann, M., Dickhuth, H. H., Schmid, P., Porzig, H., & Keul, J. (1984). Plasma catecholamines, ß-adrenergic receptors, and isoproterenol sensitivity in endurance trained and non-endurance trained volunteers. *European Journal of Applied Physiology, 52,* 362–369.

Lehmann, M., & Keul, J. (1986). Age-associated changes of exercise-induced plasma catecholamine responses. *European Journal of Applied Physiology, 55,* 302–306.

Levi, L. (1965). The urinary output of adrenalin and noradrenalin during pleasant and unpleasant emotional states. *Psychosomatic Medicine, 27,* 80–86.

Light, K. C., Obrist, P. A., James, S. A., & Strogatz, D. S. (1987). Cardiovascular responses to stress: II. Relationships to aerobic exercise patterns. *Psychophysiology, 24,* 79–86.

Manuck, S. B., & Garland, F. N. (1979). Coronary-prone behavior pattern, task incentive and cardiovascular response. *Psychophysiology, 16,* 136–147.

Matsukawa, T., Gotoh, E., Uneda, S., Miyajima, E., Shionoiri, H., Tochikubo, O., & Ishii, M. (1991). Augmented sympathetic nerve activity in response to stressors in young borderline hypertensive men. *Acta Physiologica Scandinavica, 141,* 157–165.

Mazzeo, R. S., & Grantham, P. A. (1989). Sympathetic responses to exercise in various tissues with advancing age. *Journal of Applied Physiology, 66,* 1506–1508.

McGowan, C. R., Robertson, R. J., & Epstein, L. H. (1985). The effect of bicycle ergometer exercise at varying intensities on the heart rate, EMG, and mood state responses to a mental arithmetic stressor. *Research Quarterly for Exercise and Sport, 56,* 131–137.

Morell, M. A. (1989). Psychophysiologic stress responsivity in type A and B female college students and community women. *Psychophysiology, 26,* 359–368.

Myrtek, M., & Spital, S. (1986). Psychophysiological response patterns to single, double and triple stressors. *Psychophysiology, 23,* 663–671.

Nadel, R. E. (1985). Physiological adaptations to aerobic training. *American Scientist*, 73, 334–343.

Nixon, P. A., Robertson, R. J., & Epstein, L. H. (1986). Effect of aerobic fitness level and parental history of hypertension on cardiovascular reactivity to psychological stress. *Medicine and Science in Sports and Exercise*, 18, S18(Abs).

Obrist, P. A., Gaebelein, C. J., Teller, E. S., Langer, A. W., Grignolo, A., Light, K. C., & McCubbin, J. A. (1978). The relationship among heart rate, carotid dP/dt, and blood pressure in humans as a function of the type of stress. *Psychophysiology*, 15, 102–115.

Paulev, P. E., Jordal, R., Kristensen, O., Ladefoged, J. (1984). Therapeutic effect of exercise on hypertension. *European Journal of Applied Physiology*, 53, 180–185.

Péronnet, F., Béliveau, L., Boudreau, G., Trudeau, F., Brisson, G., & Nadeau, R. (1988). Regional plasma catecholamine removal at rest and exercise in dogs. *American Journal of Physiology*, 254, R663–R672.

Péronnet, F., Blier, P., Brisson, G., Diamond, P., Ledoux, M., & Volle, M. (1986a). Plasma catecholamines at rest and exercise in subjects with high- and low-trait anxiety. *Psychosomatic Medicine*, 48, 52–58.

Péronnet, F., Blier, P., Brisson, G., Diamond, P., Ledoux, M., & Volle, M. (1986b). Reproducibility of plasma catecholamine concentrations at rest and during exercise in man. *European Journal of Applied Physiology*, 54, 555–558.

Péronnet, F., Cléroux, J., Perrault, H., Cousineau, D., de Champlain, J., & Nadeau, R. (1981). Plasma norepinephrine response to exercise before and after training in humans. *Journal of Applied Physiology*, 51, 812–815.

Péronnet, F., Massicotte, D., Paquet, J. E., Brisson, G., & de Champlain, J. (1989). Blood pressure and plasma catecholamine responses to various challenges during exercise-recovery in man. *European Journal of Applied Physiology*, 58, 551–555.

Péronnet, F., Nadeau, R., de Champlain, J., & Chartrand, C. (1982). Plasma catecholamines, heart rate and cardiac sympathetic activity in exercising dogs. *Medicine and Science in Sports and Exercise*, 14, 281–285.

Pitman, R. K., Orr, S. P., Forgue, D. F., Altman, B., & de Jong, J. B. (1990). Psychophysiologic responses to combat imagery of Vietnam veterans with post-traumatic stress disorder versus other anxiety disorders. *Journal of Abnormal Psychology*, 99, 49–54.

Plante, T. G., & Karpowitz, D. (1987). The influence of aerobic exercise on physiological stress responsivity. *Psychophysiology*, 24, 670–677.

Rajeski, W. J., Gregg, E., Thompson, A., & Berry, M. J. (1991). The effects of varying doses of acute aerobic exercise on psychophysiological stress responses in highly trained cyclists. *Journal of Sport and Exercise Psychology*, 13, 188–199.

Raven, J. C. (1965). *Advanced progressive matrices: Plan and use of the scale*. London: Lewis.

Roman, J. H., Older, H., & Jones, W. L. (1967). Flight research program: VII. Medical monitoring of Navy carrier pilots in combat. *Aerospace Medicine*, 38, 133–139.

Roth, D. L., Bachtler, S. D., & Fillingim, R. B. (1990). Acute emotional and cardiovascular effects of stressful mental work during aerobic exercise. *Psychophysiology*, 27, 694–701.

Rowell, L. B. (1980). What signals govern the cardiovascular responses to exercise? *Medicine and Science in Sports and Exercise, 12,* 307–315.

Rowell, L. B. (1986). *Human circulation regulation during physical stress* (pp. 287–327). New York: Oxford University Press.

Russell, P., Epstein, L., & Erickson, K. (1983). Effects of acute exercise and cigarette smoking on autonomic and neuromuscular responses to a cognitive stressor. *Psychological Reports, 53,* 199–206.

Seals, D. R., Victor, R. G., & Mark, A. L. (1988). Plasma norepinephrine and muscle sympathetic discharge during rhythmic exercise in humans. *Journal of Applied Physiology, 65,* 940–944.

Seraganian, P., Hanley, J. A., Hollander, B. J., Roskies, E., Smilga, C., Martin, N. D., Collu, R., & Oseasohn, R. (1985). Exaggerated psychophysiological reactivity: Issues in quantification and reliability. *Journal of Psychosomatic Research, 29,* 393–405.

Seraganian, P., Roskies, E., Hanley, J. A., Oseasohn, R., & Collu, R. (1987). Failure to alter psychophysiological reactivity in type A men with physical exercise or stress management programs. *Health Psychology, 1,* 195–213.

Sherwood, A., Allen, M. T., Obrist, P. A., & Langer, A. W. (1986). Evaluation of beta-adrenergic influences on cardiovascular and metabolic adjustments to physical and psychological stress. *Psychophysiology, 23,* 89–104.

Sherwood, A., Light, K. C., & Blumenthal, J. A. (1989). Effects of aerobic exercise training on hemodynamic responses during psychosocial stress in normotensive and borderline hypertensive type A men: A preliminary report. *Psychosomatic Medicine, 51,* 123–136.

Shulhan, D., Scher, H., & Furedy, J. F. (1986). Phasic cardiac reactivity to psychological stress as a function of aerobic fitness level. *Psychophysiology, 23,* 562–566.

Sinyor, D., Golden, M., Steinert, Y., & Seraganian, P. (1986). Experimental manipulation of aerobic fitness and the response to psychosocial stress: Heartrate and self-report measures. *Psychosomatic Medicine, 48,* 324–337.

Sinyor, D., Péronnet, F., Brisson, G., & Seraganian, P. (1988). Failure to alter sympathoadrenal response to psychosocial stress following aerobic training. *Physiology & Behavior, 42,* 293–296.

Sinyor, D., Schwartz, S. G., Péronnet, F., Brisson, G., & Seraganian, P. (1983). Aerobic fitness level and reactivity to stress: Physiological, biochemical and subjective measures. *Psychosomatic Medicine, 45,* 205–217.

Sothman, M. S., Horn, T. S., Hart, B. A., & Gustafson, A. B. (1987). Comparison of discrete cardiovascular fitness groups on plasma catecholamine and selected behavioral responses to psychological stress. *Psychophysiology, 24,* 47–54.

Steptoe, A., Moses, J., & Edwards, S. (1990a). Age-related differences in cardiovascular reactivity to mental stress tests in women. *Health Psychology, 9,* 18–34.

Steptoe, A., Moses, J., Mathews, A., & Edwards, S. (1990b). Aerobic fitness, physical activity, and psychophysiological reactions to mental tasks. *Psychophysiology, 27,* 264–274.

Stoney, C. M., Matthews, K. A., McDonald, R. H., & Johnson, C. A. (1988). Sex differences in lipid, lipoprotein, cardiovascular and neuroendocrine responses to acute stress. *Psychophysiology, 25,* 645–656.

Stroop, J. R. (1935). Studies in interference in serial verbal reactions. *Journal of Experimental Psychology, 18,* 643–662.

Sutton, J. R., Jurkowski, J. E., Keane, P., Walker, W. H. C., Jones, N. L., & Toews, C. J. (1980). Plasma catecholamine, insulin, glucose and lactate responses to exercise in relation to the menstrual cycle. *Medicine and Science in Sports and Exercise, 12,* 83–84.

Svedenhag, J. (1985). The sympatho-adrenal system in physical conditioning. *Acta Physiologica Scandinavica, 125, Supplement, 543,* 1–74.

Svedenhag, J., Henriksson, J., & Juhlin-Dannfelt, A. (1984). Beta-adrenergic blockade and training in human subjects: Effects on muscle metabolic capacity. *American Journal of Physiology, 247,* E305–E311.

Svedenhag, J., Wallin, B. J., Sundlöf, G., & Henriksson, J. (1984). Skeletal muscle sympathetic activity at rest in trained and untrained subjects. *Acta Physiologica Scandinavica, 120,* 499–504.

Szabo, A., & Gauvin, L. (1992). Reactivity to written mental arithmetic: Effects of exercise lay-off and habituation. *Physiology & Behavior, 51*(3), 501–506.

Szabo, A., Seraganian, P., Péronnet, F., Boudreau, G., Côté, L., Brisson, G., & de Champlain, J. (1990). Reactivity to mental stress following physical exercise. *Psychosomatic Medicine, 52,* 230.

Taggart, P., & Carruthers, M. (1971). Endogenous hyperlipidaemia induced by emotional stress of racing driving. *Lancet, 1,* 363–366.

Taggart, P., Carruthers, M., & Somerville, W. (1973). Electrocardiogram, plasma catecholamines and lipids, and their modification by oxprenolol when speaking before an audience. *Lancet, 2,* 341–346.

Taggart, P., Hedworth-Whitty, R., Carruthers, M., & Gordon, P. D. (1976). Observations on electrocardiogram and plasma catecholamines during dental procedures: The forgotten vagus. *British Medical Journal, 2,* 787–789.

Taylor, A. W., Schoeman, J. H., Esfandiary, A. R., & Russell, J. C. (1971). Effect of exercise on urinary catecholamine excretion in active and sedentary subjects. *Reviews in Canadian Biology, 30,* 97–105.

Tidgren, B., & Hjemdahl, P. (1989). Renal responses to mental stress and epinephrine in humans. *American Journal of Physiology, 257,* F682–F689.

Tischenkel, N. J., Saab, P. G., Schneiderman, N., Neleson, R. A., Pasin, R. D., Goldstein, D. A., Spitzer, S. B., Woo-Ming, R., & Weidler, D. J. (1989). Cardiovascular and neurohumoral responses to behavioral challenge as a function of race and sex. *Health Psychology, 8,* 503–524.

Turner, J. R., Hewitt, J. K., Morgan, R. K., Sims, J., Carroll, D., & Kelly, K. A. (1986). Graded mental arithmetic as an active psychological challenge. *International Journal of Psychophysiology, 3,* 307–309.

van Doornen, L. J. P., & de Geus, E. J. C. (1989). Aerobic fitness and the cardiovascular response to stress. *Psychophysiology, 26,* 17–28.

van Doornen, L. J. P., de Geus, E. J. C., & Orlebeke, J. F. (1988). Aerobic fitness and the physiological stress response: A critical evaluation. *Social Science and Medicine, 26,* 303–307.

Vendsalu, A. (1960). Studies on adrenaline and noradrenaline in human plasma. *Acta Physiologica Scandinavica, 49*(Suppl. 173), 1–123.

Victor, R. G., Leimbach, W. N., Jr., Seals, D. R., Wallin, B. G., & Mark, A. L. (1987). Effects of the cold pressor test on muscle sympathetic nerve activity in humans. *Hypertension Dallas, 9*, 429–436.

Ward, M. M., Mefford, I. N., Parker, S. D., Chesney, M. A., Taylor, C. B., Keegan, D. L., & Barchas, J. D. (1983). Epinephrine and norepinephrine responses in continuously collected human plasma to a series of stressors. *Psychosomatic Medicine, 45,* 471–486.

Watson, R. D. S., Hamilton, C. A., Jones, D. H., Reid, J. L., Stallard, T. J., & Littler, W. A. (1980). Sequential changes in plasma noradrenaline during bicycle exercise. *Clinical Science, 58,* 37–43.

Wilcox, R. G., Bennett, T., Brown, A. M., & McDonald, I. A. (1982). Is exercise good for high blood pressure? *British Medical Journal, 285,* 767–769.

Winder, W. W., Hagberg, J. M., Hickson, R. C., Ehsani, A. A., & McLane, J. A. (1978). Time course of sympathoadrenal adaptation to endurance exercise training in man. *Journal of Applied Physiology, 45,* 370–374.

# 8

# Experimental Versus Observational Research Methodologies

**JOHN L. JAMIESON AND KAREN R. FLOOD**

As applied to the study of exercise, the terms *experimental* and *observational* refer to the distinction between *training studies*, in which exercise is experimentally manipulated, and the study of existing exercise or fitness levels. The effects of exercise can be studied from either perspective, and this distinction is of central importance when comparing studies. The experimental method allows for a high level of control for competing explanations, thus permitting stronger conclusions about causal relationships, and is generally viewed as a superior methodology (Campbell & Stanley, 1963). However, for the study of exercise, there are several specific concerns about the experimental approach, which are described here; limitations of the observational approach also are discussed, as well as recommendations for future research directions. This chapter focuses on general design issues rather than on specific methodological concerns. However, methodological considerations relevant to a topic of particular interest to the authors of this chapter—namely, the study of physiological recovery from stress—are presented in a final section of this chapter.

Exercise psychology has been primarily guided by the question of whether exercise has psychological benefits for the individual. Investigations have generally focused on possible effects of exercise on well-being (Morgan & Goldston, 1987; Norris, Carroll, & Cochrane, 1990), and on other psychological states, such as anxiety (Long, 1985) and depression (Roth & Holmes, 1987). Research has also looked at reduced physiological response to stress (Crews & Landers, 1987) and faster recovery from stress (Cox, Evans, & Jamieson, 1979). While the question of whether exercise provides benefits (and the nature of such benefits) is of obvious importance, not enough research attention has been directed at a second, more fundamental question: What component of exercise or underlying process is responsible for any observed effects? In the study of exercise, this second question is of particular importance because of the generally assumed role of aerobic fitness level in mediating the effects of exercise. In general, research design benefits from attention to this second issue, and from reliance on explicit theoretical models of the processes that underlie or mediate any psychological benefits of exercise (Darlington, 1990; Kerlinger, 1986).

An issue central to research into the psychological effects of exercise is the role that aerobic fitness plays as a mediator or underlying cause. The focus of most exercise programs is to raise levels of physical fitness. Thus, research into the effects of exercise is very much intertwined with research into the effects of fitness. Fitness is operationalized in the literature in many ways. The most widely used index of fitness is $\dot{V}O_2$ max, a measure of the individual's ability to utilize oxygen (Astrand & Rodahl, 1986; Williams & Eston, 1989). This measure of aerobic fitness is the "gold standard"—the accepted index of the physiological benefits of exercise. However, it does not follow that this same index will optimally assess the effects of exercise that underlie either the psychological or the health benefits of exercise. In addition to changes in fitness level, exercise may produce a variety of other changes in the individual. These include improved physical competence (see Sonstroem & Morgan, 1988), increased self-confidence from being successful at adhering to the exercise program, and so on. These other consequences of exercise may underlie at least some of the psychological benefits of exercise. Also, it is possible that different types of exercise may maximally affect different psychological processes, and these effects of exercise may not all be mediated by the same mechanisms. Research to date has not directed sufficient attention toward evaluating these possible causal relationships.

## EXPERIMENTAL APPROACHES

An experimental design involves randomly assigning subjects to treatment conditions and then controlling extraneous variables that might otherwise either confound the group differences or contribute excessive variability (Kerlinger, 1986). In the experimental study of exercise, one group would undertake an exercise training program, while a control group would engage in an alternative activity. The experiment has one major advantage: control through randomization. Random assignment of subjects results in the groups being equated on all possible variables present at the time of assignment. If the remainder of the experiment is conducted properly, any group differences appearing at a later time can then be attributed to the exercise manipulation (i.e., the conclusion drawn that exercise caused the changes).

### Issues in Experimental Design

Two important decisions involved in an experiment are made in the design of the training condition and the design of the control condition. In selecting a training condition, assumptions must be made that the type, intensity, and duration of training are sufficient to modify some underlying process, such as fitness level. The experiment should include a measure of fitness change, as a means of checking the manipulation of the independent variable. However, if a different mediating process was hypothesized, this would affect both the selection of the training condition and the measures included as manipulation checks, in order to demonstrate that the hypothesized mediating process was modified by the training.

A second issue related to the design of the training condition is the nature of the relationship between exercise type or intensity and the psychological benefits of exercise. It is not established that all psychological benefits are maximally obtained from aerobic exercise, as opposed to anaerobic exercise or even less physically demanding activities, such as walking or gardening. It is also not clear whether psychological benefits continue to increase with ever-higher levels of exercise. There is some evidence suggesting that psychological benefits may be maximal at intermediate levels of exercise (Moses, Steptoe, Mathews, & Edwards, 1989; Powell, 1975). However, a caution should be raised about the conclusions from the Moses et al. paper. Their moderate-exercise group included subjects who had previously served as a waiting-list control group, and thus the design is confounded. The higher level of psychological benefit in their moderate exercise condition may in some way have been caused by this extra delay (anticipation?), which the other groups did not experience. Yet, there is also evidence that, at least for some athletes, high levels of exercise are associated with negative affect (Crossman, Jamieson, & Henderson, 1987; Steptoe & Cox, 1988). The issue of exercise type and intensity is of considerable importance because the exercise level selected for the treatment condition should reflect the optimal level, to yield benefits (Williams & Eston, 1989). Alternatively, a better design would include a variety of exercise levels, to examine the dose–response relationship.

The choice of a control condition in an experiment must address the issue of what underlying process is being controlled for by the control group. A control group should be treated identically to the experimental group except for the independent variable of interest. It is widely recognized that an experiment will be more valuable to the extent that the control and the experimental conditions are similar, other than for the independent variable (Campbell & Stanley, 1962; Cook & Campbell, 1979). For example, a waiting-list control group is unsatisfactory because it differs in so many ways from the training group (less attention is received by the subjects, etc.) and thereby leaves open many alternative explanations for any group differences. Yet, an exercise training program is such a complex enterprise that there are many aspects that the experimenter might want to incorporate into the control-group condition. In order to select which aspects to control, it is important to have a model of which aspect of training is hypothesized to underlie the effects of exercise. For example, if fitness is the postulated underlying mechanism, then a control condition that involves some exercise (e.g., anaerobic exercise) but that does not modify fitness levels might be the optimal choice. Such a control group receives an experience that is very similar to the experience received by the experimental group, leaving fitness change as the primary possible explanation for any observed change. On the other hand, if a different underlying process was assumed, then a different control-group condition might be required (Rodin & Plante, 1989).

## Factors Affecting Experimental Validity

If an experiment is well designed and well conducted, it should yield clear conclusions about the effect of the independent variable. However, a variety of factors may threaten the validity of an experiment (Campbell & Stanley, 1963; Cook & Campbell, 1979). For the study of exercise, three threats are particularly serious: attrition, which threatens internal validity; expectation effects, which threaten construct validity; and the use of volunteers, which affects external validity. These three problems are discussed next and are followed by a consideration of their impact on two particular types of experiment: clinical trials and the study of the acute effects of exercise.

**Attrition.**    Dropouts occur more frequently in the exercise group. Dropouts are not random, being more likely in those who initially were more unfit, more obese, heavier smokers, from lower socioeconomic levels, and having less-positive psychological profiles (Dishman, 1988). Subject attrition negates the equivalence created by the initial random assignment. This problem should not be ignored because the attrition creates a serious confounding difference between the two samples. Later differences may reflect the different types of subjects remaining in the two groups, rather than the effect of training. Whenever any attrition occurs, the experiment loses the advantage created by random assignment, and routine inferences about causality are not appropriate.

An interesting reverse side to the attrition issue should also be considered. Conventional exercise programs, such as those offered at community centers, and so forth, normally experience 50% or so attrition during the first 6 months (Dishman, 1988). If an experiment is successful in preventing any attrition, it probably achieved this result because the subjects were treated to a very high level of experimenter attention and support. Such an experiment would have internal validity (i.e., attrition would not be a threat to causal inferences) but would have limited external validity (ability to draw inferences beyond this particular training situation) because it is so unlike more conventional exercise programs.

**Expectation Effects.**    It is impossible for subjects to be blind to their treatment condition. Those in the experimental group are acutely aware of their group assignment and of how much effort is required by the exercise program. Also, subjects assigned to a nonexercise condition surely volunteered initially for an exercise program (to satisfy ethical requirements) and may resent not receiving the training they expected. The experiment is thus very susceptible to a confound produced by the differing demand characteristics of the two conditions (Wuebben, Straits, & Schulman, 1974).

Exercise has been generally accepted by the population as something that is beneficial to do. Popular magazines contain articles about the therapeutic benefits of exercise and about the positive psychological changes (improved mood, etc.) achieved through exercise (Rodin & Plante, 1989). Subjects in the exercise group are very likely to be aware of the benefits that they expect to be experiencing (Folkins & Sime, 1981). These expectations may affect their responses to questionnaires concerning their psychological state, especially if the questionnaires are administered by someone associated with the training program, and if the purpose of the questionnaires is apparent to the subjects. In addition, those assigned to the nonexercise condition may have expected initially to participate in an exercise program and may have anticipated certain benefits, and they may also bias their responses in a way that reflects their disappointment.

Hence, it is necessary to design the control condition in such a way that subjects have expectations of equivalent benefits from both the exercise and the control conditions (Folkins & Sime, 1981). Few experiments pay sufficient attention to this important issue. A waiting-list control condition does not control for expectation effects. Many experiments control for some superficial aspect of the treatment, such as amount of contact time with the experimenter. Thus, control subjects may meet three times a week for a discussion of some kind. However, it is unlikely that subjects expect to achieve the same benefits from these meetings as they would from exercise. A better design uses a treatment that is a plausible source of benefits for the subject, such as a program of anaerobic exercise (Norris et al., 1990), a therapy program such as relaxation training (Berger, Friedmann, & Eaton, 1988; Roth & Holmes, 1987), or a support group (Berger et al., 1988).

In addition to designing a control condition that minimizes differential expectations of benefits between conditions, the experimenter should also check that the groups do, in fact, have comparable expectations of benefits. Several methods are available for doing this. One example is the concept of a quasi control (Orne, 1969). This is carried out by presenting each randomized group of subjects with descriptions of one of the conditions and then asking them to respond to the dependent variables (e.g., questionnaires) as if they had just completed this condition—that is, to imagine how they would feel if they had just completed the condition described. If significant differences in the questionnaire responses are found, it indicates that these different conditions create different expectations of benefits.

Another general concern about expectation effects is whether the dependent measures are particularly susceptible to such effects. The measures and data-collection techniques should be designed to unobtrusively and accurately tap the psychological factors of interest (Wuebben et al., 1974).

A fortuitous finding that may minimize the need for concerns about expectation effects in some designs is that the benefits of exercise appear to be maximal at moderate, not high intensities of exercise (e.g., Moses et al., 1989). If it could be shown that expected benefits increase monotonically with increasing exercise intensities, then observed curvilinear benefits could not be attributed to expectation effects.

**External Validity.** In addition to the aforementioned problems, there is also concern about external validity—that is, whether the findings from an experiment can be generalized. Experiments use volunteers. It is possible that those who volunteer for a training program have a more positive attitude toward exercise, greater education about the effects of exercise, or possess greater self-esteem and self-confidence than those who do not volunteer. Individuals may also volunteer for this sort of program because of a desire to make a change in their lives (Folkins & Sime, 1981; Taylor, 1987), and it is possible that such individuals would benefit from any of a wide range of interventions. Whether exercise has comparable benefits for the general population (including nonvolunteers) cannot be assessed from such a sample.

Whether findings from an experiment can be generalized may also depend on the exercise condition itself. Until recently, most experiments involving training have used only one intensity of aerobic exercise. Findings therefore cannot be generalized to different intensities of, or other types of, aerobic or anaerobic exercise. Focusing mainly on aerobic exercise, the experimental approach has not provided much information about psycho-logical benefits of other types of exercise. There is some evidence that anaerobic exercise may be just as effective in enhancing psychological func-tioning (Doyne, Ossip-Klein, Bowman, Osborn, McDougall-Wilson, & Neimeyer, 1987; Sime, 1987). It is important to ascertain whether equivalent psychological benefits can be derived from less physically demanding ac-tivities, because they may be ones at which more individuals would persist.

## Clinical Trials

Experiments designed to evaluate the therapeutic value of exercise for specific clinical populations (clinical trials) involve additional consider-ations. Such programs have investigated the benefits of exercise for coro-nary heart disease patients (Stern & Cleary, 1982), and for individuals suffering from clinical depression (Doyne et al., 1987). These designs are clearly most concerned with possible health benefits of exercise. However, the health of each individual client is also of supreme importance, and it is very difficult to sustain a randomized experiment if a particular individual appears to be experiencing difficulties with the treatment condition (either exercise or control). Thus, attrition (or other modifications of treatment resulting in nonrandom assignment) is a particularly serious problem in this situation. Further, because of the degree of concern for the patient's welfare, the actual treatment program may involve excessive attention, resulting in decreased generalizability of the findings to other exercise programs. In the design of the control condition, the experimenter must carefully control for the possibility that this attention is partially mediating the benefits.

## Experiments Assessing the Acute Effects of Exercise

While most studies are concerned with the effects of long-term exercise, the psychological effects of a single exercise session have also been studied (see Chapter 4 by Tuson & Sinyor). This sort of experiment involves random assignment of subjects to either a single exercise session or a control condi-tion of comparable time duration. Psychological measures are collected at fixed times following termination of the exercise or control conditions. This design is concerned with a short-term phenomenon that may or may not be related to the benefits expected from long-term exercise. It is unlikely to be affected by subject attrition, but it is especially susceptible to demand characteristics. Because the psychological measures are administered shortly after the exercise session, it is difficult to disguise the purpose of the questionnaires.

The design of the control condition must be tailored to consider the component of the exercise session that is hypothesized to underlie the benefits, so that other factors can be held constant between the control and experimental conditions. A single exercise session involves a great number of components, and appropriate control groups are needed to identify which components are responsible for any changes observed. For example, an exercise session involves what may be called "time-out" from everyday activities, active participation in a project, and receiving attention from a trainer; it may also involve socializing with others, and so forth. The control group should include these components but not the single component of exercise hypothesized to be responsible for its benefits.

## OBSERVATIONAL APPROACHES

### Relative Advantages

In general, the experiment is widely accepted as the more scientifically valuable approach. However, the experimental approach to the study of exercise has several disadvantages that make observational (nonexperimental) methods appear increasingly attractive. Experiments are very costly to conduct because they require supervised exercise programs (and comparable sessions with the control group), which are generally conducted at least three times per week for a duration of 3 months or more. There are also interpersonal stresses that may result from the ethical requirement that subjects be aware that exercise is one of the treatment options, which may lead to disappointment experienced by those not receiving this condition. In addition, the changes in aerobic fitness resulting from a training program lasting about 3 months are of quite small magnitude relative to existing variation in fitness levels.

Observational studies can involve the use of interview or self-report questionnaires to assess existing exercise behaviors and existing fitness levels. They may also include laboratory measures of fitness. These exercise and/or fitness measures are then examined for their relationship to the psychological factors of interest. Observational studies are much less time-consuming and less costly to conduct than experiments, and they provide a large amount of information, often from a large sample. They also permit an evaluation of the actual state of affairs, without the artificiality of experiments.

### Problems Regarding Interpretation

Unfortunately, two problems plague the interpretation of nonexperimental research: the third-variable problem and the directionality problem (Neale & Liebert, 1980).

**Third-Variable Problem.**   The main advantage of using an experiment is the control of potentially confounding variables through randomization.

This control is not present in observational studies because subjects choose their own level of exercise. There are many possible reasons for subjects deciding whether to exercise, and it is probable that many differences exist between those who choose to exercise and those who choose not to do so. Consequently, many competing explanations may exist for the observed relationships. A positive correlation between exercise and a psychological variable such as mood could be the direct result of one of these other differences (the third variable)—for example, socioeconomic status. Thus, high socioeconomic status may cause people both to feel good and to exercise. A simple correlation between exercise and mood does not provide sufficient evidence to infer a causal link between exercise and mood because many other factors may have caused this relationship.

**Directionality Problem.**    While a unidirectional causation is generally assumed (i.e., that exercise causes psychological benefits), a plausible case can be made for the reverse causation (i.e., that exercise may be initiated *because of* a general feeling of well-being and interest in preparing for future endeavors). For example, professionals working with the elderly frequently express the view that those who take part in exercise programs do so because they feel good about life. With younger adults, it is equally plausible that exercise may be initiated because of a general feeling of well-being. For different individuals, the causality may go in either direction. Also, it is quite possible that, at least in some cases, there is reciprocal causation, in which exercise produces good feelings, which motivate more exercise, and so on, without implying that either the good feelings or the exercise came first.

These reverse and reciprocal causation possibilities have not received research attention. It should be noted that the experimental approach could detect only a unidirectional effect of exercise on psychological processes. An experiment cannot detect either reverse causation or reciprocal causation, even though both of these may operate in the real world. While the observational approach is capable of detecting that a relationship exists, it is not capable of resolving the issue of the direction of the causation.

## Alternative Uses and Benefits of Observational Studies: Path Analysis

Because of the preceding two problems, observational studies are not capable of answering the question of whether exercise produces (causes) psychological benefits. Observational studies have value for describing the current state of affairs—that is, existing relationships in the population. They also have value for suggesting possibilities that can be further studied using experimental methods. However, observational studies may also be valuable for evaluating possible explanations for the process responsible for mediating the relationship between exercise and psychological factors. The method for making such inferences is called "path analysis" (Darlington, 1990; Pedhazur, 1982). Because path analysis fits well with the recommendation of this chapter for more attention to the factors underlying the relationship between exercise and psychological factors, it is illustrated in some detail in the following section.

**Path Analysis Methodology.**   In observational research, the existence of other possible explanations is not an overwhelming obstacle and can even be viewed as a valuable feature of this type of research. This is so if it forces us to consider the issue of causality in more depth; that is, rather than just asking whether exercise affects a psychological characteristic such as the feeling of well-being, we question what underlies the relationship between exercise and well-being. The general approach used to address this issue is (a) to identify what factors are plausible mediators of the relationship, (b) to include measures of these factors in the study, and (c) to use statistical methods to evaluate whether these factors can account for the relationship.

A variety of statistical methods can be used to achieve the goal of statistically controlling for (partialling out) the effect of the potentially confounding third variable. These methods include multiple regression, analysis of covariance, partial correlation, and analysis of residual scores, all of which produce numerically identical solutions. This approach is sometimes called "path analysis" because the goal is to identify the most plausible causal pathway between exercise and psychological benefits (i.e., Is the link direct, or is it mediated by another variable?).

The following example (see Figure 8.1) illustrates the logic behind the path-analysis approach. Two possible models for the role of socioeconomic level in the relationship between exercise and well-being might be considered: In Model 1, both exercise and socioeconomic level have independent influences on well-being (i.e., Model 1 is consistent with a direct psychological benefit of exercise). In Model 2, exercise does not have an independent effect on well-being—that is, Model 2 denies any direct psychological benefit of exercise. A simple correlation between exercise and well-being does not provide a basis for evaluating these models. However, if the third variable, socioeconomic level, is also measured, then the researcher can determine which model is most likely to be correct.

The statistical analysis underlying the decision between the two models involves an examination of the partial correlation between exercise and well-being, controlling for socioeconomic level. (One of the other aforementioned methods could be used instead; the answer would be identical.) There are two possible outcomes. If the partial correlation was significant, Model 1 would be supported. This finding would indicate a relationship between exercise and well-being not due to (or mediated by) socioeconomic level. On the other hand, if the partial correlation was not significant, then

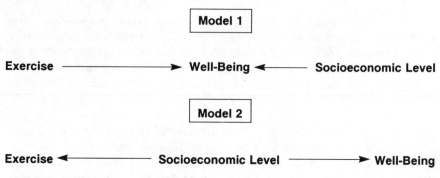

Figure 8.1.   Illustration of two possible causal models for the relationship of exercise to well-being.

Model 2 would be supported. The conclusion would be that there was no evidence for any effect of exercise independent of socioeconomic level.

**Strengths of Path Analysis.**   The strength of this approach is that any variable that can be measured can be tested as a possible mediator of the relationship. A particularly important application is the evaluation of a suspected mediator of the relationship between exercise and well-being, such as aerobic fitness. If the partial correlation of exercise and well-being was not significant when controlling for fitness, this would indicate that no relationship between exercise and well-being existed other than that accounted for by fitness level. In this case, fitness level would be a plausible mediator of the benefits of exercise. On the other hand, if the partial correlation of exercise and well-being still was significant when controlling for fitness, then fitness level would be ruled out as the sole mediator because at least some of the relationship between exercise and well-being was not accounted for by fitness level alone.

In observational research, a variety of measures reflective of the postulated mediating process (e.g., fitness) can be measured, in addition to exercise levels. Path-analysis methods may be used to evaluate whether these measures can explain any relationship between exercise and psychological variables—that is, whether these other variables are plausible mediators of the relationship. Three examples illustrating different applications of path analysis to the study of exercise are given next.

Roth, Wiebe, Fillingim, and Shay (1989) studied the interrelationships of exercise, fitness, stress, hardiness, and illness in a sample of 373 college students. Using a linear-modeling program (LISREL IV), they concluded that variation in illness was accounted for by independent effects of stress and fitness, and they rejected a model that also included an independent effect of hardiness on illness. Exercise was not found to have any relationship with illness, independent of fitness levels.

Ross and Hayes (1988), using a regression approach, found that exercise level was related to depression, anxiety, and malaise, even after variation in socioeconomic level, obesity, and instrumentalism were controlled for. Some, but not all, of the association between exercise level and well-being was explained by subjective physical health. They concluded that the association between exercise and well-being was not mediated by any of these factors.

Path analysis can also be used in experimental research. Darlington (1990, p. 409) provides an example of the application of path analysis to an experimental study of the effects of exercise. The exercise variable was experimentally manipulated through random assignment of subjects to groups. By measuring changes in fitness level in each group, it was possible to test whether the effects of exercise on the outcome measures were mediated by changes in fitness. Exercise was found to have effects on state anxiety, trait anxiety, and Type A behavior scores, which were not mediated by changes in fitness level.

**Limitations of Path Analysis.**    A limitation of the path-analysis approach is that all potential mediators must be accurately measured, or they cannot be ruled out (Pedhazur, 1982). For example, if socioeconomic level or aerobic fitness were imperfectly measured, they could not be conclusively ruled out as mediators. More detailed considerations of other factors that may affect path analysis is beyond the scope of this chapter, and the reader is referred to more advanced sources (Cohen & Cohen, 1983; Darlington, 1990; Pedhazur, 1982). One should also remember that causality is only relative—that is, a mediator is not necessarily an ultimate cause, and some other mechanism may underlie the mediation. Science proceeds by gaining an understanding of causality at progressively deeper levels (Darlington, 1990).

## METHODOLOGICAL CONSIDERATIONS IN THE STUDY OF PHYSIOLOGICAL RECOVERY FROM STRESS

There is currently considerable interest in faster physiological recovery from stress as a possible benefit of exercise (Long, 1991; Steptoe, Moses, Mathews, & Edwards, 1990). However, some of the methodological issues relevant to the study of the recovery period are not generally addressed. In particular, the recovery period can be viewed from two quite different perspectives, and there are two corresponding methods for studying factors related to recovery. To date, few studies explicitly state which approach they are taking, thereby making cross-study comparisons difficult. Also, in many cases, researchers may not be using the most sensitive methodology to study the relationship of exercise to physiological recovery from stress.

From one perspective, the recovery period can be seen as an extension of the stress response. Thus, interest is directed at individuals who show *exaggerated and sustained* physiological responses. The alternative perspective focuses on speed of recovery, independent of the magnitude of response to the stressor. The rationale for this second perspective can be seen from a statement by Dillbeck and Orme-Johnson (1987) who proposed that "the most adaptive response to stress would probably not be absence of physiological response to a threatening situation, but rather rapid recovery after stress" (p. 880). A similar view has been expressed by Dienstbier (1989), who proposed that individuals best suited to deal with stress ("physiologically tough individuals") would exhibit a strong sympathetic response to stress, followed by rapid recovery. These authors focus on speed of recovery as the important dimension and deemphasize the importance of differences in the magnitude of the stress response.

The foregoing two viewpoints differ in whether the recovery period is seen as an extension of the stress response, or as a separate phenomenon to be studied in isolation from the stress response. There are also two methods for studying the recovery period. The most common method, corresponding to the first viewpoint, has been to examine a difference score (or residual score), which compares the physiological level at a certain time following stressor termination to a single resting baseline level (Holmes & Roth, 1985; Sinyor, Schwartz, Péronnet, Brisson, & Seraganian, 1983; Steptoe et al., 1990). Recovery differences are thus reflected in how close the level is to baseline (i.e., full recovery). Individuals showing slower recovery will have larger difference (or residual) scores. Thus, in part, the recovery differences being studied reflect differences in magnitude of response to the stressor. This method for indexing recovery is particularly appropriate when the recovery period is viewed as an extension of the stress response. It is appropriate when studying factors that have an effect on the magnitude of the physiological response to the stressor, in order to determine the duration of time for which such effects persist following stressor termination.

The alternative method involves partialling out two factors: resting baseline and arousal level (Cox et al., 1979; Jamieson & Lavoie, 1987). This yields a measure of recovery that is independent of the magnitude of response to the stressor. This second method views variation in response magnitude as extraneous variation, which is partialled out to yield a more sensitive index of recovery differences. In this case, the index of recovery reflects differences in physiological levels during the recovery period that are independent of the magnitude of the response to stress. This second method is therefore useful for identifying factors that have an effect on recovery that is not mediated by differences in magnitude of response to the stressor. Thus, the second method might be viewed as yielding a purer index of recovery.

In cases where exercise does not have a clear effect on the stress response, failure to employ the second approach results in a loss of statistical power because a large source of extraneous variability (i.e., individual differences in magnitude of response to the stressor) is not removed. In general, the second approach will be more powerful.

## SUMMARY

A decade ago, when Folkins and Sime (1981) reviewed the literature on the psychological effects of exercise, they concluded that studies in this area were generally poorly designed, and "with a candid appeal for scientific rigor" (p. 386), they emphasized the need for control groups. Since then, well-designed experiments have proliferated, and the emphasis in this chapter is on where we need to go from here. The issue now requiring attention is clarification of the process by which psychological benefits result from exercise. Explicit models of hypothesized underlying processes are needed. For the experimental approach, such models can be tested through the design of the control condition. Observational research can also evaluate various causal models through path-analysis techniques.

## REFERENCES

Astrand, P., & Rodahl, K. (1986). *Textbook of work physiology.* New York: McGraw-Hill.

Berger, B. G., Friedmann, E., & Eaton, M. (1988). Comparison of jogging, the relaxation response, and group interaction for stress reduction. *Journal of Sport and Exercise Psychology, 10,* 431–447.

Campbell, D. T., & Stanley, J. C. (1963). *Experimental and quasi-experimental designs for research.* Chicago: Rand-McNally.

Cohen, J., & Cohen, P. (1983). *Applied multiple regression/correlation analysis for the behavioral sciences* (2nd ed.). Hillsdale, NJ: Erlbaum.

Cook, T. D., & Campbell, D. T. (1979). *Quasi-experimentation, design and analysis issues for field settings.* Chicago: Rand-McNally.

Cox, J. P., Evans, J. F., & Jamieson, J. L. (1979). Aerobic power and tonic heart rate response to psychosocial stressors. *Personality and Social Psychology Bulletin, 2,* 160–163.

Crews, D. J., & Landers, D. M. (1987). A meta-analytic review of aerobic fitness and reactivity to psychosocial stressors. *Medicine and Science in Sport and Exercise, 19,* S114–S120.

Crossman, J., Jamieson, J., & Henderson, J. (1987). Responses of competitive athletes to lay-offs in training: Exercise addiction or psychological relief. *Journal of Sport Behavior, 10,* 28–38.

Darlington, R. B. (1990). *Regression and linear models.* New York: McGraw-Hill.

Dienstbier, R. A. (1989). Arousal and physiological toughness: Implications for mental and physical health. *Psychological Review, 96,* 84–100.

Dillbeck, M. C., & Orme-Johnson, D. W. (1987). Physiological differences between transcendental meditation and rest. *American Psychologist, 42,* 879–881.

Dishman, R. K. (1988). *Exercise adherence.* Champaign, IL: Human Kinetic Books.

Doyne, E. J., Ossip-Klein, D. J., Bowman, E. D., Osborn, K. M., McDougall-Wilson, I. B., & Neimeyer, R. A. (1987). Running versus weight lifting in the treatment of depression. *Journal of Consulting and Clinical Psychology, 55,* 748–754.

Folkins, C. H., & Sime, W. E. (1981). Physical fitness training and mental health. *American Psychologist, 36,* 373–389.

Holmes, D. S., & Roth, D. L. (1985). Association of aerobic fitness with pulse rate and subjective responses to psychological stress. *Psychophysiology, 22,* 525–529.

Jamieson, J., & Lavoie, N. F. (1987). Type A behavior, aerobic power, and cardiovascular recovery from a psychosocial stressor. *Health Psychology, 6,* 361–371.

Kerlinger, F. (1986). *Foundations of behavioral research* (3rd ed.). New York: Holt Rinehart and Winston.

Long, B. C. (1985). Stress-management interventions: A 15 month follow-up of aerobic conditioning and stress inoculation training. *Cognitive Therapy and Research, 9,* 471–478.

Long, B. C. (1991). Physiological and psychological stress recovery of physically fit and unfit women. *Canadian Journal of Behavioural Science, 23,* 53–65.

Morgan, W. P., & Goldston, S. E. (Eds.). (1987). *Exercise and mental health.* Washington, DC: Hemisphere.

Moses, J., Steptoe, A., Mathews, A., & Edwards, S. (1989). The effects of exercise training on mental well-being in the normal population: A controlled trial. *Journal of Psychosomatic Research, 33,* 47–61.

Neale, J. M., & Liebert, R. M. (1980). *Science and behavior* (2nd ed.). Englewood Cliffs, NJ: Prentice-Hall.

Norris, R., Carroll, D., & Cochrane, R. (1990). The effects of aerobic and anaerobic training on fitness, blood pressure, and psychological stress and well-being. *Journal of Psychosomatic Research, 34,* 367–375.

Orne, M. T. (1969). Demand characteristics and the concept of quasi-controls. In R. Rosenthal & R. L. Rosnow (Eds.), *Artifact in behavioral research* (pp. 147–179). New York: Academic Press.

Pedhazur, E. J. (1982). *Multiple regression in behavioral research* (2nd ed.). New York: Holt Rinehart and Winston.

Powell, R. R. (1975). Effects of exercise on mental functioning. *Journal of Sports Medicine and Physical Fitness, 15,* 125–131.

Rodin, J., & Plante, T. (1989). The psychological effects of exercise. In R. S. Williams & A. G. Wallace (Eds.), *Biological effects of physical activity.* Champaign, IL: Human Kinetics.

Ross, C. E., & Hayes, D. (1988). Exercise and psychologic well-being in the community. *American Journal of Epidemiology, 127,* 762–771.

Roth, D. L., & Holmes, D. S. (1987). Influence of aerobic exercise training and relaxation training on physical and psychologic health following stressful life events. *Psychosomatic Medicine, 49*, 355–365.

Roth, D. L., Wiebe, D. J., Fillingim, R. B., & Shay, K. A. (1989). Life events, fitness, hardiness, and health: A simultaneous analysis of proposed stress-resistance effects. *Journal of Personality and Social Psychology, 57*, 136–142.

Sime, W. E. (1987). Exercise in the prevention and treatment of depression. In W. P. Morgan & S. E. Goldston (Eds.), *Exercise and mental health*. Washington, DC: Hemisphere.

Sinyor, D., Schwartz, S. G., Péronnet, F., Brisson, G., & Seraganian, P. (1983). Aerobic fitness level and reactivity to psychosocial stress: Physiological, biochemical, and subjective measures. *Psychosomatic Medicine, 45*, 205–217.

Sonstroem, R. J., & Morgan, W. P. (1988). Exercise and self-esteem: Rationale and model. *Medicine and Science in Sport and Exercise, 21*, 329–337.

Steptoe, A., & Cox, S. (1988). Acute effects of aerobic exercise on mood. *Health Psychology, 1*, 329–340.

Steptoe, A., Moses, J., Mathews, A., & Edwards, S. (1990). Aerobic fitness, physical activity, and psychophysiological reactions to mental tasks. *Psychophysiology, 27*, 264–274.

Stern, M. J., & Cleary, P. (1982). The National Exercise and Heart Disease Project: Long term psychosocial outcome. *Archives of Internal Medicine, 142*, 1093–1097.

Taylor, J. (1987). A review of validity issues in sport psychological research: Types, problems, solutions. *Journal of Sport Behavior, 10*, 3–13.

Williams, J. G., & Eston, R. G. (1989). Determination of the intensity dimension in vigorous exercise programmes with particular reference to the use of the rating of perceived exertion. *Sports Medicine, 8*, 177–189.

Wuebben, P. L., Straits, B. C., & Schulman, G. I. (1974). *The experiment as a social occasion*. Berkeley, CA: Glendessary Press.

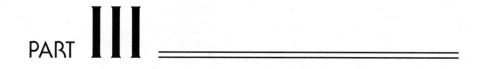

PART **III**

# APPLICATIONS

# 9

# Psychological Effects of Exercise Among the Elderly

## ROGER B. FILLINGIM AND JAMES A. BLUMENTHAL

Advancing age is associated with declines in cardiac performance. Elderly persons also tend to show impairments in psychological functioning, including greater prevalence of mood disturbance (Pfeiffer, 1977) and decrements in cognitive performance (Botwinick, 1977; Craik, 1977). Across all ages, increased physical activity has been shown to be related to decreased risk of cardiovascular events (Leon, Connett, Jacobs, & Rauramma, 1987; Paffenbarger, Hyde, Irving, & Steinmetz, 1984), and increased maximal oxygen uptake (Astrand & Rodahl, 1986). Studies of younger people have shown that exercise also appears to improve mood (Blumenthal, Williams, Needels, & Wallace, 1982; Morgan & Goldston, 1987; Roth, 1989) and may enhance cognitive performance (Spirduso, 1980; Tomporowski & Ellis,

1986). Thus, exercise could be an especially important health-promoting activity in elderly individuals.

The majority of exercise research has been conducted on younger adults; however, investigation of the effects of exercise among the older population recently has received increased attention. The purpose of this chapter is to examine the research on the psychological and psychophysiological effects of exercise in the elderly. First, we briefly summarize the changes in cardiovascular functioning associated with normal aging, followed by a discussion of methodological issues and barriers to research in this area. Then, we examine the physiological and psychological effects of acute and chronic exercise in the elderly.

## PHYSIOLOGICAL CHANGES ASSOCIATED WITH AGING

A number of cardiovascular indices decline with age. Specifically, maximal heart rate during exercise decreases steadily after the first decade of life (Astrand & Christensen, 1964). Also, progressive declines in cardiac output and heart rate (Brandfonbrenner, Landowne, & Shock, 1955; Strandell, 1976a, 1976b) as well as stroke volume and left ventricular ejection-fraction during exercise have been found to occur with aging (Port, Cobb, Coleman, & Jones, 1980). However, a more recent study of healthy subjects between the ages of 25 and 79 reported that during exercise, cardiac output did not change with age, and stroke volume increased (Rodeheffer et al., 1984). These authors suggested that, with advancing age, cardiac output during exercise is maintained more by the Frank–Starling mechanism rather than by catecholamine-mediated effects. These changes in cardiovascular response to exercise may be related to the decreased ability of beta-adrenergic stimulation to increase heart rate, myocardial contractility, and arterial vascular tone that occurs with age (Lakatta, 1980). However, with the exception of maximal heart rate, all of the parameters of cardiovascular function that decrease with age have been shown to be improved with exercise training in younger populations (Rerych, Scholz, Sabiston, & Jones, 1980; Scheuer & Tipton, 1977).

Maximal oxygen uptake ($\dot{V}O_2$ max), which represents the capacity of an individual's cardiovascular system to meet the metabolic requirements of physiological work, also declines progressively with age (Bruce, 1984). According to cross-sectional research, the rate of change in $\dot{V}O_2$ max with age is –0.4 mL/minute/kg/year (Dehn & Bruce, 1972). However, longitudinal studies, which provide a much more reliable description of changes in $\dot{V}O_2$ max over time, suggest a rate of change approximately twice that of cross-sectional research (Bruce, 1984). It has also been demonstrated that physically active persons show half the age-related reductions in $\dot{V}O_2$ max, compared to sedentary individuals (Dehn & Bruce, 1972). It has been suggested that elderly individuals are less physiologically responsive to physical exercise training, and little improvement in $\dot{V}O_2$ max can be expected when training begins late in life (Hogdson & Buskirk, 1977). Consistent with this prediction, some studies have failed to demonstrate training effects in the elderly (Benestad, 1965; deVries, 1970). In contrast, a number of longitudinal studies have demonstrated that exercise may increase aerobic power from 18% to 30% (Seals, Hagberg, Hurley, Ehsani, & Holloszy, 1984). In a 1991 study, Blumenthal et al. showed that a 14-month program of aerobic exercise increased $\dot{V}O_2$ max by 18%, and some individuals may achieve more than a 58% improvement.

The foregoing data suggest that many of the physiological adaptations to exercise that occur in young persons also occur in the elderly; however, the psychological adaptations to exercise that have been studied in young people have only recently been examined in older subjects. This review next discusses a number of methodological issues relevant to research on exercise and psychological changes in the elderly.

## METHODOLOGICAL ISSUES AND BARRIERS TO RESEARCH

A number of methodological issues are relevant to research on the psychological benefits of exercise in the elderly. These include experimental design and selection of control conditions, subject population (e.g., clinical vs. nonclinical), fitness assessment, exercise parameters, and choice of outcome measures.

Two designs are frequently used to examine the psychological effects of exercise in the elderly: cross-sectional and interventional. *Cross-sectional studies* assess levels of aerobic fitness or physical activity levels at one point in time and then investigate the relationship of these variables of psychological functioning. Cross-sectional studies examine the relationship between aerobic fitness or physical activity and psychological functioning. However, their value is often limited by selection bias and imprecise measures of fitness and activity levels. Additionally, these studies do not permit causal conclusions. In order to determine whether exercise training produces psychological changes, interventional studies are needed. *Interventional studies* involve the assessment of psychological functioning before and after an aerobic exercise program. With proper randomization and experimental control, longitudinal studies can address the question of whether exercise causes changes in psychological functioning.

To reduce selection bias and improve generalizability, longitudinal studies must employ randomized designs. In a simple pre–post design, the psychological functioning of a subject population is compared before and after a physical training program. Though psychological changes may be observed, the absence of a control group prevents investigators from attributing these changes specifically to exercise, as nonspecific factors (e.g., demand characteristics, regression to the mean, practice effects) may influence outcome measures. Random assignment of subjects to either an exercise or a control condition can overcome many of these interpretive problems. A control condition should be matched to the exercise condition on important variables such as subject expectations and experimenter contact. Suitable control conditions include meditation or relaxation (e.g., Roth & Holmes, 1987), nonaerobic exercise (Blumenthal, Fredrikson, Kuhn, Ulmer, Walsh-Riddle, & Applebaum, 1990), or a waiting-list nonexercise condition (Blumenthal et al., 1988). Ideally, subjects believe that these alternative treatment control conditions are effective at improving psychological functioning. Assessment of subject expectations before and after interventions can provide a manipulation check to determine the effectiveness of the control conditions.

The selection of a subject population is another important design issue. In their review of the literature on exercise and mental health, Folkins and Sime (1981) found that most studies were performed on clinical populations. Findings of improved psychological functioning following exercise in psychiatric patients may have limited generalizability to nonclinical subjects. It has been reported that in healthy subjects, those with the greatest mood disturbance prior to exercise show the greatest improvements (Simons & Birkimer, 1988). In other words, a subject will more likely become less depressed following exercise if he or she is somewhat depressed beforehand. This may be an artifact of the outcome measures rather than an interpretable finding. Regardless of whether preexisting psychological dysfunction is present, it is possible that the mechanisms that mediate potential psychological changes and the changes themselves are different for clinical versus nonclinical populations. Therefore, it may be difficult to compare findings across these types of studies.

Adequate evaluation of aerobic fitness is an important methodological issue because assessment of aerobic capacity is the basis for exercise prescription, and it is a critical manipulation check in longitudinal exercise training studies. An abundance of methods to estimate aerobic fitness is available, and no one method is optimal for all purposes. Questionnaires that inquire as to subjects' physical activity patterns have been used as gross measures of physical fitness (e.g., Fillingim, Roth, & Haley, 1989; Light, Obrist, James, & Strogatz, 1987). However, even if subjects accurately report their exercise habits, these self-report measures are based on the assumption that compared to inactive people, more active people are more physically fit, which is not necessarily true. For example, genetic factors may be an important determinant of physical fitness (Bouchard & Malina, 1983). Therefore, paper-and-pencil instruments ideally should be used only for mass screening.

Exercise testing is necessary to accurately measure aerobic fitness. Submaximal exercise tests require the subject to exercise to a specified submaximal endpoint (e.g., 70% of age-predicated maximum heart rate), and these methods are often used for nondiagnostic purposes (e.g., with healthy persons) or when financial and/or equipment limitations prevent the use of maximal tests. Several submaximal bicycle ergometer tests use a standard nomogram to predict $\dot{V}O_2$ max and are relatively easy to perform (see Åstrand & Rodahl, 1986, for a discussion). However, submaximal tests are far less accurate at estimating $\dot{V}O_2$ max than maximal tests, and they also are less sensitive for detecting underlying coronary disease.

Ideally, a multistage maximal or symptom-limited exercise test on a treadmill or bicycle ergometer with an electrocardiogram (ECG) and measurement of oxygen consumption is performed to provide the most accurate measure of aerobic fitness. Obviously, this must be performed under adequate professional supervision, and the American College of Sports Medicine (ACSM) guidelines for exercise testing should be followed (ACSM, 1986). Several protocols for maximal exercise testing are available. For example, the Bruce treadmill protocol (Bruce, 1971) increases the speed and slope every third minute, while the Balke protocol (Balke, 1954) keeps treadmill speed constant and increases the slope by 2.5% either every minute or every other minute. Other treadmill testing protocols provide similar assessments of maximal aerobic power (Pollock, Willmore, & Fox, 1978).

In addition to the assessment of aerobic fitness, the exercise training regimen is an important consideration for research in this area. Exercise programs can vary significantly along the dimensions of the type, intensity, duration, and frequency of exercise. In designing an exercise program, ACSM guidelines for exercise prescription should be observed (ACSM, 1986). Briefly summarized, these guidelines recommend the use of exercise involving large muscle groups, which is relatively continuous in nature (e.g., running, cycling, swimming). Exercise intensity should be 70% of $\dot{V}O_2$ max or maximum heart rate reserve {i.e., [(HR max – HR rest) 0.7 + HR rest]}, should be performed 3 to 5 times per week for 15 to 60 minutes per day. The length of the exercise program necessary to produce a conditioning effect will vary with the frequency, duration, and intensity of exercise sessions. Studies on exercise and mood have used exercise training ranging from 3 to 104 weeks in duration (see Hughes, 1984). In general, a minimum of 8 to 12 weeks of exercise should be used (ACSM, 1986), and in the elderly, somewhat longer programs may be needed to produce a training effect.

The outcome measures used are of paramount importance, and in his review of the psychological effects of aerobic exercise, Hughes (1984) cited poor choice of psychological measures as a consistent methodological problem. Most studies have relied on self-report measures, many of which assess only mood disturbances. These measures are highly susceptible to subject bias, and their reliability and validity are often questionable. Additionally, these measures have often developed normative scores based on young populations. Further research is needed to assess the reliability and validity of current measures for use with elderly individuals. Frequently used psychometric instruments often tap predominantly negative emotional states, and the assessment of both positive and negative mood dimensions is important (King, Taylor, Haskell, & DeBusk, 1990). Moreover, in addition to self-report, the use of psychophysiological (e.g., Fillingim, Roth, & Cook, 1990; Roth, 1989) and behavioral (see Zillmann, 1983) measures of psychological functioning is warranted.

## MOOD EFFECTS OF AEROBIC EXERCISE IN THE ELDERLY

Psychological improvements that have been reported following aerobic exercise training in young and middle-aged subjects include reductions in depression (Greist et al., 1979; Roth & Holmes, 1987) and anxiety (Blumenthal et al., 1982; Goldwater & Collins, 1985), improved self-esteem (Sonstroem, 1984), and improved cognitive functioning (Tomporowski & Ellis, 1986). Research on the mood effects of exercise in the elderly has yielded less consistent results. In a cross-sectional study, Perri and Templer (1984–1985) found less depression and anxiety and greater internal locus of control in exercisers, compared to nonexercisers. Stacey, Kozma, and Stones (1985) showed that 6 months of exercise led to increased happiness in older individuals who were just beginning, compared to those who were continuing to exercise. Valliant and Asu (1985) reported reduced depression in elderly subjects following a 12-week exercise program, and males in this study showed improved self-esteem.

In contrast, Buccola and Stone (1975) found few changes on a test of personality characteristics in older male joggers. Relatedly, Stamford, Hambacher, & Fallica (1974) and Powell (1974) found no improvements in mood or personality following exercise training in geriatric psychiatric inpatients. In an uncontrolled pre–post design, psychological changes following an 11-week conditioning program were examined in young-old (65–69) and old-old (70–85) volunteers (Blumenthal, Schocken, Needels, & Hindle, 1982). While significant aerobic training effects were observed, improvements in mood were small and generally nonsignificant. In 1990, Emery and Gatz found few improvements in psychological functioning in elderly subjects who participated in a 3-month exercise program.

Several recent randomized controlled trials of exercise in the elderly have been conducted. Gitlin (1985) reported no mood benefits of a 4-month exercise program, compared to a lecture/discussion control condition. In a study of 43 sedentary individuals ages 55–70 years, aerobic exercise was compared to strength and flexibility training, and a no-treatment control group (Dustman et al., 1984). The exercise program consisted of three 1-hour sessions per week for 4 months, during which subjects engaged in fast walking or jogging. The aerobic-exercise group showed greater increases in $\dot{V}O_2$ max than the other two groups (a 27% increase); however, depression scores were not improved following the exercise program.

In the Duke Aging and Exercise Study of 101 older individuals (mean age = 67), the cardiovascular and psychological effects of aerobic exercise were compared to those of a yoga and flexibility group, and those of a waiting-list control condition (Blumenthal et al., 1989). The aerobic exercise program lasted 4 months, and subjects participated in three weekly exercise sessions, during which they performed cycle ergometry, walking/jogging, and arm ergometry. The aerobic-exercise group showed significant improvements in aerobic capacity (11.6% increase) and anaerobic threshold (13% increase). Men in the aerobic-exercise group showed significant reductions in depression, compared to women in the same group and all control subjects. Also, in the aerobic group, there was a tendency for men to show lower trait anxiety and for women to show less state anxiety, compared to the control groups. A follow-up report assessing these subjects after 14 months of exercise indicated no additional beneficial effects of exercise on mood (Blumenthal et al., 1991). These data from controlled experimental studies lend little support to the hypothesis that exercise training improves mood in elderly non-depressed subjects; however, the paucity of well-controlled empirical research in clinical populations makes it difficult to draw definitive conclusions.

## NEUROPSYCHOLOGICAL EFFECTS OF AEROBIC EXERCISE

It has been suggested that, in addition to its possible mood benefits, exercise may also enhance some aspects of cognitive functioning (Spirduso, 1980; Tomporowski & Ellis, 1986). Additionally, there are age-related declines in cognitive functioning (Botwinick, 1977; Craik, 1977), and it has been proposed that these changes may be due, in part, to lower levels of physical activity in old as compared to young persons (Botwinick & Thompson, 1968). It has been noted that young active subjects showed faster simple reaction times (RTs) than did older subjects; however, young inactive individuals did not show faster RTs than the elderly group. Further cross-sectional research has lent additional support to the notion that age-related changes in cognitive functioning may relate to physical fitness.

Spirduso (1975, 1980) compared the RTs of groups of old and young subjects who were either physically active or inactive. While the old-inactive men showed slower RTs than the young men, the old-active men had RTs comparable to the younger groups. Similarly, age differences in mean RT have been found to be smaller for physically active versus inactive men (Spirduso & Clifford, 1978). Rikli and Busch (1986) found a similar pattern of results in women. Perri and Templer (1984–1985) found that exercisers showed better performance on the Rey Auditory Training Test, compared to nonexercisers. More recently, Stacey et al. (1985) showed that aerobic exercise also improved performance on the Digit Symbol subtest of the Wechsler Adult Intelligence Scale (WAIS). Shay and Roth (1991) found that active elderly subjects showed better performance on visuospatial tasks compared to inactive elderly subjects. These data suggest that the maintenance of a physically active life-style may attenuate age-related declines in information-processing speed; however, interpretation of these studies must be tempered by an awareness of their significant methodological shortcomings. These studies have generally relied on self-report measures of physical activity, which have questionable reliability and validity. Also, the cross-sectional nature of the design renders the data highly susceptible to self-selection bias and third-variable effects (e.g. an additional variable, such as genetic endowment or health status may predispose people toward both high physical activity levels and enhanced cognitive functioning).

Several recent longitudinal studies examining the effects of aerobic exercise training on cognitive performance in the elderly have been conducted. In a study with younger men (mean age 43), Blumenthal and Madden (1988) found that, after a 12-week aerobic-exercise program, memory-search performance was related to initial level of fitness and age but not to the amount of change in fitness resulting from the training program. In a study of older subjects, Elsayed, Ismail, and Young (1980) found that a 4-month aerobic exercise program improved performance on speed-related psychometric tests, but not on an untimed assessment of the subject's general fund of knowledge. However, this study did not include a control group.

In a longitudinal study among older subjects, Dustman et al. (1984) compared the effects of 4 months of aerobic exercise, strength/flexibility training, or no treatment on neuropsychological function in older individuals (ages 55–70). The aerobic exercise group showed greater improvements in simple RT and the Stroop color test than did either control group, but the aerobic exercisers did not improve on two-choice-RT tasks. Stones and Kozma (1988) reported that an aerobic-exercise program produced greater improvements in neuropsychological test performance compared to control conditions. In this study, however, aerobic-capacity measures and neuropsychological test data were not reported in sufficient detail to allow accurate interpretation.

Other well-controlled studies have demonstrated no effects of aerobic training on neuropsychological functioning. The Duke Aging and Exercise Study (see Blumenthal et al., 1989, 1991; Madden, Allen, Blumenthal, & Emery, 1989) randomly assigned 101 older adults (mean age 67) to one of three conditions: (1) 16 weeks of aerobic exercise, (2) 16 weeks of nonaerobic exercise (yoga), or (3) a waiting-list control. Assessments at the beginning and the end of the 16 weeks included measures of depression, anxiety, psychiatric symptoms, and a wide range of neuropsychological measures. It was found that subjects in all three groups experienced decreases in psychiatric symptoms at posttest. Also, males in the aerobic-exercise group reported fewer symptoms of depression at posttest. However, there were no other significant effects of exercise on psychological well-being. On the measures of neuropsychological functioning, improvements occurred for all three groups on several of the measures, which appeared to be the result of practice effects, rather than attributable to the exercise intervention. Even after 14 months of exercise, no substantial improvements in psychological well-being or neuropsychological functioning were observed (Blumenthal et al., 1991).

In a report on a subsample ($n$ = 85) of older subjects and 24 younger (mean age = 22 years) adults, Madden et al. (1989) reported that older adults were slower than the younger subjects on RT tests of attention and memory retrieval, and older subjects showed no improvements in cognitive function as a result of aerobic-exercise training, despite a significant increase in aerobic fitness. Similar results were reported after 14 months of exercise in this cohort (Blumenthal et al., in press). Another recent investigation compared a 6-month aerobic exercise program to a strength-training program and to a no-treatment condition over the same time period, in a group of 49 older (ages 70–79) individuals (Panton, Graves, Pollock, Hagberg, & Chen, 1990). The aerobic-exercise group showed significant improvements in aerobic capacity; however, they showed no increase in RT performance. In spite of achieving few objective improvements in psychological well-being and cognitive functioning following exercise, older exercise participants often report subjective benefits of exercise (Emery & Blumenthal, 1990). Further research, using standardized measures of fitness, training, and psychological and cognitive functioning, is necessary to further explicate the basis for perceived benefits of exercise.

The findings of these longitudinal studies are inconsistent. Although the designs are similar, there are noteworthy differences among these experiments. First, Dustman et al. reported a greater increase in $\dot{V}O_2$ max than did the Blumenthal et al. and Panton et al. studies, and this may have produced a stronger effect on neuropsychological functioning. Additionally, both the Dustman et al. research and the Stones and Kozma studies pooled the neuropsychological test data in their analyses, which may have affected the statistical outcome. Due to the inconsistent findings and differences among studies, the question of whether aerobic exercise enhances cognitive performance in the elderly merits further research. Additional longitudinal studies assessing specific cognitive abilities (e.g., visuospatial tasks, fractionated RT) before and after aerobic conditioning would be useful. Also, designs that combine cross-sectional and longitudinal methodologies to assess the cognitive effects of exercise throughout the life span could address the question of whether exercise can prevent or retard cognitive declines before they occur, or even reverse them.

## PSYCHOLOGICAL EFFECTS OF ACUTE EXERCISE IN THE ELDERLY

It has been suggested that many of the psychological benefits of chronic exercise may be attributable to the cumulative effects of individual bouts of exercise (Haskell, 1987). In young subjects, acute exercise has been found to improve mood (Berger & Owens, 1983; Roth, 1989); however, little research has examined the effects of single exercise sessions in older individuals. In one study comparing the affective responses of young (mean age 26 years) and old (mean age 66 years) persons to a graded exercise test on a bicycle ergometer, neither group showed improved mood following acute exercise (Hatfield, Goldfarb, Sforzo, & Flynn, 1987).

Another study compared the mood and cognitive performance of 15 older subjects (mean age 66) before and after both exercise and rest over a 45-minute period (Molloy, Beerschoten, Borrie, Crilly, & Cape, 1988). Mood did not change significantly in either condition, but the authors reported that subjects showed improved performance on several neuropsychological tests following exercise. However, this experiment has several method-ological limitations. First, the sample size is quite small and consists solely of active people; therefore, the generality of the findings is limited. Also, the exercise performed was not of aerobic intensity, and it offered social inter-action in some cases; hence, the nonspecific effects of exercise may have outweighed its physiological impact. Finally, the statistical analyses were not thoroughly presented, and they may have capitalized on chance find-ings due to multiple statistical tests. Much more research on the acute effects of exercise in the elderly is needed.

## PSYCHOPHYSIOLOGICAL EFFECTS OF EXERCISE IN THE ELDERLY

A large body of research concerning the psychophysiological effects of exercise in younger subjects has accumulated. Cross-sectional research lends some support to the notion that aerobic fitness is related to attenuated cardiovascular responses to psychological stress (see Crews & Landers, 1987, for a review; Van Doornen & de Geus, 1989). The results of longitudi-nal studies have been more inconsistent. Only three studies report differ-ences in reactivity, one of which found differences only in borderline hypertensives (Sherwood, Light, & Blumenthal, 1989), a second among Type A men (Blumenthal et al., 1988), and the third used nonrandom group assignment and showed differences only in subjects with low fitness levels (Holmes & McGilley, 1987).

Some studies report more rapid post-stress recovery or lower absolute levels of cardiovascular activity during stress, and the potential clinical and conceptual merit of these findings requires further investigation (e.g., Blumenthal et al., 1988). Finally, a few studies found no differences (e.g., Roskies et al., 1986; Sinyor, Golden, Steinert, & Seraganian, 1986).

Additionally, several studies have addressed the effects of acute exercise on physiological responses to stress, (e.g., Fillingim et al., 1989; McGowan, Robertson, & Epstein, 1985; Peronnet, Massicotte, Paquee, Brisson, & de Champlain, 1989; Roth, 1989), and these results have been mixed. Unfortu-nately, there are no published studies examining the psychophysiological effects of exercise in the elderly; however, one cross-sectional study found that fitness was related to smaller cardiovascular stress responses only in subjects over 40 years old (Hull, Young, & Ziegler, 1984). To date, only one study has examined the relationship of aerobic exercise and cardiovascular stress reactivity in the elderly. Roth and Shay (1990) compared the cardio-vascular responses of active versus inactive old and young subjects to the Stroop color-word test. They reported less vasoconstriction in both old and young active subjects, compared to inactive subjects. Thus, research into the psychophysiological effects of both acute and chronic exercise in the elderly seems warranted.

## CONCLUSIONS AND FUTURE DIRECTIONS

The research discussed herein is characterized by methodological incon-sistencies and by a small number of studies, which yield mixed results; therefore, a general summary is difficult to provide. Declines in aerobic capacity occur with aging; however, it has been demonstrated that physical activity can slow this decline (Bruce, 1984; Dehn & Bruce, 1972). Addition-ally, aerobic training programs have been found to substantially improve $\dot{V}O_2$ max in the elderly (Blumenthal et al., 1991).

Despite the physiological changes that exercise produces, research has not consistently borne out that exercise holds psychological benefits for the elderly. Studies examining the mood benefits of aerobic training in the elderly have reported few significant effects. With regard to the effects of exercise on cognitive functioning, cross-sectional studies have suggested that physical activity relates to attenuation of age-related cognitive declines. However, longitudinal research on this topic has yielded mixed results, with some studies reporting improvements on some measures of cognitive performance following an aerobic training program (e.g., Dustman et al., 1984; Elsayed et al., 1980), and others reporting no cognitive changes follow-ing exercise (e.g., Blumenthal et al., 1991; Madden, Blumenthal, Allen, & Emery, 1988; Panton et al., 1990). There has been insufficient research con-ducted on the psychological effects of acute exercise, as well as on the psychophysiological effects of exercise in the elderly, to make reliable generalizations.

Several considerations should guide future research in this area. First, improved dependent measures that have been psychometrically validated in older subjects are needed. Despite the fact that currently employed measures show few mood benefits of exercise in the elderly, these subjects often perceive subjective benefits of exercise (Emery & Blumenthal, 1990). It is possible that our dependent measures are insensitive to these exercise-induced changes. Additionally, the mechanisms whereby exercise may improve mood and cognitive functioning merit attention.

Three questions are important for geriatric exercise psychology. First, does physical activity throughout the life span enhance psychological functioning and attenuate age-related declines in cognitive performance and mood? Second, can exercise training beginning later in life produce improvements or prevent further declines in psychological functioning in the elderly? Third, are there specific subgroups of older adults (e.g., patients who are depressed, have hypertension, or have pulmonary disease) who may benefit most from exercise? Large-scale prospective longitudinal studies are needed to directly address these questions.

If future research indicates that exercise can attenuate or reverse psychological declines that occur with aging, this provides a strong case for the clinical utility of exercise in the elderly. However, a thorough examination of the cost–benefit ratio of exercise for older adults will be necessary before exercise is universally prescribed for physical and psychological health promotion.

## ACKNOWLEDGMENTS

This chapter was supported in part, by grants from the National Heart, Lung and Blood Institute (HL30675 and HL43028). The authors wish to thank Ms. Janet Ivey for her secretarial assistance.

## REFERENCES

American College of Sports Medicine. (1986). *Guidelines for exercise testing and prescription* (4th ed.).

Åstrand, P.O., & Christensen, E. H. (1964). Aerobic work capacity. In F. Dickens, E. Neil, W. F. Widdas (Eds.), *Oxygen in the animal organism* (p. 295). New York: Pergamon Press.

Åstrand, P. O., & Rodahl, K. (1986). *Textbook of work physiology* (3rd ed.). New York: McGraw-Hill.

Balke, B. (1954). Optimale korperliche leistungfahigkeit, ihre messung und veranderung infolge arbeitsermudung. *Arbeitsphysiology, 15,* 311.

Benestad, A. M. (1965). Trainability of old men. *Acta Medica Scandinavica, 178,* 321–327.

Berger, B. G., & Owen, D. R. (1983). Mood alteration with swimming: Swimmers really do "feel better." *Psychosomatic Medicine, 45,* 425–433.

Blumenthal, J. A., Emery, C. F., Madden, D. J., Coleman, R. E., Riddle, M. W., Schniebolk, S., Cobb, F. R., Sullivan, M. J., & Higginbotham, M. D. (1991). Effects of exercise training on cardiorespiratory function in men and women >60 years of age. *American Journal of Cardiology, 67,* 633–639.

Blumenthal, J. A., Emery, C. F., Madden, D. J., George, L. K., Coleman, R. E., Riddle, M. W., McKee, D. C., Reasoner, J., & Williams, R. S. (1989). Cardiovascular and behavioral effects of aerobic exercise training in healthy older men and women. *Journal of Gerontology, 44,* M147–M157.

Blumenthal, J. A., Emery, C. F., Madden, D. J., Schneibolk, S. S., Walsh-Riddle, M. W., George, L. K., McKee, D. C., Higginbotham, M., Cobb, F. R., & Coleman, R. E. (1991). Long term effects of exercise on psychological functioning in older men and women. *Journal of Gerontology, 46,* 352–361.

Blumenthal, J. A., Emery, C. F., Walsh, M. A., Cox, D. R., Kuhn, C. M., Williams, R. B., & Williams, R. S. (1988). Exercise training in healthy Type A middle-aged men: Effects on behavioral and cardiovascular responses. *Psychosomatic Medicine, 50,* 418–433.

Blumenthal, J. A., Fredrikson, M., Kuhn, C., Ulmer, R. L., Walsh-Riddle, M., & Applebaum, M. (1990). Aerobic exercise reduces levels of cardiovascular and sympathoadrenal responses to mental stress in subjects without prior evidence of myocardial ischemia. *American Journal of Cardiology, 65,* 93–98.

Blumenthal, J. A., & Madden, D. J. (1988). Effects of aerobic exercise training, age, and physical fitness on memory-search performance. *Psychology and Aging, 3,* 280–285.

Blumenthal, J. A., Schocken, D. D., Needels, T. L., & Hindle, P. (1982). Psychological and physiological effects of physical conditioning on the elderly. *Journal of Psychosomatic Research, 26,* 505–510.

Blumenthal, J. A., Williams, S., Needels, T. L., Wallace, A. G. (1982). Psychological changes accompany aerobic exercise in healthy middle-aged adults. *Psychosomatic Medicine, 44,* 529–536.

Botwinick, J. (1977). Intellectual abilities. In J. E. Birren & K. W. Schaie (Eds.), *Handbook of the psychology of aging* (pp. 580–605). New York: Van Nostrand Reinhold.

Botwinick, J. E., & Thompson, L. W. (1968). Age differences in reaction time: An artifact? *Gerontologist, 8,* 25–28.

Bouchard, C., & Malina, R. M. (1983). Genetics of physical fitness and motor performance. *Exercise and Sport Sciences Reviews, 11,* 306.

Brandfonbrenner, M., Landowne, M., & Shock, N. W. (1955). Changes in cardiac output with age. *Circulation, 12,* 557–566.

Bruce, R. A. (1971). Exercise testing of patients with coronary heart disease. *Annals of Clinical Research, 3,* 323.

Bruce, R. A. (1984). Exercise, Functional aerobic capacity, and aging: Another viewpoint. *Medicine and Science in Sports and Exercise, 16,* 8–13.

Buccola, V. A., & Stone, W. J. (1975). Effects of jogging and cycling program on physiological and personality variables in aged men. *Research Quarterly, 46,* 134–139.

Craik, F. I. M. (1977). Age differences in human memory. In J. E. Birren & K. W. Schaie (Eds.), *Handbook of the psychology of aging* (pp. 384–420). New York: Van Nostrand Reinhold.

Crews, D. J., & Landers, D. M. (1987). A meta-analytic review of aerobic fitness and reactivity to psychosocial stressors. *Medicine and Science in Sports and Exercise, 19*(Suppl.), S114–S120.

Dehn, M. M., & Bruce, R. A. (1972). Longitudinal variations in maximal oxygen intake with age and activity. *Journal of Applied Physiology, 33,* 805–807.

deVries, H. A. (1970). Physiological effects of an exercise training program upon men aged 52–88. *Journal of Gerontology, 25,* 325–336.

Dustman, R. E., Ruhling, R. O., Russell, E. M., Shearer, D. E., Bonekat, W., Shigeoka, J. W., Wood, J. S., & Bradford, D. C. (1984). Aerobic exercise training and improved neuropsychological function of older individuals. *Neurobiology of Aging, 5,* 35–42.

Elsayed, M., Ismail, A. H., & Young, R. J. (1980). Intellectual of adult men related to age and physical fitness before and after an exercise program. *Journal of Gerontology, 35,* 383–387.

Emery, C. F., & Blumenthal, J. A. (1990). Perceived change among participants in an exercise program for older adults. *Gerontologist, 30,* 516–521.

Emery, C. F., & Gatz, M. (1990). Psychological and cognitive effects of an exercise program for community-residing older adults. *Gerontologist, 30,* 184–188.

Fillingim, R. B., Roth, D. L., & Cook, E. W. (1989, October 19–22). *The effects of aerobic exercise on subjective and psychophysiological responses to emotional imagery.* Paper presented at the meeting of the Society for Psychophysiological Research, New Orleans, LA.

Fillingim, R. B., Roth, D. L., & Haley, W. E. (1989). The effects of distraction on the perception of exercise-induced symptoms. *Journal of Psychosomatic Research, 33,* 241–248.

Folkins, C. H., & Sime, W. E. (1981). Physical fitness training and mental health. *American Psychologist, 36,* 373–389.

Gitlin, L. N. (1985, March 7). *Psychological effects of physical conditioning in the well elderly.* Paper presented at the second National Forum on Research in Aging: Health, Wellness and Independence, University of Nebraska.

Goldwater, B. C., & Collins, M. L. (1985). Psychological effects of cardiovascular conditioning: A controlled experiment. *Psychosomatic Medicine, 47,* 174–181.

Greist, J. H., Klein, M. H., Eischens, R. R., Faris, J., Gurman, A. S., & Morgan, W. P. (1979). Running as treatment for depression. *Comparative Psychiatry, 20,* 41–54.

Haskell, W. L. (1987). Developing an activity plan for improving health. In W. P. Morgan & S. E. Goldston (Eds.), *Exercise and mental health* (pp. 37–55). Washington, DC: Hemisphere.

Hatfield, B. D., Goldfarb, A. H., Sforzo, G. A., & Flynn, M. G. (1987). Serum beta-endorphin and affective responses to graded exercise in young and elderly men. *Journal of Gerontology, 42,* 429–431.

Hodgson, J. L., & Buskirk, E. R. (1977). Physical fitness and age, with emphasis on cardiovascular function in the elderly. *Journal of the American Geriatric Society, 25,* 385–392.

Holmes, D. S., & McGilley, B. M. (1987). Influence of a brief aerobic training program on heart rate and subjective response to a psychologic stressor. *Psychosomatic Medicine, 49,* 366–374.

Hughes, J. R. (1984). Psychological effects of habitual aerobic exercise: A critical review. *Preventive Medicine, 13,* 66–78.

Hull, E. M., Young, S. H., & Ziegler, M. G. (1984). Aerobic fitness affects cardiovascular and catecholamine responses to stressors. *Psychophysiology, 21,* 353–360.

King, A. C., Taylor, C. B., Haskell, W. L., & DeBusk, R. F. (1990). Influence of regular aerobic exercise on psychological health: A randomized controlled trial of healthy, middle-aged adults. *Health Psychology, 8,* 305–324.

Lakatta, E. G. (1980). Age-related alterations in the cardiovascular response to adrenergic mediated stress. *Federation Proceedings, 39,* 3173.

Leon, A. S., Connett, J., Jacobs, D. R., & Rauramma, R. (1987). Leisure-time physical activity levels and risk of coronary health disease and death: The multiple risk factor intervention trial. *Journal of the American Medical Association, 258,* 2388–2395.

Light, K. C., Obrist, P. A., James, S. A., & Strogatz, D. S. (1987). Cardiovascular responses to stress: II. Relationships to aerobic exercise patterns. *Psychophysiology, 24,* 79–86.

Madden, D. J., Blumenthal, J. A., Allen, P. A., & Emery, C. F. (1989). Improving aerobic capacity in healthy older adults does not necessarily lead to improved cognitive performance. *Psychology and Aging, 4,* 307–320.

McGowan, C. R., Robertson, R. J., & Epstein, L. H. (1985). The effect of bicycle ergometer exercise at varying intensities on the heart rate, EMG and mood state responses to a mental arithmetic stressor. *Research Quarterly for Exercise and Sport, 56,* 131–137.

Molloy, D. W., Beerschoten, D. A., Borrie, M. J., Crilly, R. G., & Cape, R. D. T. (1988). Acute effects of exercise on neuropsychological function in elderly subjects. *Journal of the American Geriatric Society, 36,* 29–33.

Morgan, W. P., & Goldston, S. E. (Eds.) (1987). *Exercise and mental health.* Washington, DC: Hemisphere.

Paffenbarger, R. S., Hyde, R. T., Irving, A. S., & Steinmetz, C. H. (1984). A natural history of athleticism and cardiovascular health. *Journal of the American Medical Association, 252,* 491–495.

Panton, L. B., Graves, J. E., Pollock, M. L., Hagberg, J. M., & Chen, W. (1990). Effect of aerobic and resistance training on fractionated reaction time and speed of movement. *Journal of Gerontology, 45,* M26–M31.

Peronnet, F., Massicotte, D., Paquee, J. E., Brisson, G., & de Champlain, J. (1989). Blood pressure and catecholamine responses to various challenges during exercise–recovery in man. *European Journal of Applied Physiology, 58,* 551–555.

Perri, S., & Templer, D. (1984–1985). The effects of an aerobic exercise program on psychological variables in older adults. *International Journal of Aging and Human Development, 20,* 167–172.

Pfeiffer, E. (1977). Psychopathology and social pathology. In J. E. Birren & K. W. Schaie (Eds.), *Handbook of the psychology of aging* (pp. 650–671). New York: Van Nostrand Reinhold.

Pollock, M. L., Wilmore, J. H., & Fox, S. M., III (1978). Health and fitness through physical activity. *American College of Sports Medicine Series.* New York: Wiley.

Port, S., Cobb, F. R., Coleman, R. E., & Jones, R. H. (1980). Effect of age on the response of the left ventricular ejection fraction to exercise. *New England Journal of Medicine, 303,* 1133–1137.

Powell, R. R. (1974). Psychological effects of exercise therapy upon institutionalized geriatric mental patients. *Journal of Gerontology, 29,* 157–161.

Rerych, S. K., Scholz, P. M., Sabiston, D. C., & Jones, R. H. (1980). Effects of exercise training on left ventricular function in normal subjects: A longitudinal study by radionuclide angiography. *American Journal of Cardiology, 45,* 244–252.

Rikli, R., & Busch, S. (1986). Motor function of women as a function of age and activity level. *Journal of Gerontology, 41,* 645–649.

Rodeheffer, R. J., Gerstenblith, G., Becker, L. C., Fleg, J. L., Weisfeldt, M. L., & Lakatta, E. G. (1984). Exercise cardiac output is maintained with advancing age in healthy human subjects: Cardiac dilatation and stroke volume compensate for a diminished heart rate. *Circulation, 69,* 203–213.

Roskies, E., Seraganian, P., Oseasohn, R., Hanley, J. A., Collu, R., Martin, N., & Smilga, C. (1986). The Montreal Type A intervention project: Major findings. *Health Psychology, 5,* 45–69.

Roth, D. L. (1989). Acute emotional and psychophysiological effects of aerobic exercise. *Psychophysiology, 26,* 593–602.

Roth, D. L., & Holmes, D. S. (1987). Influence of aerobic exercise training and relaxation training on physical and psychologic health following stressful life events. *Psychosomatic Medicine, 49,* 355–365.

Roth, D. L., & Shay, K. A. (1990). Effects of regular aerobic exercise on acute cardiovascular responses to a mental stressor in young and older adults. *Psychophysiology, 27,* S61.

Scheuer, J., & Tipton, C. M. (1977). Cardiovascular adaptations to physical training. *Annual Review of Physiology, 39,* 222–251.

Seals, D. R., Hagberg, J. M., Hurley, B. F., Ehsani, A. A., & Holloszy, J. O. (1984). Endurance training in older men and women: I. Cardiovascular responses to exercise. *Journal of Applied Physiology, 57,* 1024–1029.

Shay, K. A., & Roth, D. L. (1991). *The association of aerobic fitness and visuospatial performance in healthy older adults.* Manuscript submitted for publication.

Sherwood, A., Light, K. C., & Blumenthal, J. A. (1989). Effects of aerobic exercise on hemodynamic responses during psychosocial stress in normotensive and borderline hypertensive Type A men: A preliminary report. *Psychosomatic Medicine, 51,* 123–136.

Simons, C. W., & Birkimer, J. C. (1988). An exploration of factors predicting the effects of aerobic conditioning on mood state. *Journal of Psychosomatic Research, 32,* 63–85.

Sinyor, D. S., Golden, M., Steinert, Y., & Seraganian, P. (1986). Experimental manipulation of aerobic fitness and the response to psychosocial stress: Heart rate and self-report measures. *Psychosomatic Medicine, 48,* 324–337.

Sonstroem, R. J. (1984). Exercise and self-esteem. In R. L. Terjung (Ed.), *Exercise and sports sciences reviews* (Vol. 12, pp. 123–155). Lexington, MA: The Collamore Press.

Spirduso, W. W. (1975). Reaction and movement time as a function of age and physical activity level. *Journal of Gerontology, 30,* 435–440.

Spirduso, W. W. (1980). Physical fitness, aging, and psychomotor speed: A review. *Journal of Gerontology, 35,* 850–865.

Spirduso, W. W., & Clifford, P. (1978). Replication of age and physical activity effects on reaction and movement time. *Journal of Gerontology, 33,* 25–30.

Stacey, C., Kozma, A., & Stones, M. J. (1985). Simple cognitive and behavioral changes resulting from improved physical fitness in persons over 50 years of age. *Canadian Journal on Aging, 4,* 67–74.

Stamford, B. A., Hambacher, W., & Fallica, A. (1974). Effects of daily physical exercise on the psychiatric state of institutionalized geriatric mental patients. *Research Quarterly, 45,* 34–41.

Stones, M. J., & Kozma, A. (1988). Physical activity, age and cognitive motor performance. In M. L. Howe & C. I. Brainerd (Eds.), Cognitive development in adulthood (pp. 293–321). NY: Springer.

Stones, M. J., & Kozma, A. (1989). Age, exercise, and coding performance. *Psychology and Aging, 4,* 190–194.

Strandell, T. (1976a). Cardiac output in old age. In F. T. Caird, J. L. C. Doll, & R. D. Kennedy (Eds.), *Cardiology in old age* (pp. 81–99). New York: Plenum.

Strandell, T. (1976b). Circulatory studies on healthy old men. *Acta Medica Scandinavica , 414*(Suppl.), 1–43.

Tomporowski, P. D., & Ellis, N. R. (1986). Effects of exercise on cognitive processes: A review. *Psychological Bulletin, 99,* 338–346.

Valliant, P. M., & Asu, M. E. (1985). Exercise and its effects on cognition and physiology in older adults. *Perceptual and Motor Skills, 63,* 955–961.

Van Doornen, L. J. P., & de Geus, E. J. C. (1989). Aerobic fitness and the cardiovascular response to stress. *Psychophysiology, 26,* 17–28.

Zillmann, D. (1983). Transfer of excitation of emotional behavior. In J. T. Cacioppo & R. E. Petty (Eds.), *Social psychophysiology: A sourcebook* (pp. 215–240). New York:

# 10

# Social-Psychological Aspects of Fitness Promotion

**LAWRENCE R. BRAWLEY AND WENDY M. RODGERS**

## FITNESS PROMOTION: IS THERE A NEED?

Physical fitness has become a more visible social phenomenon than ever before in North America. Some indicators, such as the growth of recreational and health facilities over the past 15 years, the increased media coverage of fitness and of sport events, might give most people the impression that physical fitness is news, of societal importance as an aspect of leisure, and is self-promoting. Participation in exercise as leisure appears to be on the rise. Why discuss the promotion of fitness when the phenomenon is apparently selling itself?

However, is this leisure-time phenomenon really affecting that many people? Although participation in physical fitness activities is more visible in the popular media and is having a large commercial impact, it is questionable as to whether more people are really more active. Reviews by Wankel (1988) and epidemiological studies by Sallis and Hovell (1990) provide sobering evidence to the contrary. For example, 70–80% of American adults are sedentary (Dishman, 1988). In cases where greater rates of participation in fitness activities are reported by adults, it is often those who are already active who are increasing their physical activity, not those who are sedentary (Wankel, 1988). Powell, Spain, Christenson, and Mollenkamp (1986) report cross-age-group comparisons of participation rates where the current levels of physical activity in 1986 were contrasted with the U.S. Public Health Service's goals for physical activity in 1990. Not only do these comparisons show a tremendous decline in physical activity with age (i.e., from 65% participation at ages 10–17 to 15% at ages 18–64, with the same or lower rates beyond age 50), they also show that rates in 1986 were between 25 and 45% less than the goal rates for 1990. There is little evidence to suggest that participation rates have improved drastically since 1986.

Statistics about participants' adherence to various forms of physical activity in both normal and clinical settings are equally sobering. An often-cited statistic about most of these programs is that the dropout rate can be as high as 50% within the first 6 months of participation (Dishman, 1988). There is also evidence that the rate can equal or exceed this in community-based fitness programs within 10–12 weeks (e.g., Brawley & Horne, 1987). These nonadherence rates are not unique to normal adult programs of structured exercise. When exercise program rates are considered across activity types and settings, normal and clinical groups, as well as when exercise is a treatment modality, statistics on dropout are similar. Furthermore, the dropout rate and pattern is similar to others observed in programs of change for other health behaviors, such as weight loss, smoking cessation, control of hypertension, and psychotherapy (cf. Dishman, 1988; Meichenbaum & Turk, 1987). On the basis of exercise, health, and leisure dropout statistics, it is reasonable to question whether the efforts to promote physical fitness have been successful. These data force scientists interested in exercise both as a leisure activity and as a health activity to conclude that much more should be done. For the nonactive segment of the population, the goal should be to have more of these people initiate exercise and thereby decrease the number of sedentary individuals in the population. The second goal should be to increase the rate of participation for those individuals who are only sporadically active (e.g., 1–4 times per month). Efforts to promote fitness activities address both of these goals.

However, reasons for fitness-promotion efforts go beyond altering the scope of the public's rate of leisure-time involvement in exercise. The health-related outcomes associated with physical-fitness involvement are more important from a societal perspective than ever before. If positive health outcomes lessen the treatment demand on a struggling primary health-care system, then fitness and its promotion become part of society's effort to change health care from being a sole responsibility of governments to the responsibility of the individual (Matarazzo, 1980).

To illustrate, consider the following health benefits thought to be accrued as a result of exercise participation. Physical fitness has been associated with the positive outcomes of better *mental* health and well-being (Morgan & Goldston, 1987); for example, lowered mental stress has been associated with increased exercise (Morgan & O'Connor, 1988). Also, increased physical fitness is now commonly acknowledged as desirable for *physical* health reasons (Powell, 1988), such as reduced risk of cardiovascular disease. Powell (1988) discussed a variety of important health conditions related to habitual exercise from an epidemiological perspective; he noted that the available evidence suggested that habitual exercise not only reduced the risk of cardiac arrest but also helped to lower hypertension. He also reported positive signs that habitual physical activity (a) may be inversely related to osteoporosis, (b) may provide some benefit for diabetic children, (c) may aid in the management of lower-back pain, and (d) may beneficially affect weight control. Adverse effects of exercise, such as injuries, are potential risks, but they are largely outweighed by the potential individual health benefits to be gained.

Powell (1988) further noted that the relation of exercise to health should be considered not only for the individual (i.e., the clinical or medical concern) but also in terms of its impact on a community or society (i.e., the public health concern). Just as the various aforementioned health conditions (e.g., cardiovascular disease) have a large impact on the community and demand the attention of public-health advocates, so also does habitual exercise because it seems to prevent or slow the progress of these negative health conditions.

It is therefore apparent that there are health reasons for individuals to exercise and for society to adopt exercise as a disease prevention, health-promotion activity. However, the benefits to be gained are not likely to be realized through current rates of participation. The promotion of fitness is obviously required at both the individual and the community or societal level if such benefits are to be achieved. How might promotion be attempted from a social-psychological viewpoint?

## CHAPTER OBJECTIVES: PSYCHOLOGICAL ASPECTS OF PROMOTION

From a psychological perspective, the approaches to physical-fitness promotion for an individual and for a community of individuals are quite different. At the individual level, behavior-change strategies such as stimulus control and positive reinforcement have been used. At the community or mass-change level, mass-media campaigns (e.g., Canada: "Participation") are used in attempts to promote normative expectancy change, to educate regarding the benefits or outcomes of exercise, and to offer exercise as a leisure alternative. This chapter cannot serve as a review of all the efforts that have been attempted to promote fitness from a psychological perspective. A number of authors have compiled the evidence about efforts geared to individual physical-fitness promotion (e.g., Wankel, 1987). Others have written articles suggesting what could be done but has not yet been attempted. One of the most recent that has compiled research evidence and made thoughtful suggestions has been a well-organized chapter by Knapp (1988) in Dishman's (1988) landmark text on exercise adherence. The present chapter does not reinvent the wheel by reiterating all of Knapp's points. Instead, the objective of this chapter is first to review Knapp's individualized approach to fitness promotion, and second to extend the discussion of fitness promotion by addressing mass-promotion approaches that Knapp considers important but admittedly ignores.

The title of the chapter indicates that it concerns social-psychological aspects of fitness promotion. The reader will find that some of the topics discussed would more probably be categorized as behavioral, cognitive-behavioral, or clinical in other psychology texts. However, all of the techniques to change behavior primarily occur in a social context, where change regimens either have been assigned by others or are attempted with others. The adherence to or compliance with these regimens becomes a social-psychological phenomenon because of this social involvement. Readers should keep this underlying idea in mind as they consider the ideas throughout the chapter.

## THE DYNAMIC EXERCISE CYCLE AND FITNESS PROMOTION

Promotion of exercise and physical activity in general must be considered in the context of three phases in the dynamic cycle of exercise. These are Phase 1, the sedentary phase; Phase 2, exercise initiation and adoption, then dropout or relapse followed by exercise resumption; and Phase 3, exercise maintenance. These three phases of the exercise cycle are similar to Sallis and Hovell's (1990) epidemiological description of a person's exercise history and includes Knapp's (1988) three-stage habit-acquisition process of (1) the decision to start exercising, (2) the early stages of behavior change, and (3) maintenance of the new behavior. From a psychological perspective, promotion strategies in each phase should be related. Ideally, each successive phase of people's exercise histories should build on the previous phase, from the time people start a program through the period where they consistently maintain it by self-regulation. From a psychological perspective, that period of time allows for substantial social learning to occur. This social learning involves the experience of various forms of exercise as people move from being relatively sedentary, to exercise initiation and adoption, to maintenance/dropout, to once again resuming exercise (see Figure 10.1).

This cycle occurs over time and describes an exercise behavior pattern that may characterize a large proportion of the people who normally would be involved in exercise at levels of varying intensity over a period of months or years. For example, people wishing to become involved for the first time may maintain a steady level of exercise when they first begin, but for a variety of reasons, they may choose to stop exercising. Unless the experience is totally unpleasant, individuals resume exercising at some later point, perhaps becoming a bit more consistent in their exercise behavior. The cycle continues to be observed, although its duration may wax and wane, according to other demands in each individual's life. Evidence of this pattern can be found in epidemiological reviews (e.g., Sallis & Hovell, 1990) and has also been illustrated in Dishman's (1988) text on exercise adherence.

Why is it important to acknowledge this cycle and take it into account relative to fitness promotion? One important reason is that the specific contents of individualized behavior-change approaches (see Knapp, 1988) or mass-promotion efforts would need to be adjusted in response to this cycle. This adjustment would involve both content and social-psychological dimensions in order to be relevant to the particular stage of the exercise

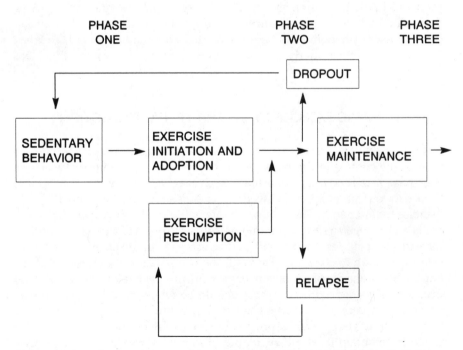

**Figure 10.1.**   The dynamic exercise cycle (adapted from Sallis & Hovell, 1990).

cycle in which target individuals are involved. For example, the specific content of the social-persuasion techniques used to encourage a beginning exerciser to take part would differ from the content used to persuade individuals at other phases of the exercise cycle. This is discussed further later in this chapter.

## ADHERENCE OR COMPLIANCE?

Before beginning the discussion of the two broad categories of fitness promotion (i.e., for individuals and for communities), it is important to define and thus distinguish between two behavioral concepts often used interchangeably: *adherence* and *compliance*. The basic idea behind fitness promotion is to encourage a greater degree of adherence to, or compliance with, physical activity. However, these concepts are not synonymous. The promotion approach used may differ, depending on whether the individual *chooses to adhere to* or *must comply with* ongoing physical activity. To understand the significance of differentiating between these terms, it is probably best to focus on the motivational difference.

### Compliance

As discussed by Meichenbaum and Turk (1987) in their book *Facilitating Treatment Adherence, compliance* concerns the extent to which people obey and follow the instructions or prescriptions of health or exercise care providers. Motivationally, it connotes a more passive role on the part of the participant, where he or she faithfully follows advice. *Noncompliance* is often the view taken by the exercise or health-care provider that the participant is at fault when failing to comply. This view may have impact on the motivational and individual behavioral techniques that the exercise provider decides to impose in order to remedy apparent problems of compliance. The view that the participant is at fault may encourage the provider to be even more behaviorally controlling or constraining so that the participant has no choice but to comply.

An example may help to illustrate. The well-intentioned exercise leader attempts to get an overweight, 50-year-old male, advised by his doctor to exercise, to follow American Congress of Sport Medicine (ACSM) guidelines in order to develop an exercise training effect. Substantive research evidence suggests that compliance with these guidelines produces desired outcomes of weight loss, improved cardiac output, and increased muscular endurance and strength. The guidelines specify that the graded exercise regimen include specific frequency, intensity, and duration aspects, tailored to the individual's level of age, health, and fitness. The formula, tested in controlled conditions, *works*.

However, our 50-year-old male was not consulted as to how difficult he perceives it will be to follow the exercise prescription. With good intentions, the exercise leader concludes that this regimen is best to produce outcomes quickly. The 50-year-old initially tries hard to comply but finds it too difficult to adjust the prescription to fit with his busy schedule, travel, and varying levels of start-up fatigue. A later fitness test reveals that compliance to ACSM exercise guidelines has been poor because the expected exercise outcomes are not evident. The exercise provider suspects that a lack of willpower and time conflicts among work, exercise, and famiiy are the problems. He prescribes further change, by suggesting other techniques, that would help to manage the behavior if they were followed. He recommends an early morning workout bout, to help avoid scheduling problems, and a health-and-exercise diary, to log the degree of compliance with the nutrition-and-exercise regimen. On the surface, it looks good. Our 50-year-old male will still have a full work day after exercise, and the diary will help provide both feedback and an awareness of progress to the exerciser.

One month later, after a second fitness test, the same fitness levels still exist, and it is obvious that the exerciser did not comply. What happened? A simple behavioral analysis reveals that even though the 50-year-old believed that the exercise regimen would work within his current life-style, it was too hard. There was no reevaluation of the compliance regimen between provider and exerciser when difficulties arose. The social role of the provider was to *provide* and the social role of the 50-year-old was to *follow* in terms of frequency (times per week), intensity (130+ heart rate), and duration (30–40 minutes/session). Also, the exerciser was to train early in the morning and to record everything on a daily basis. Generally, this involved at least *five* types of behavior to follow, without guidance regarding what to adjust, and without provider–participant discussion regarding the level of motivational and behavioral difficulty for each of the five types.

The unwritten philosophy was *"Just Do It"* because it's good for you and you know it. While this makes the exercise provider sound unfeeling and the participant unthinking, the noninteractive nature of this compliance example illustrates a situation where the exerciser is just *not* motivated to "do it." This behavioral attempt at fitness promotion failed because the motivational aspects of the compliance social situation were not well understood by either the exercise provider or the participant.

### Adherence

What qualities would this situation have had if we had discussed *adherence*? According to Meichenbaum and Turk (1987), *adherence* implies a person's freely chosen involvement. Thus, adherence would involve following one's own exercise regimen or choosing to follow one provided by someone else. At minimum, it concerns a perceived choice about action, and an acceptance of performing specified actions. Adherence to behaviors or plans based on provider–adherer collaboration may be higher than those simply specified by others. This is because the adherer may be more committed to actions that they perceive to be partly their own ideas (e.g., Marlatt & Kaplan, 1972). In the case of our 50-year-old male example, *collaboration with* the well-intentioned exercise provider would have created conditions for exercise adherence rather than complying with prescribed exercise.

While the social-situational conditions that would characterize adherence seem desirable from a fitness-promotion perspective, the dynamic nature of adhering to or complying with behavior in stages of the exercise cycle can vary. Perceptions of freely chosen action may be altered or overridden by failures to quickly achieve desired exercise outcomes (e.g., weight loss). The adherer's initial confidence or self-efficacy for following a freely chosen exercise regimen may be dashed after experiencing initial muscle soreness. The relative difficulty of adherence is quickly revealed when considering the incidence of nonadherence. As noted earlier in this chapter, nonadherence rates exceeding 60% for freely chosen exercise programs (cf. Dishman, 1988) show that even though trying to adhere may be more motivating than trying to comply, it is still difficult for most people. If exercise was a behavior characterized by a uniquely high level of nonadherence, perhaps our approaches to and concern for this problem would be different. However, many health behavior-change programs have similar nonadherence rates. These rates cut across factors such as race, complexity of treatment, duration of therapy, and exercisers' beliefs in the effectiveness of health-promotion actions (cf. Epstein & Masek, 1978). Is there any hope for reducing these rates? A qualified "yes" is the answer.

## APPROACHES TO FITNESS PROMOTION

As mentioned previously, two broad approaches have been taken toward promoting fitness and reducing rates of nonadherence and noncompliance: (1) individual and small-group behavioral- and cognitive-change strategies, and (2) promotion and change through mass-media social-psychological strategies. The first approach has received far more attention in the exercise-psychology literature than the second. For example, Knapp (1988) and others have discussed the first approach extensively, and the success of similar strategies have been thoroughly analyzed in reviews of other health-promotion topics (e.g., obesity: Kirschenbaum, 1992; general treatment adherence: Meichenbaum & Turk, 1987).

In most cases, the discussion on the following pages presumes that the individual has voluntarily chosen to exercise. A number of the topics discussed can also apply to the situations requiring compliance. However, for many people the decision to begin or maintain exercise will be made under *voluntary* conditions. Therefore, the fitness promoter will be attempting to encourage either exercise initiation and/or *adherence* to the goal of increased involvement.

## THE PROCESS OF INCREASING EXERCISE: BEHAVIORAL-MANAGEMENT TECHNIQUES

Knapp (1988) discussed various approaches to the behavioral management of increasing exercise by indicating which approaches are appropriate to each of the various stages of the exercise cycle.

### The Decision to Start Exercise

**Education.** Techniques used at this stage have had an educational focus. Two major educational models have been suggested for use. These are the health-belief model (Becker, 1976) and the self-regulation model (Meyer, Leventhal, & Gutmann, 1985). A common approach in using these models is to educate exercisers about the benefits of exercise.

In the case of the health-belief model, beliefs about susceptibility to disease, the severity or evaluation of the consequences of contracting the disease, beliefs about barriers to health actions against the disease, and beliefs about the effectiveness of a particular health action are the major belief factors. For those individuals concerned about health problems (e.g., cardiac-rehabilitation patients), the education to change beliefs and to initiate a step toward exercise would be a reasonable place to focus efforts to encourage exercise initiation. The model has had limited success at predicting adherence in an exercise context (see Sonstroem, 1988). This may be because it emphasizes the motivation to avoid illness, and there are many reasons other than this why exercisers wish to begin exercising.

The self-regulatory model assumes that regulation involves two facets that occur simultaneously and that often are in conflict within the individual. These self-regulatory processes involve health, physical fitness, resistance to disease, and affect (e.g., fear). The presumption is that if some negative aspect about a health-risk factor is made clear via education this may get people to understand and know what is at risk. As a result of the initiate exerciser understanding, the fitness promoter hopes that if exercise is perceived as a deterrent to the health risk, people will logically self-regulate behavior by increasing exercise in order to reduce the risk. They also reduce any fear associated with the risk by taking this action.

Unfortunately, simply providing nonexercisers with education based on either of these models has been ineffective in promoting exercise initiation unless a number of conditions are met. Knapp (1988) suggests that the following belief conditions are necessary for prompting the initiation of exercise: (a) perceived vulnerability to a health problem that can be countered by exercise, (b) belief in the negative consequences of the health problem so that reinforcement salience to avoid the problem is high, (c) belief that exercise will counter the problem, (d) belief that negative perceived exercise side effects (e.g., muscle soreness) do not outweigh the perceived personal benefits of exercise, and (e) belief in the personal ability to carry out the exercise regimen. The problems with the self-regulation approach (at least in using vulnerability to disease as a key belief) is that many individuals view themselves as invulnerable to risk. Weinstein (1984) points out that an individual's optimistic biases about health risk relative to similar others may counter simple education attempts to promote self-regulation of health behaviors (e.g., exercise).

The attention given both the health-belief and the self-regulation models as applied to exercise is minimal. In both cases, changes for their success would be increased (1) by directing their use toward fitness promotion for specific target groups having a health risk, and (2) by ensuring that a variety of secondary, but equally important exercise-related beliefs are met.

**Decision Strategies.**   Decisions to initiate exercise have also been influenced by a number of strategies designed to facilitate effective decision-making. These procedures, Knapp (1988) suggests, may promote the salience of the costs and benefits of exercise, as well as the salience of personal health vulnerability for diseases where exercise is thought to reduce health risk.

Two techniques that appear to be useful are the decision-balance sheet (Hoyt & Janis, 1975), and the decision matrix (Marlatt & Gordon, 1985). Both procedures require the individual to record anticipated positive and negative consequences of exercise participation in terms of gains and losses. In the case of the decision-balance sheet technique for the initiate exerciser, the gains and losses to self and important others as well as self and others' approval and disapproval are considered. Wankel (see review, 1987) has used both this technique and variations of it to produce short-term adherence-rate increases among female exercisers.

In the case of the decision-matrix technique, while the approach was designed with respect to countering relapse in smoking cessation, Knapp (1988) believes that it may be useful for initiating exercise. Individuals are asked to list short- and long-term positive and negative consequences of regular participation in exercise and of not participating in exercise (either not initiating it or, for relapse, dropping out of it). The individual not only considers the gains/losses as in the decision-balance procedure, but also differentiates among various short- and long-term positive and negative consequences of exercising and of failing to exercise.

Both decision-making procedures require that potential exercise initiates discuss their decisions with a leader or a counselor. Depending on the procedure, desired responses are reinforced and various coping strategies that encourage initiation and discourage exercise problems are discussed. Thus, the procedures require some initial collaboration that may enhance commitment. The question that may be raised, however, is whether the exerciser is sufficiently knowledgeable to do collaborative decision making. Collaboration and listing of pluses and minuses may be more motivational at the initial decision-making stage.

**Self-Efficacy Enhancement.** Also useful in promoting the decision to start exercise are strategies for enhancing *self-efficacy* (situation-specific self-confidence). Knapp (1988) discusses these strategies from a behavioral-management perspective. The theoretical basis for self-efficacy has been outlined elsewhere by Bandura (1977, 1986). There is a growing body of evidence that suggests that the impact of a variety of different treatment modalities is partly a function of the influence of perceived self-efficacy. This includes exercise as a health-behavior modality (see Bandura, 1991). Basically, Bandura postulates (if we use the exercise context as the example) that an individual's motivation to undertake exercise is a function of two beliefs. These are the person's perceived self-efficacy for actually doing the behaviors associated with various aspects of the exercise context *and* the person's perception of the possible outcomes that might be expected as a result of completing exercise-related behavior (i.e., outcome expectancy). An individual might have the self-efficacy to complete exercise behaviors, but without a foreseeable, valued outcome, there is little incentive to engage in exercise. An individual's self-efficacy for personal exercise skills and abilities are the beliefs that she or he can perform various aspects of exercise (including beliefs about personal level of proficiency). Outcome expectancy, as defined by Bandura, is not simply the completion of the exercise itself, but rather expectancies about eventual outcomes, such as weight loss, praise for exercise achievements from others, or self-acknowledgment of improved appearance.

Self-efficacy and outcome expectancies are a function of past social learning, and therefore, such beliefs and expectancies may be modified or enhanced through behavior management. In the case of those deciding to initiate exercise, the increased belief in exercise self-efficacy and/or attaining a valued outcome may make the decision easier and may tip the scales in favor of exercise.

Direct or vicarious experience with exercise activity are two aspects of social learning thought to enhance both self-efficacy and outcome expectancies (see Bandura, 1986). Accordingly, the use of behavioral-management techniques of modeling and behavioral rehearsal may encourage changes in self-efficacy or outcome expectancies. Using the example of the 50-year-old male discussed earlier, the modeling approach would encourage vicarious experience of this person via observation of other similar 50-year-olds exercising at a level the observer thinks that he could achieve. Self-efficacy is indirectly encouraged through the notion, "If they can do it, I can do it." By contrast, a poor modeling situation may be having this same 50-year-old observer watch the fit 20- to 30-year-old, in tight-fitting spandex, exercise to the latest "rap" or "rock n' roll" music.

Behavioral rehearsal allows the exercise initiate to actually try the exercise in a manner that maximizes successful performance accompanied by reinforcing feedback. Self-efficacy is encouraged because it is obvious to the 50-year-old that he has completed the exercise behavior and knows what he did right and wrong. Research evidence exists for these strategies. For example, Ewart, Taylor, Reese, and DeBusk (1983) demonstrated that post-myocardial-infarction patients who completed exercise testing (e.g., treadmill test) early in their rehabilitative program (i.e., direct experience and behavioral rehearsal) had increased their perceived self-efficacy for related forms of exercise such as stair-climbing, running, or walking. In the case of a university sample, Rodgers and Brawley (1991b) found that persons who were beginning weight training had, after exposure to a 2-day "how to weight-train" clinic, increased their self-efficacy beliefs about their ability to succeed in weight training on their own, as well as outcome expectations for their increased strength. Both efficacy and outcome expectations predicted these beginners' future intentions to engage in weight training on their own.

One of the more neglected aspects of fitness promotion is understanding *why* people begin exercising. About this, we know very little, according to Sallis and Hovell (1990). Although various educational and behavior-management strategies can encourage the first steps toward exercise, actual investigation of why people begin has not, until recently, received systematic attention. In most cases, where it has received attention (e.g., participation motivation research: Gould, 1987; exercise goals: Canada Fitness Survey, Fitness and Lifestyle in Canada, 1983; Miller Brewing Company, Miller Lite Report of American Attitudes Toward Sport, 1983), there has been no theoretical basis for the examination of the phenomenon. This has been the case even though there have been existing theories that could easily have served as a basis for the beginning of investigations as to why people begin to exercise.

One approach that has been suggested as a basis for future investigation of the participation-motivation literature is the use of a modified version of self-efficacy theory (see Rodgers & Brawley, 1991a). The modification is one proposed by Maddux, Norton, and Stoltenberg (1986). Essentially, they postulate that both the value and the likelihood of an outcome are important, in order for the outcome to have any impact on the intent to behave. Value of outcome has also been emphasized by Lau, Hartman, and Ware (1986) with respect to linking beliefs about health outcomes to behavior. They note that desirable health behaviors are unlikely to occur without the anticipated outcomes or consequences being valued by the individual.

Rodgers and Brawley (1991a) proposed the use of outcome likelihood (OL) and outcome value (OV) as a conceptual combination and operational definition of outcome expectancy in the study of participation motivation.

Evidence for the use of self-efficacy theory and the combined OL and OV version of outcome expectancy has been shown in the aforementioned setting for beginners at a weight-training clinic. In this case, intentions to begin weight training independently at the outset of the clinic was related to initial outcome expectations for an increase in strength as a result of training. Although the variable most predictive of later intent to train was self-efficacy, an outcome expectation for increased strength was the initial motivating variable (Rodgers & Brawley, 1991b).

Desharnais, Bouillon, and Godin (1986) also examined the use of outcome expectancy (OV x OL) and self-efficacy in predicting future intentions to exercise among participants in an exercise setting. Although these participants were not beginners, both outcome expectancy and self-efficacy acted in linear fashion to predict exercise intention. While these studies are only suggestive of the impact of outcome expectations in the initial decision to begin exercise (or to maintain exercise), they do offer a theoretical and methodological basis for systematically investigating why people begin to exercise (also see Dzewaltowski, 1989). Self-efficacy theory can also be a useful model to consider for mass-promotion efforts, and this is discussed more later in this chapter.

Concerning the second (adoption) and third (maintenance) phases of the exercise cycle, many of the individualized approaches to promoting fitness activity have to do with encouraging an increase in the amount of activity and the transition to maintaining this level of activity. Some of these strategies are examined next.

## Promotion Strategies for Exercise Adoption

Knapp (1988) argues that behavior patterns are sustained because they are both cued and socially reinforced by environmental factors. She breaks the behavior chain into an antecedent–behavior–consequence sequence, in which habit modification and environmental change are targeted. With respect to antecedents or competing cues (e.g., exercise versus eating), stimulus-control techniques are advised. As to the behavior (exercise) itself, skill training or type of exercise prescription is the focus. Finally, in regard to consequences, techniques such as contingency management or contracting are advised. As the reader will no doubt recognize, many of these suggestions are rooted in a behavior-therapy tradition.

**Managing Behavioral Antecedents.** Two categories of management strategies are those in which (a) the objective is to increase exercise cues, and (b) the objective is to decrease competing behavioral cues. Strategies for increasing exercise cues have been to ensure that the behavioral and environmental cues are consistent for every bout of exercise (e.g., time, location, warm-up pattern). Also, the use of logs for recording exercise behavior is an example of *self-monitoring*, a technique that heightens awareness of major exercise cues. Simply attending a structured exercise class supplies the participant with many of the initial stimulus controls. However, this provision does not encourage development of self-managed exercise programs beyond the limits or duration of the structured program. For this purpose, Knapp (1988) suggests building a means for generalizing stimulus control into the teaching of the formal program. The purpose of the suggestion is to wean the participants to a self-regulated pattern of exercise, where they adjust the various antecedents to their own exercise. Examples of controlled studies of these suggestions are those by Keefe and Blumenthal (1980) in managing consistency of time, location, warm-up; Nelson, Haynes, Spong, Jarrett, and McKnight (1983) for exercise self-monitoring; and Martin and numerous colleagues (1984) in a series of studies designed to prepare subjects for self-regulating exercise after a structured program.

Strategies for decreasing the cues for behaviors competing with and/or problematic to exercise appear to be less well investigated. Competing behaviors could be various family obligations, time and work demands, other attractive leisure pursuits, or social obligations. The suggested strategies Knapp describes are choosing an exercise location and time away from competing behaviors—for example, exercising in the morning prior to work. Another example would be taking exercise gear to work, in order to avoid coming home to exercise, where numerous competing behaviors await.

Unfortunately, as a means of reducing inconsistent exercise behavior or dropout, only the logic of this strategy is apparent, and no empirical evidence supports it. Also, although some of the competing cues have been discussed in the literature as barriers to ongoing participation, the difficulty with this conceptualization is that the degree to which something is an obstacle or barrier as opposed to whether it is an attractive, competing cue is open to question. The ways in which the researchers obtained the subjects' responses about barriers or competing cues in adherence studies may leave questions as to whether these alternative cues are (a) simply attributions for why individuals dropped out of a program rather than the real causes, (b) actually available in sufficient quantity and strength to compete with exercise, and (c) of sufficient importance to the subject for them to adopt an alternative behavioral strategy in response to the competing cues. Only empirical evidence will give a clear answer. Both the measurement of competing alternatives/barriers and the testing of behavioral strategies is required to ascertain an answer. In addition, if successful strategies are developed, there will also be the question about the target audience most receptive to the strategies. It is interesting to note that in the Canada Fitness

Survey, when people were asked about potential changes in life that would increase their activity, there was a much greater percentage of those already active who said that changes would further encourage their activity than of those who were sedentary (see Wankel, 1988).

**Managing Behavioral Consequences.** Knapp (1988) discusses a variety of consequences in terms of those that are reinforcing and those that are punishing. The former type is thought to increase the likelihood of a behavior when repeated in similar situations, and the latter is thought to decrease it.

Reinforcement can be discussed from both a negative and positive viewpoint. Both negative and positive reinforcers enhance the probability that behavior following either type of reinforcement will be repeated in future. When a person wishes to positively reinforce a behavior, some kind of rewarding stimulus follows the behavior. These reinforcements could be simple knowledge of the results, positive encouragement, the receipt of a T-shirt or other tangible reward acknowledging goal attainment (i.e., performance-contingent reward), self-reinforcement, or social support. The techniques that may be effective in increasing positive reinforcement are provisions of social support, self-monitoring, goal setting, provision of material rewards, and self-reinforcement.

Negative reinforcers are things that are withdrawn following a behavior. The everyday method of doing this involves escaping from stimuli perceived as unpleasant. Repetition of this tactic often leads to avoidance behavior. In the exercise context, examples of aversive reminders that people seek to avoid (i.e., thus reducing their exercise behavior) would be the exercise partner or leader making remarks perceived as critical, threatening, or overly controlling. The exerciser may seek to avoid the source of the remarks, which in turn, leads to not exercising in that context.

Punishment is another behavioral consequence that may require management. Evidence regarding learning theory shows that punishment alone has been ineffective in reducing frequent undesirable behavior unless matched with immediate positive reward for the correct behavior (see Knapp, 1988). However, the exerciser may often have to deal with the punishing consequences of initiating or increasing exercise (e.g., muscle discomfort, fatigue, soreness, minor injury; stress due to giving up attractive competing alternative activities; perceived negative attention or harassment from others). In particular, those who are inexperienced with exercise, overweight, older, and pressed for time, such as persons with coronary-prone, Type A behavior pattern, may have to deal with the real and perceived punishing consequences of exercise. One of the main ways in which investigators have examined a reduction of the punishing consequences in a subject's experience is through individualized exercise prescription, education, and cognitive restructuring of maladaptive thoughts. Thus, levels of exercise intensity and frequency appropriate to the target group's characteristics and wants (as opposed to strictly applying the ACSM guidelines) plus education on how to deal with the aches and pains of exercise initiation are a first step. As to cognitive restructuring, Martin et al. (1984) successfully used dissociative techniques, in which perception was focused toward the exercise environment and away from the physiological cues that initially cause discomfort.

Environmental changes or alterations have also been suggested as a means of removing the punishing aspects of negative arousal created by the presence of other people. Thus, a participant can be encouraged to choose exercise locations that minimize anxiety and promote personal safety.

The evidence regarding the management of behavioral consequences has been summarized by Wankel (1987) and by Knapp (1988). In general, varying levels of support have been found for the numerous techniques. Examples where adherence enhancement has been claimed following the management of exercise-related consequences are

1.  *Social support*—Wankel, Yardley, and Graham (1985) found that a spirit of camaraderie and the support of the fitness leader promoted continued involvement in a structured program. Spousal support also has often been associated with increased compliance in exercise rehabilitation programs (Erling & Oldridge, 1985).

2.  *Goal setting*—Keefe and Blumenthal (1980) had a small sample of subjects set weekly distance goals just slightly above the distance walked the previous week. These specific, achievable goals both helped exercisers to progress at a realistic rate and promoted their adherence.

3.  *Self-monitoring*—Self-monitoring is commonly included in exercise interventions in conjunction with other behavioral techniques. For example, Nelson et al. (1983) included self-monitoring with another behavioral-antecedent procedure and found that the combined technique promoted more exercise among subjects in that condition than among exercisers who only self-monitored.

4.  *Self-reinforcement*—This procedure entails consciously rewarding oneself for achieving self-set exercise criterion levels. Keefe and Blumenthal (1980) used this procedure successfully in conjunction with other techniques. What is most interesting, however, is that the procedure was initially effective but decreased in effectiveness as time went on among adherers. Apparently, they no longer needed this form of reinforcement after 2 years in their maintenance of exercise, but it was helpful in promoting adherence during the learning stages of developing their personal exercise program.

5.  *Material rewards*—Rewards of this sort apparently have the most success in programs where there may not be much social reinforcement. When these rewards are performance contingent, they serve to

emphasize competency in some exercise-related behavior. The relative successfulness of such strategies is open to question because there are few controlled studies of their effects in the exercise context. Behavioral contracts and attendance lotteries are examples where program-related rewards are provided and serve to aid adherence during the course of a program (e.g., Epstein, Wing, Thompson, & Griffin, 1980). However, when follow-up studies are done on self-regulated exercise following the program participation, such program-related contracts do not have a lasting effect (Knapp, 1988).

## Promotion Strategies for Exercise Maintenance

Once the initiate exerciser begins to follow some pattern of regular exercise (e.g., once to twice per week or more), the promotion of exercise must still continue. Of the various techniques attempted, most have been used in situations other than exercise (e.g., weight control, smoking cessation) in order to encourage adherence. Because little research has been done on the effectiveness of these approaches in the exercise context, they are only mentioned briefly.

**Gradual Withdrawal of Reinforcement.**    In structured exercise programs for the initiate, there is often a high degree of reinforcement provided for the desired behavior (e.g., Baun & Bernacki, 1988). However, individuals may become satiated with reinforcement to the extent that it has little impact on encouraging desired adherence. On the basis of learning theory, Knapp (1988) recommends gradual withdrawal of the reinforcements. Thus, the reinforcement schedule moves from constant to variable, while all other factors remain relatively constant. This may happen to the initiate exerciser who graduates from a small class with a low student-to-leader ratio to a class of intermediate difficulty, where the class size is larger and the reinforcement and feedback less frequent. This would be an abrupt change unless the instructor in the beginner class provides a schedule of variable reinforcement to wean the initiate exerciser from constant to variable reinforcement. However, there is little evidence to determine whether such transition practices are in place in structured programs of exercise.

**Self-Control and Attribution Techniques.**    The basic idea for maintaining exercise is to use strategies that aid the person in the self-regulation of exercise and/or in regular class attendance. In moving from dependence on the exercise class and/or staff to self-dependence for exercise, there may be some question in the initiate's mind about what and who is primarily responsible for making exercise and associated physical changes happen. Beginners may explain their initial exercise success through statements such as "If everyone else like me wasn't trying so hard and our exercise leader wasn't so good, I'd never be able to keep exercising." Such explanations about the causes of exercise adherence being outside the exerciser are called "external attributions." *Attributions* are our explanations for everyday actions and in this example, they are external because the control, as perceived by the beginner, is partly a function of social influences other than the individual's effort to exercise (i.e., the support of other class members and the exercise leader).

The self-control approach to maintenance involves teaching the exerciser a number of strategies that require self-regulation of exercise so that the attributions made for completing the exercise actions will be to their own personal efforts and strategies. It is generally recognized that such attributions lead to beliefs about personal ability and effort and therefore indirectly encourage self-regulated exercise (see Meichenbaum & Turk, 1987). Some of the strategies for self-regulation have already been discussed, and these are, for example, self-monitoring, goal setting, stimulus control, and others. Essentially, the practice of these strategies is thought to encourage self-determined behavior and to engender adherence to a level of exercise beyond the beginner's first exercise experiences.

There is some evidence for the short-term effectiveness of these strategies with very small classes. In discussing this evidence, Wankel (1987) cites examples of their short-term success in encouraging adherence for both beginners and continuing exercisers. However, little research has been done to examine whether such strategies encourage long-term exercise maintenance.

**Relapse Prevention.**    Marlatt (1985) proposed a model that encompasses the pattern of behavior characteristic of the dynamic cycle of exercise. This model was derived from health-behavior and drug-addiction research. The pattern of continuing to try to avoid engaging in health-destructive behavior, becoming inconsistent in or stopping that effort, and then resuming it a later time is not unlike the characteristic exercise pattern of starting to exercise, maintaining this for a series of weeks/months, dropping out for a period of weeks/months, then resuming exercise again. Unlike the addiction-relapse situation where cessation of a behavior is desired and then relapse to old destructive behavior resumes, the exercise example appears to be a mirror opposite. That is, the exerciser maintains or increases exercise for better health, and the relapse is usually to exercise cessation (i.e., relapse to nonexercise). The lapse in this case may not be as obviously destructive to health as a return to addictive behaviors. The idea behind relapse prevention as applied to exercise is to prevent the patterns of lower exercise frequency and temporary dropout that occur. In addictive behavior, prevention focuses on maintaining cessation of destructive behavior and avoiding its return.

A key point to be made is that the model applies to the starting–stopping behavior of individuals engaged in voluntary efforts to control their exercise. Consistent with the definitions provided earlier in this chapter, the model concerns adherence behavior (i.e., in freely chosen, self-selected activity). The differences between this model and the strategies to prevent relapse from discrete exercise initiation or adoption or maintenance situations is that the relapse model considers the ongoing exercise cycle prospectively. This contrasts with the promotion efforts focused on discrete phases of the exercise cycle without a view to the future behavior of the exerciser.

A brief scenario may serve to illustrate how relapse occurs in an exercise context. According to the relapse model, an exerciser who is a potential candidate for relapse experiences a high-risk situation. For example, a mother who exercises just before her children return from school suddenly finds that the children are released to her care earlier in the school term than expected because the season for their school's team sport has ended. Her exercise time is now in conflict with child care, and a potential high-risk situation for nonadherence now exists. The mother can exhibit either a positive coping response (e.g., asking a neighbor to provide the child care for the exercise hour) or a negative coping response, in which efficacy for coping with the child care problem is low, no alternatives seem available, and it is easier to give up on exercise than to try to manage the time conflict. At the same time, positive outcome expectancies for this slip in exercise behavior may include more time to spend with her children. This combination of events leads to her avoidance of exercise class that week.

At this point, the first exercise violation effect has occurred. The combined lack of efficacy to manage the conflict plus the positive outcomes that this conflict affords may allow the individual an opportunity to attribute good reasons for not attending exercise class (i.e., to relapse). This temporary dropout would continue until some later date, when the time conflict may be resolved by forces beyond the mother's control (e.g., more school activities available for the children later in the afternoon) and the mother can resume exercise class. While this all-too-brief description does not do justice to Marlatt's model, it gives the reader some idea of how one might conceptualize the reasons for the ebb and flow in exercise adherence. The ultimate purpose of knowing whether this relapse model is correct is that such a model would pinpoint key times when the targeted prevention of a relapse could occur.

How successful has exercise relapse prevention been? Unfortunately, in the exercise context, relapse prevention exists as more of an idea than a well-investigated intervention. There may be practical reasons for this absence of evidence. The first is that the relapse model and relapse prevention have only recently been introduced to the exercise community as a whole (e.g., in Dishman's 1988 text). The second is that relapse prevention is a comprehensive program that must, by model definition, be implemented over time, involve many behavioral-management strategies, and from a funded research perspective, be relatively costly to investigate.

Nonetheless, some researchers have attempted to examine aspects of relapse prevention. Two examples are studies by Martin et al. (1984) and by King and Frederiksen (1984). Regardless of flaws in these initial studies of nonexercise relapse prevention, they represent attempts to consider prevention of nonadherence from a more dynamic perspective. The King and Frederiksen study provided some evidence that nonexercise relapse prevention worked within the specific context of their study involving 5 weeks of jogging plus a follow-up. In the Martin et al. studies, exercising individuals were taught procedures to counter relapse and then were given a "planned relapse" day so they could counter the relapse, using learned prevention techniques. However, initial success was compromised by later procedural errors. The authors of both studies caution about the interpretation of their results. Such cautious perspectives about investigation of comprehensive prevention approaches is commendable. It also begs the question of whether we need to investigate the *nonexercise relapse process* rather than just assume a direct parallel to other health-behavior relapse situations (e.g., smoking cessation or weight control). Perhaps adaptation of the relapse model is needed. This essentially requires fitness-promotion experts to take a step backward and to critically reexamine what is known. Such a critique would require a major review, which is not this chapter's purpose. However, characteristics of the studies concerning the behavioral-management approach to individual and group fitness promotion may allow the reader to consider the limits to what we know. A summary of these characteristics is considered now.

### Research Characteristics: Individual and Group Fitness Promotion

**The Studies.**    In considering the current literature reviews of exercise-adherence interventions (i.e., Dishman, 1988; Knapp, 1988; Wankel, 1987), common features of the studies quickly become apparent. For the most part, the following list "of five typical problems" typifies those in the literature.

First, subjects are from both clinical and normal samples. Very often, discussions of the effectiveness of a specific promotion technique do not distinguish among types of samples and settings, although these individual characteristics may moderate the effect of the intervention on fitness promotion. Also, in controlled studies of promotion techniques, sample sizes tend to be small, for the most part, thereby raising questions about the studies having sufficient statistical power to detect a true treatment difference in affecting either an adherence or compliance rate.

Second, conceptual definitions of adherence and compliance are mixed, and the motivational difference between the two types of behavior is often ignored. In so doing, these studies also ignore the interaction between person and situation when a person is required to comply versus when they have chosen to adhere. As a result, explanations for why an intervention succeeded or failed are not forthcoming, and the reasons for equivocal results remain unclear. Operational definitions of adherence and compliance are often highly variable, again limiting generalizability across studies. For example, some investigations have used a variety of frequency behavioral measures as adherence, while others have used outcome measures as adherence indicators. Methodological and conceptual questions have been raised about many of these definitions (see Perkins & Epstein, 1988).

Third, promotion techniques are often examined either individually, relative to a control group, or in a single sample, within-subjects design with no control condition. Few studies compare several different techniques against a control group or include conditions where techniques are successively added together and compared to one another, as well as to a control (e.g., the addition of successive techniques: Perri, Nezu, McAllister, Gange, Jordan, & McAdoo, 1988).

Fourth, there is evidence of some success with a variety of techniques at each of the phases of the exercise cycle. However, the reliability of success for any given technique is not clear. Beginning a comparison of techniques across studies is difficult because sample and setting inconsistencies can be claimed even before other methodological criticisms are raised.

Finally, very few studies have long-term follow-ups of greater than 6 months. It is difficult to conclude anything about the longevity of adherence treatment effects after subjects completed the program in which adherence/compliance was enhanced. In most cases, then, demonstration of increased adherence has only been as a relatively short-term effect.

**The Strategies.** The following characteristics of the strategies were discussed earlier in this chapter:

1. The strategies are generally both behavioral or cognitive-behavioral in approach.
2. They are designed to affect individuals and small groups in particular settings.
3. They reach relatively few individuals at any single point in time.
4. Each of the individual techniques and comprehensive techniques mentioned herein demand a professional's time and expertise to convey the technique to the exerciser. Also, effort is required on the part of both the professional and the exerciser to apply the technique over successive weeks of a program.

**Comments on Individualized Promotion Efforts.** There appear to be modest but encouraging signs that cognitive-behavioral techniques can facilitate exercise adoption and maintenance. However, a lesson could be taken from the use of many of the same procedures in the obesity/weight-control literature—an enormous literature on ·the effectiveness of techniques used to encourage people to lose weight (i.e., hundreds of studies over 30+ years). Kirschenbaum (1992) recently drew a parallel between this literature and efforts to promote adherence and performance enhancement in exercise and sport. He suggested that a major lesson for those interested in exercise-adherence interventions could be obtained from research on the treatment of obesity. This lesson might best be captured by the single word *humility*. By trying to avoid some of the mistakes made in the weight-loss literature in designing intervention research and in applying behavioral techniques, exercise-adherence investigators may be able to benefit when exploring fitness-promotion and exercise-adherence questions. In addition to Kirschenbaum's advice, it is important to pay close attention to Perkins and Epstein's (1988) discussion of adherence methodology. It details many of the problems typical of adherence research in various areas of health promotion, including exercise. Before beginning another intervention study, exercise-adherence investigators should attempt to follow many of Perkins and Epstein's recommendations.

As Knapp (1988) pointed out in her review of behavioral-management techniques for exercise promotion, these individualized approaches are not the only avenue to encourage the adoption and maintenance of exercise. Mass-change strategies may be able to reach more people. While they have the limitation of less intimate contact with the individual, they provide another means to promote fitness.

## MASS-CHANGE APPROACHES

### Goals of Mass-Change Strategies

As with the goal of more individualized promotion strategies, one of the goals of mass change is to encourage initiation and then maintenance of some level of involvement in exercise. Where the mass-change approach differs, however, is in the goal of trying to influence large numbers of specifically targeted people at any one time. This second goal is characterized by mass-media communications as a visible part of the attempt to influence people to become more involved in exercise (e.g., in Canada: "Participation" messages; in the United States: "President's Council on Sport and Fitness" messages).

Mass-media attempts to promote behavior change are not unusual. In the health-promotion field, magazine and television campaigns regarding smoking cessation, "just [saying] no" to drugs, and avoidance of drinking and driving are quite visible efforts to discourage one type of behavior while trying to promote a healthier alternative behavior. It seems reasonable to argue that some behavioral change should occur, given the visibility and logic of the message, as well as its repetitive exposure to the public. Fitness practitioners have certainly adopted this idea, given the mass-change efforts that are currently being made (see examples noted earlier). Given that such attempts at mass change are already underway, the logical question as to their effectiveness arises. How many people do they reach? What are the resulting changes in both the behavioral and the psychological aspects of exercise? Is there increased participation in fitness activities as a result?

If we address the question of increased participation, one indicator (although admittedly confounded) may be a historical view of increased participation in exercise activities. Wankel (1988) reports that "minimal" levels of exercise involvement (i.e., participation at least once in the past year, as considered in the 1983 Canada Fitness Survey) were reported by 66% of respondents (e.g., aerobics, jogging, biking). A much more active level of involvement was reported for 56% of the sample (i.e., 3 hours per week for at least 9 months of the year). The report of the 1983 Miller Lite survey on U.S. sport indicated that among Americans over 14 years of age, 44% reported being active on an almost daily basis. When these results are compared to reports of participation 20 years earlier, there appears to be a definite increase in activity (e.g., in 1961, 24% of Americans reported they were active daily; in 1976, 54% of Canadians reported that they were this active; Wankel, 1988).

Another indicator of effectiveness of mass-media campaigns concerns their goal of developing *awareness* of the need for physical activity. Various surveys conducted in Australia (e.g., "Australian Life Be In It" campaign), in Canada (e.g., "Participation"), and in West Germany (e.g., "Trimm") all reveal high rates of public awareness of their country's fitness/sports promotion campaigns (Wankel, 1988; e.g., range of 79-97% of the samples were aware in the years of 1976-1977).

Public awareness, however, does not equal participation. Some of the same 1977 samples, in responding to questions regarding the influence of the message on their involvement had response rates of only 38% who increased activity due to the message (e.g., Australia). These rates also varied, depending on the city sampled (e.g., Canada: 27% in one city and 10% in another, Jackson, 1979).

Thus, there seems to be a major difference in impact between awareness achieved and involvement observed. The evidence becomes even more contradictory when, as Wankel (1988) points out, data from countries without mass-media promotion campaigns are considered. The activity increase observed in recent years in these countries parallels the increase that occurred in campaign countries. Thus, the impact of such campaigns seems to be mainly in creating public awareness, not in directly increasing participation.

## Limitations of Promotion Messages

From a social-psychological viewpoint, there are good reasons why such campaigns may not be promoting involvement. In 1987, Olson and Zanna elaborated on some of these reasons and suggested how messages might be altered to improve their impact on psychological and behavioral factors. Not unlike public health campaigns, fitness-promotion campaigns have assumed an educational focus. Fitness campaigns tend to educate on the general consequences of exercising, such as improved cardiovascular health, fitness, more energy, mental alertness, and so on. Thus, such promotion emphasizes general rather than specific concepts and consequences. This does not help the individual message recipient. It seems to be expected that it is intuitive for the individual to transfer from the general message consequences to something more personally relevant. As pointed out by Knapp (1988) and by Olson and Zanna (1987), the relation between such general concepts or general beliefs at which these campaigns are directed and individuals' behavior is weak.

Promotion messages often show healthy, attractive people doing exciting activities that are appealing on the surface. Watching a healthy individual ski, skate, play tennis, swim, or cycle makes the activity attractive and creates an awareness of various things one might do to be active. What does the message not tell the observer, however? The observer is not told about the personal outcomes of their specific efforts to become involved. The message discussion is general, in order to appeal to anyone watching, and therefore the personal consequences of exercise for an individual cannot be evaluated. The absence of a more explicit discussion that causes the individuals to personally evaluate a specific form of exercise forces them (if they are motivated to try to extrapolate beyond the message in order to attempt these activities—something about which initiate exercisers are unlikely to know. This raises another major limitation noted by Olson and Zanna (1987).

Fitness-promotion messages do not encourage an increase in perceived behavioral control. That is, initiate exercisers or those resuming exercise again after a sedentary period must believe that they have the means to organize their time, have the skills to do the activity, and have the ability to control other aspects of their daily lives (e.g., business or home commitments) in order to exercise. Messages rarely stress these how-to aspects of either the activity or the time/planning needed for it. Without this information, people are left to their own devices. People who are not overly self-efficacious about their skills and abilities to carry out the physical activity are unlikely to become involved (see Bandura, 1986; McAuley, 1992).

## A Social-Psychological Approach to Mass-Media Promotion

The social-psychological approach taken by Olson and Zanna (1987) suggests the following strategies for developing effective fitness-promotion messages for mass-media dissemination:

1.  The message developers should have a *theoretical basis* for the development of messages and for the variables being targeted for change. Having a model to follow in this regard not only gives direction for the variables to attempt to alter and change but also provides a basis for reexamination of the promotion attempt in the case of failure.
2.  The messages should emphasize a more detailed discussion of the personal consequences of *specific* exercise behaviors so that a personally relevant evaluation of these consequences can occur for these behaviors.
3.  The message should contain *simple how-to* advice rather than assume that individuals receiving the message will know how to modify their behavior, based on observation. The messages should highlight simple, not complex skills, with actions that are easy to complete and that help to heighten the novice's perceived control of exercise.
4.  The messages should further enhance perceived control through the provision not only of general how-to information about exercise, but also of more specific information about forms of exercise compatible with different life-styles and about variations and types of exercise—thereby allowing nearly anyone to adapt exercise to suit individual health, fitness, and age needs.

**Theoretical Basis: An Overview.**   A recognized limitation in the adherence/compliance and the physical-fitness promotion literature is the absence of guiding theory (see Dishman, 1988; Olson & Zanna, 1987; Rejeski, 1992). Sonstroem (1988) and Rejeski (1992) have recently noted the use of various theories as beginnings of a more systematic approach to examining adherence and fitness-promotion questions. For the remainder of the present chapter, the social-psychological basis for mass-change fitness promotion is specifically focused on three compatible psychological perspectives that have been used to understand and affect the determinants of fitness behavior. These perspectives are attitudes and attitude change, self-efficacy, and social persuasion. Each of these are related to the recommendations made for improving fitness-promotion campaigns by Olson and Zanna (1987).

The major theories considered herein concern attitudes toward actions: the theory of reasoned action (Fishbein & Ajzen, 1975), and its extension, the theory of planned behavior (Ajzen, 1985; Ajzen & Madden, 1986); Bandura's (1977, 1986) self-efficacy theory; and Petty and Cacioppo's (1981, 1986) elaboration likelihood model of persuasion in regard to attitude formation and change. The obvious question the reader may ask is, Why choose these theories as a basis for fitness promotion? While the answers to such questions are never simple, there are some basic reasons that are important for this choice. First, these attitudinal theories and self-efficacy theories provide for a more comprehensive examination of behavioral determinants across different social settings (see Ajzen & Fishbein, 1980; Bandura, 1986) than does the simple altering of external environmental cues, external reinforcements or material rewards, and self-monitoring discussed earlier in the chapter.

Second, the reasoned action/planned behavior and the self-efficacy models acknowledge social learning as the process by which attitudes and self-efficacy are formed. Given that these constructs can be socially learned, they can also be changed through interventions and promotional strategies based on aspects of social learning.

Third, there is evidence that both models predict exercise intentions and behavior in different fitness contexts. This evidence supports the notion that these models may be useful in promotional campaigns. Also, there is preliminary evidence for the use of the elaboration-likelihood model in a fitness-promotion context, lending support to considering its future use in fitness-promotion efforts using messages.

While it is not within the scope of this chapter to critically review all of the exercise-related evidence concerning these models, some examples are presented along with a brief description of the theories. These examples illustrate the supportive evidence available to justify research efforts using these models for fitness promotion.

### Reasoned Action and Planned Behavior

*Theories.*    Briefly explained, both the reasoned action and the planned behavior theories concern attitude–behavior relations. The theory of reasoned action was developed by Fishbein and Ajzen to explain volitional or freely chosen behavior. Using exercise as the behavioral example, the theory would propose that it is determined by intentions to carry out (or not) exercise-related behavior. Exercise intentions are jointly determined by one's attitudes toward exercise and by subjective norms. *Attitudes* are a person's evaluative feelings toward aspects of exercise (i.e., their likes and dislikes). *Subjective norms* are the social pressures to behave in specific ways. The attitudes refer to people's feelings about themselves performing an action. This is distinguished from other psychological theories concerning attitudes toward objects or issues. The subjective norm is an individual's view that important other people—such as family, friends, doctor, or spouse, with whom the person is motivated to comply—think that the individual should exercise. These determinants of exercise intention are not proposed to affect intent with equal weight. The weight these determinants bring to bear on intention is partly a function of the person's experience and the situation. Thus, in some cases, such as exercise, attitudes may more greatly influence intent, whereas for other health behaviors, such as birth control, subjective norms may be very influential. In the former case, one individual may choose to exercise, while in the latter, two people may be required to make a decision.

The determinants of both attitudes and subjective norms are an individual's salient beliefs about the personal consequences of exercising (attitudes) and about what that person believes are the views of significant others toward the individual engaging in exercise (subjective norm). Thus, the beliefs concern what exercise provides for an individual, from either a positive or a negative view (i.e., evaluation of the exercise consequence) and how strongly the individual feels that others wish him or her to participate. As an example, I may prefer the structured exercise offered from an aerobics class, whereas my friend hates the structure and prefers running for the same amount of time. Both of us evaluate the outcomes of the class differently (e.g., "fitness, being with friends" in my case versus "too much order, not enough aerobics" for my friend). This would also apply to running, but the evaluations would be opposite for both parties. Therefore, although both people exercise and do so for similar reasons, the activities chosen by both parties differ because of the beliefs and evaluations of some of the personal consequences associated with the specific form of exercise.

Usually the attitude–behavior relationship examined by the theory is specified in terms of time, context, and action. Consider a personal future intention—for example, "I'm going to try to *attend* my *fitness class twice* per *week* for the next *month*." This intention, plus my attitudes and subjective norms will concern this time, context, and action. The behavior intended and predicted will be regular attendance as specified in the example.

The basic assumption of the theory is that people make their voluntary choices about exercise behavior rationally. To do this, they systematically use information, much of which concerns their own belief and feeling about a type of exercise and the context in which it occurs. This may be fine for the person with more concrete beliefs and feelings (i.e., either positive or negative), but what about the inexperienced person without enough information to decide on an action (e.g., to initiate a certain type of activity)? These people may be neutral to mildly positive about specific types of activity and may represent one of the key target groups at which the mass promotion message must be directed. More is written about this later in this chapter. The theory has been supported in many behavioral contexts (see Ajzen & Fishbein, 1980), notably including both public health and exercise behavior.

What about those situations, however, where our behavior is not as voluntary? For example, we are forced to work over the noon hour rather than attending our exercise sessions because we have to meet a job deadline. In this case, the individual's choice for exercising is constrained and that behavior, at that time, and in that context is not available (if the individual wants to remain employed). This time, the individual's personal control over exercise has been limited, and if this happens often, the personal control over this form of exercise is reduced. For behavior in this fairly common example (e.g., exercise-barrier literature), the theory of reasoned action does not predict well. Promotions based on the theory must be targeted toward contexts that offer free choice or toward people who have free choice over their actions. Alternatively, the promotion strategy would be to help the individual develop strategies or beliefs that enhance personal control over other forms of exercise.

Recently, however, Ajzen (1985) and Ajzen and Madden (1986) proposed an extension of the reasoned action model, called the "theory of planned behavior." How this differs from reasoned action is through the inclusion of a perceived behavioral control construct. In the 1986 version of the model, perceived behavioral control functions in two different ways. The first way in which perceived behavioral control functions is, in addition to attitudes and subjective norms, as a third determinant of intention to exercise (still using exercise as the example behavior). That is, intentions are stronger when perceived behavioral control over exercise is high. When choices are constrained and less personal behavioral control is perceived, the theory would allow for the explanation of accordingly lower exercise intentions and subsequent behavior. Thus, perceived behavioral control would help to predict variability in exercise intention and is considered to be on a continuum rather than assuming that the individual is always in control, as required by the theory of reasoned action. As with the other determinants of intention (i.e., attitudes and subjective norms), perceived behavioral control would vary in its impact on exercise intent for an individual.

The second way in which perceived behavioral control is proposed to function is to affect exercise behavior directly. If self-efficacy is considered an indicator of perceived behavioral control (see Ajzen & Madden, 1986), then this prediction becomes quite compatible with existing self-efficacy theory (addressed later). While there is less overall evidence for the newer theory of planned behavior (in contrast to reasoned action), there is support for the theory in the exercise-science literature.

*Evidence for Reasoned Action/Planned Behavior.*   The discussion of this evidence is limited to the exercise context, although support has been demonstrated for both theories in other domains (e.g., Ajzen & Madden, 1986; Schifter & Ajzen, 1985). Critical reviews of the exercise literature concerning the theory of reasoned action have been presented elsewhere (e.g., Rejeski, 1992; Sonstroem, 1988). Some of the more reliable findings are that attitude generally predicts exercise/fitness/physical activity intentions better than subjective norms do, and in some cases, it is the only predictor. The range of explained variance in intention as predicted by attitudes and subjective norms is as little as 5% (Dzewaltowski, 1989) and as great as 55% (Riddle, 1980), with attitudes being the better predictor by a substantial margin. Shared variance between intentions and self-reported exercise behavior has been between 9% and 32% (see Rejeski, 1992). Godin and his colleagues have been the most frequent investigators of this model in exercise-related contexts (e.g., Godin & Shephard, 1990; Godin, Valois, Shephard, & Desharnais, 1987).

Regarding the theory of planned behavior, support is limited but positive when design strength and measurement considerations are taken into account. Many previous studies of the reasoned-action model tended either to be retrospective (i.e., relating predictor variables to recalled exercise behavior) or to be prospective but with program onset measures as the only predictors of self-reported behavior. Recently, investigators have become more rigorous in their examinations of the planned-behavior model than was the case when examining the reasoned-action model.

In these newer studies, (a) the designs used were prospective; (b) greater account was taken of the way in which at least some of the theoretical variables were carefully operationalized; (c) actual behavior—rather than self-reported data—was collected; and (d) in some studies more than exercise program onset assessment was made (i.e., mid program and end program assessments). Studies offering support for the theory of planned behavior have concerned both a common structured physical activity (e.g., exercise classes) and a variety of self-regulated physical activities.

Brawley and Horne (1988) followed the participation of 250 adults in community-based programs in three different municipalities for 12 weeks. Planned-behavior-model variables were assessed at three equal intervals throughout the duration of the program (Weeks 2, 6, and 10), and these measures were used to predict the exercise attendance of the weeks that followed their assessment (e.g., Week 2 variables predicted attendance in weeks 3, 4, and 5). The typical rate of greater than 50% dropout (i.e., 2 consecutive weeks of absence with no return) occurred. Attitudes and perceived behavioral control (i.e., assessed by attendance self-efficacy) predicted attendance intentions and actual behavior at the last two assessment points for adherers (Weeks 6, 10). In the case of dropouts, attitude predicted their intentions to attend at all three assessment points while perceived behavioral control predicted the declining attendance of dropouts. Attitudes and perceived behavioral control successfully discriminated between adherers and dropouts at the various program assessment points.

In a similar design examining a social-support intervention, the same investigators used the planned-behavior model to examine exercise attendance of 117 participants in six coed community-based programs, again in different municipalities. Attendance (thus, adherence) was high for both the control and the intervention groups. Ajzen (1985) suggests that the predictions of the planned-behavior model should be essentially the same as for the theory of reasoned action when perceived behavioral control is high and consistent with actual behavior. In such cases, predictor variables in the theory of reasoned action should account for variations in exercise intent and attendance. What Brawley and Horne (1988) found was that attitude was the most consistent predictor of attendance intent and behavior for both intervention and control groups. These predictions were strongest at the midpoint of the program.

Dzewaltowski, Noble, and Shaw (1990) prospectively considered the activity of 254 coed undergraduates over a 4-week period. Although the study only used onset measures to predict recalled exercise participation, it is interesting that attitude–behavior measures were able to predict unstructured, freely chosen physical activity. The purpose of the investigation was to compare two different theories relative to their predictive capabilities. What is also interesting is that although support was found for the theory of reasoned action (i.e., attitudes predicted intention and extent of recalled participation), support for self-efficacy was also evident, in that it predicted recalled participation. Although the theories were contrasted, the findings do not argue against the planned-behavior model because Ajzen and Madden (1986) have proposed that self-efficacy is a reasonable indicator of perceived behavioral control. Thus, the findings seem to be partially supportive of planned-behavior variables predicting exercise-related intent and self-reported participation. With respect to physical activity regardless of exercise setting, Godin and Gionet (1991) have recently reported support for variables consistent with the planned behavior model in the prediction of exercise intentions of work site employees for a variety of physical activities ($R^2 = .41$). Both attitudes and perceived barriers (as an indicant of perceived behavioral control) were strong predictors.

Finally, in a recent exercise psychology symposium, Wankel and his colleagues (1991) presented the results of a large national survey on self-reported physical activity participation in the Canadian population (i.e., the Campbell Survey on Well Being, Stephens & Craig, 1988). The theory of planned behavior was used to examine physical-activity intentions and recalled behavior. Data from 4000 individuals of differing age, gender, income, and education were analyzed. Mummery and Wankel (1991) found support for the inclusion of perceived behavioral control in a regression model that added this variable after first considering variance explained in intention via the reasoned-action model. They found that perception of behavioral control added significantly to the prediction of physical-activity-participation intentions ($R^2 = .25$, $p < .001$). The theory of planned behavior also predicted recalled physical-activity involvement better than the theory of reasoned action.

In the same symposium, Horne (1991) used the theory to examine the physical activity of an interesting and, from a scientific viewpoint, neglected sample—rural mothers of preschool children—a population identified as having a low incidence of exercise activity. From 600 women in small towns in the Canadian province of Alberta (population 4600–6000), 473 participants and 157 nonparticipants were obtained. The participation criterion was moderate physical activity (e.g., twice per week in easy walking, social dancing). In this study, the combination of all three determinants of intention (i.e., attitude, subjective norm, and perceived behavioral control) significantly predicted activity intentions for participants ($R^2 = .26$). For nonparticipants, the prediction was significantly determined by attitudes and perceived behavioral control ($R^2 = .13$). In a difference test of the model variables, participants had significantly more positive feeling, were more motivated to comply with others' wishes for them to exercise, and perceived greater personal control over their ability to be active at this level than did nonparticipants.

### Self-Efficacy

*Theory.* This theoretical perspective was described earlier in this chapter, and supporting evidence for it has been reviewed elsewhere (see Bandura, 1986). Efficacy expectations are a person's belief that he or she can perform a particular behavior, such as attending an exercise activity. These beliefs concern the perceived capability to carry out the behavior in a specific context. The outcome-expectancy aspect of self-efficacy theory concerns the person's estimate that these behaviors may lead to specific outcomes/consequences.

For example, people can believe that their attending exercise class will lead to outcomes such as a better body shape, praise from their friends, or self-satisfaction independent of having the belief (confidence) that they can regularly attend exercise class several times per week. Although these beliefs are related, Bandura (1986) emphasizes that they are different. In Bandura's theory, both self-efficacy and outcome expectancy can operate as determinants of behavior. Bandura also notes that self-efficacy is unlikely to strongly motivate individuals in the absence of adequate incentives. Outcomes provide the incentive, and individuals vary in their level of efficaciousness regarding their abilities to engage in actions necessary to achieve such outcomes. Self-efficacy has been clearly identified as playing an influential role in health behavior (see Strecher, DeVillis, Becker, & Rosenstock, 1986) as well as numerous other domains of endeavor (Bandura, 1986). As Dishman (1988) emphasizes, no individual variable alone determines exercise initiation or adherence; however, self-efficacy has clearly been related to a variety of physical-activity and exercise behaviors (cf. Bandura, 1991; McAuley, 1991). By contrast, few studies have examined the role that outcome expectancies might play relative to exercise intentions and behavior (see Rodgers & Brawley, 1991a).

In general, individuals who are highly efficacious about their abilities to exercise would tend to be physically active and perceive that they have sufficient capabilities and resources to make exercise a part of their lifestyle. They would persist with or initiate exercise even in the face of obstacles to do so. Less exercise-efficacious individuals would not be likely to initiate activity or to maintain their activity patterns. Dropout or irregular activity would be more characteristic of their behavior. While this pattern of exercise behavior would be predicted using self-efficacy theory as a model, is there evidence to support self-efficacy's relationship to such behavior?

*Evidence for Self-Efficacy.* Some of the evidence on self-efficacy cited earlier in this chapter reflects the efficacy–behavior relationship. There is also evidence of a relationship in some of the following exercise contexts when subjects were initiating or maintaining physical activity. For example, Sallis, Haskell, Fortmann, Vranizan, Taylor, and Solomon (1986) considered the predictors of self-reported physical activity in 1411 adults. Adoption of vigorous activity among young males was predicted by self-efficacy, and maintenance of moderate activity for females was predicted by specific exercise knowledge and self-efficacy.

In a prospective design, sedentary coed university-level students ($n = 98$) who were starting a structured aerobics class were assessed by McAuley and Rowney (1990). Baseline and end-of-program measures were taken. Initial levels of efficacy at baseline predicted attendance during the program, while perceived exercise performance best predicted postprogram efficacy. This finding not only illustrated the relationship of self-efficacy to later exercise-class attendance but also suggests that postprogram efficacy was developed by direct experience with the program.

Exercise initiation was examined in an older sedentary female sample ($n = 58$) by McAuley and Jacobson (1991). They studied overall exercise levels of subjects who initiated an 8-week low-impact structured exercise class. Preprogram efficacy for barriers best predicted overall exercise level. Aspects of self-efficacy differentiated good and poor exercise-class attenders in these initiate exercisers. Rodgers and Brawley (1991b) also examined the self-efficacy and outcome expectancy of initiates. Their study concerned the exercise intentions of beginning weight trainers exposed to a 2-day "learn to weight train" clinic. They found that both outcome expectancy and self-efficacy predicted the exercise intentions of those who were beginning weight training. Outcome expectancy was a preclinic predictor of intent, while self-efficacy predicted postclinic intent. McAuley (1991) reported one other prospectively designed study of self-efficacy with elderly persons initiating exercise. Previously sedentary elderly persons who had been exercising over a 5-month period were assessed on exercise frequency, self-efficacy, attributions, and affect. More-frequent exercisers who were more efficacious about their 5-month progress, attributed the cause of their progress to themselves and were positively affective when making such attributions. This finding with initiate exercisers underscores social-learning experiences as the determinant of exercise-related cognitions.

Dzewaltowski et al. (1990) examined the predictors of unstructured, freely chosen physical-activity participation. The self-reported physical activity of 254 university undergraduates of both sexes was followed over 4 weeks. A program-onset measure of self-efficacy was one of two significant predictors of recalled participation.

Self-efficacy has also been studied with other cognitive predictors of exercise behavior. In a prospective study by Poag-DuCharme and Brawley (1991a), self-efficacy and goal influence were the significant indicators of exercise-class intentions of undergraduate university students who were engaged in structured exercise classes three times per week. Also, Poag-DuCharme and Brawley (1991b) predicted the exercise intentions of 63 exercising elderly persons. They were engaged in a twice-per-week, structured, moderate-intensity exercise program. Their intentions to regularly attend were a function of their in-class social support and their scheduling and planning self-efficacy.

Finally, with respect to longer-duration studies of adherence, in a recent prospective clinical trial with 74 sedentary, healthy, elderly persons, Garcia and King (1991) considered the adherence of subjects for 1 year and compared groups of varying exercise intensity, either supervised in a group or home based with some supervision. Three assessments (onset, 6 months, and 12 months) were conducted. Self-efficacy was the strongest predictor of exercise adherence at 7–12 months.

Thus, there have been demonstrations of support for self-efficacy theory in a variety of exercise contexts. While these are not the only exercise studies, they are representative examples of those supporting efficacy as a predictor of exercise. Results of several of the prospective investigations support the development of self-efficacy as a function of direct or vicarious experience. As with the consideration of other reliable, single-variable, theory-based predictors, self-efficacy for exercise is able to explain between 8 and 20% of variance in behavior and to explain higher amounts of variance in intention (e.g., $R^2$ adj = .35, Poag-DuCharme & Brawley, 1991b). Like the attitude–behavior evidence, studies vary in the strength of design, and although prospective in a number of cases, they also vary in their use of multiple assessments over the duration of an exercise program. However, although the evidence is still growing in the exercise domain, there is substantive evidence of a link between perceived self-efficacy and an individual's *adoption* of health practices. From a persuasive communications standpoint, the effectiveness of such health communication is partly a function of an individual's perceived self-efficacy that they can *stick with* the health prevention regimen advocated (Bandura, 1991). Other "motivators" such as fear arousal (i.e., risk of disease) have not encouraged regimen adoption with the same reliability.

**Social Persuasion.**    A traditional approach to persuasion has sometimes been called the "Yale approach" (where much of the research was done). Investigators were interested in *when* persuasion should occur and *when* associated attitude change would occur. Also, their practical interests were in *how* such change could be produced. However, their attention did not focus on *why* attitude change occurred. Without the answer to the *why* question, insights into reasons for failures and successes of persuasion attempts are lacking. Essentially, the Yale approach was captured by the phrase, "Who says what to whom, and with what effect?" Thus, a credible source must present an appealing, attention-grabbing argument to a specific audience. Both the message and its delivery must encourage the target audience to remember the message and, as a result of all these factors, act on the message (i.e., the marketing aspects: Olson & Zanna, 1987). While the importance of these factors is acknowledged, the use of a theoretical model to guide the development of a message may help to produce more durable attitude change that leads to eventual action. In other words, a theoretically based mass-change campaign may be more likely to alter attitudes and encourage the initiation or maintenance of physical activity.

The elaboration likelihood model (ELM) proposed by Petty and Cacioppo (see 1986) concerns the degree to which people think about a persuasive message. It is what the message encourages people to think about, they argue, and not the message itself, that persuades individuals to change their attitudes. However, we do vary greatly in our efforts to process message information, depending upon how relevant it is to us. Thus, persuasion approaches may differ because of this.

According to the ELM, persuasion operates through two different processes. The process selected for persuasion depends on the amount of elaboration or close scrutiny a person directs toward a persuasive message. If a great deal of attention is paid to the message arguments, then persuasion occurs through the *central route*. This is where the individual carefully and thoughtfully considers the issue and its arguments. To the extent that the arguments are convincing and the facts are strong, attitude change will result. No change occurs when facts are weak.

The second route to persuasion is the *peripheral route*. Individuals respond mainly to persuasive cues such as the status or expertise of the person delivering the message. They accept the message at face value without carefully processing the information. In this case, if attitude change occurs, it is mainly because of the source's status or credibility.

It quickly becomes apparent that it would be important to assess any target group's existing beliefs in order to tailor a message designed to encourage exercise participation. If salient beliefs are assessed prior to a message campaign, arguments in the persuasive message can be made salient and relevant. This would be the strategy used to encourage persuasion by the central route. If individuals do not hold salient beliefs, they may be more open to attitude change via persuasive cues. Of the two routes to persuasion, the central route is the one associated with the most durable attitude change.

This model of persuasion fits well with the recommendations of Olson and Zanna (1987) for developing messages designed to persuade people to start or to maintain exercise. The following series of recommendations describe their suggestions for promotion. First, select a target audience who will receive the message. The target audience is neither so negative that they will never try exercise, nor so positive that all the arguments have been heard before and the message is "preaching to the converted." In both cases, the persuasiveness of the message is wasted because the attitude is either further polarized in the case of the negative target or wasted because the very positive are already exercising regularly.

Thus, the target individuals are neutral to moderately positive in their attitudes toward *specific* forms of exercise (e.g., swimming, bicycling, running, aerobics). Because the specific exercise is relevant to these individuals, they will pay more attention to and think about the following information. The type of information to be included in the message is presented first and is accompanied, where appropriate, by the variable it promotes, from a theoretical perspective.

1.  Emphasize positive personal consequences of exercise (i.e., attitudes and valued outcomes).

2.  Emphasize how to minimize negative personal consequences of exercise (e.g., muscle aches/pains). For example, encourage initiate exercisers to stretch before and after exercise (i.e., the development of self-efficacy to control such consequences).

3.  Emphasize negative outcomes of not exercising (e.g., cardiovascular risk: fear appeal) and how to avoid these consequences. Information and teaching should involve "how to begin exercise" (i.e., self-efficacy development).

4.  Create social pressure to exercise. Communicate that other important people want these individuals to perform specific types of exercise. Getting these individuals, as well as doctors, teachers, employers, involved in spreading the message is another tactic to make the behavior more normative (i.e., subjective norm development).

5.  Emphasize increasing perceptions of perceived control over exercise-related behavior. This would entail the provision of information that exercise can fit into any life-style and can be a variety of different activities (i.e., perceived behavioral control is developed).

6.  Provide the most basic and detailed information about how to do the activity, and provide resource people/groups where such information can be obtained. Sedentary people may know little about how to get started with respect to seeking an exercise facility for their specific interest, finding out the cost of joining, beginning a program, and so forth (i.e., development of efficacy and perceived behavioral control).

## Evidence for Mass-Change Fitness Promotion

At present, little evidence for this approach has been suggested. Although there is either psychological or exercise-science evidence for each of the theories that would serve as a basis for a mass-change approach, exercise science has concerned itself mainly with direct efforts to behaviorally manage initiation and maintenance of exercise, and the mass-change approach is not hands-on exercise intervention. Also, such interventions have been attempted with what may be called "captive" audiences (e.g., research or clinical samples) rather than with larger groups of people. Investigations of mass-change fitness promotion with large numbers of people might be a problem when this research is in its infancy. How can the process of studying fitness promotion by message delivery be started and investigated?

First, it is important to note that attitude change has been demonstrated in nonexercise domains using the ELM social-persuasion approach mentioned (Petty & Cacioppo, 1986). Second, preliminary exercise-science evidence for this approach does exist. Brawley and his colleagues (Brawley, Rodgers, & Horne, 1990; Rodgers, Horne, & Brawley, 1989; Rodgers, Brawley, Horne, & Cargoe, 1990) have investigated the approach recommended by Olson and Zanna (1987). In two studies concerned with persuasive messages, they used the theories of planned behavior and self-efficacy to guide message development. The messages were targeted toward individuals who would use the central route to persuasion and was tested on these select individuals after assessing their premessage beliefs and attitudes (i.e., to ensure both that the correct target audience was identified and that the message was salient). Olson and Zanna's (1987) recommendations were used to develop both the written message in Study 1 and the audiovisual message in Study 2. Message-content categories were centered around the variables in the theories of planned behavior and self-efficacy.

The basic promotion dilemma for mass change is that it is often difficult to assess increased participation as a result of message-induced attitude change. The fitness promoter or investigator must wait to observe some outcome. However, some of the other objectives of the message delivery are to have the audiences (a) pay attention to the message, (b) thoughtfully consider the message content, (c) remember some of the message content, and finally, (d) act on the basis of both the changed attitude and the information provided in the message. A research strategy would be to examine whether at least one of these objectives is actually achieved. One logical objective that allows for controlled investigation of message impact is whether individuals retain the message information. If people do not retain the message information, will their attitudes change? How can they act on the message without remembering some of it? The examination of message recall was one of the key objectives in the two studies described in the previous paragraph.

In both studies, subjects were exposed to the systematically developed message. These individuals were sedentary office workers ($n = 25$) in Study 1 and sedentary adults from the community in Study 2 ($n = 21$). A key feature of the design of the studies was a week's delay following message exposure before subjects' recalled the message. No advance notice of the recall was given, so subjects were not motivated to memorize at the time of exposure. In both studies, planned behavior variables significantly predicted intent to participate twice per week in a self-stated activity of the subjects' choice immediately after presentation and after recall 1 week later. Prior to receiving the message, the theoretical variables did not predict the exercise intentions of the sedentary individuals in either study. Some change in the ability to predict postmessage intentions appears to have been the result of initial exposure to and later recall of the persuasive messages.

In Study 1, where the written message was examined, there were significant changes in attitude and in perceived control when premessage levels were compared with those at immediate postmessage and post recall. Both measures increased after exposure to the message, and these increases were maintained at post recall. As to the retention of the written-message information, scheduling of exercise, how-to information, and exercise benefits were the categories of relevant material that were well recalled. Interestingly, the behavioral-control information of how-to and scheduling were best recalled, and the variable of perceived behavioral control (i.e., scheduling self-efficacy) best predicted exercise behavioral intention at post recall.

In Study 2, subjects were examined as to their premessage attitude, then were divided into those with highly positive attitudes and those with neutral to moderately positive attitudes. The latter group was the target audience for attitude change after being persuaded by the audiovisual message. Modest differences in the predicted direction for attitude and scheduling efficacy were obtained at post recall. Subjects were more positive in their attitudes about getting involved twice a week in activity, and they perceived that they had greater behavioral control in scheduling exercise bouts. Scheduling information was the category of information best recalled.

The important conclusions to draw from both studies about message retention are as follows. Free recall was selective, not random. In cued recall, subjects remembered more than 60% of the material on which they were questioned. Therefore, recall was not simply a function of remembering more about information that appeared most frequently in the message. Selective message information was retained for at least 1 week following each persuasive message.

Thus, several of Olson and Zanna's (1987) recommendations for developing a mass-change fitness promotion message received some support. The studies represent one of the first fitness-promotion messages studied where some degree of success was observed in message recipients' change of attitude via the central route to persuasion and where memory for the message was selective (also see Rimer & Glassman, 1984). Although these results are encouraging, further research is necessary to show reliable attitude change and extent of recall. In addition, as recommended in the attitude-change literature (see Olson & Zanna, 1981), it would be wise to provide the opportunity for message recipients to engage in a relevant behavior (e.g., sign up to observe or partake in a free introductory fitness class; report more active life-style behavior, such as taking stairs vs. the elevator; engage in more gardening or walking; or purchasing and using a bike). This direct experience may further or maintain the changed attitude and may increase commitment to initiating or increasing exercise. There is also social-persuasion evidence suggesting that if messages are repeated, change is more probable (Olson & Zanna, 1981). This is important because it suggests that several message inoculations may be important for durable change.

It is important to note that several health communication attempts reviewed by Bandura (1991) point to the use of a number of Olson and Zanna's (1987) social psychological recommendations for fitness promotion. For this health-related literature, Bandura (1991) suggests that a strong preexisting perceived self-efficacy will encourage further persuasion by messages designed to foster self-regulative efficacy. If this is done, adoption of behaviors targeted for change is suggested as more likely. Bandura also emphasizes the same basic points made by Olson and Zanna; enhance self-efficacy beliefs and tell people *how to* alter behavior. As well, he emphasizes making people realize repeated attempts to change are necessary for enduring change.

## Beyond Message Construction

The future of the mass-change approach to fitness promotion is not certain. The application of the systematic, theory-based approach described still requires more evidence to clearly ascertain the degree of attitude and behavior change that can be created. However, the approach suggested has much greater potential for creating exercise attitude–behavior change than current applied approaches, which only create public awareness. At the research level, the future requires more investigation using the theories suggested in order to accurately fine-tune persuasive fitness-promotion messages to affect target audiences. A great deal of attitude-change and persuasion research can be utilized to help develop research plans to meet this goal.

At the message-delivery level, a communication process called "the two-step flow of communication" is recommended (see Sherif & Sherif, 1969). That is, information from various forms of mass media, once presented, should also be transmitted through community opinion leaders to the target audience within the general public. Although mass-media messages are systematically designed, they only provide opportunities for one-way communication. Exercise novices or persons receptive to increasing their level of regular exercise are passive recipients of the message. When community opinion leaders reiterate aspects of the message, the target individual gains an opportunity for face-to-face interaction and either thoughtful consideration of message arguments or answers to related questions. These situations provide conditions ripe for interpersonal influence.

The two-step flow of message information is consistent with Olson and Zanna's (1981, 1987) recommendations for increasing the normative pressure for an individual to exercise (cf. subjective norm: theory of planned behavior) and provides knowledgeable others to which the target person can turn as how-to information sources.

The contexts in which the face-to-face delivery of the message occurs should be those that the target audience encounters regularly. Thus, Olson and Zanna (1981) recommend contact with fitness practitioners, doctors, and similar others who are successfully fitting exercise into a busy life. For example, these contacts should occur at (a) the work setting (i.e., guest speakers), (b) free advertised group or panel discussions, (c) information desks or displays at shopping centers, (d) telephone advice services, and (e) fitness experiences for the target audience.

However, from both a scientific and an applied perspective, exercise scientists and fitness practitioners are still several steps away from executing the mass-change fitness-promotion efforts discussed. Until research efforts are made to understand the process behind fitness-promotion strategies (i.e., why it works) or to evaluate their effectiveness, the potential for mass-change fitness promotion to increase exercise initiation, level of involvement and to change attitudes toward fitness behavior will not be realized.

## CONCLUDING COMMENTS: FITNESS-PROMOTION STRATEGIES

The title of this chapter is "Social-Psychological Aspects of Fitness Promotion." Upon reading its content, it could be argued that behavioral-management strategies are not the focus of attention of those studying the social psychology of exercise. However, the fact that the majority of promotion efforts require interaction between an exercise behavior provider and a client, a fitness promoter and the lay public, and a rehabilitation/health-care provider and a patient underscores the point that fitness promotion occurs in a context of social interaction. This point has implications for the social-psychological aspects of fitness promotion, adherence, and compliance. Not all the theories behind behavioral-management aspects of promotion are social-psychological but the implementation of the strategies by the exerciser has social-psychological consequences (e.g., changes in motivation, beliefs, attitudes, attributions, self-efficacy, and behavioral intentions). The basic premise of the social-psychological perspective is that the exerciser, in any part of the exercise cycle (see Figure 10.1) is not a passive recipient of promotion efforts. It is the exerciser's perception of the promotion tactic and interaction with the others providing it that partially dictates the success or failure of fitness-promotion strategies.

What, therefore, is the overall social-psychological and research perspective for the two fitness-promotion approaches discussed? First, research designs examining the long-term effect of sustained effort at fitness promotion are required. That is, promotion may be required at each phase of the exercise cycle, as the individual encounters the new experiences with that state (e.g., increased intensity and frequency, time commitment). Thus, designs examining promotion effects and associated adherence need to be longitudinal and prospective.

Second, both mass-change and behavioral-management promotion strategies can complement each other (see Olson & Zanna, 1987). Some examples are (a) offering a message that includes in its how-to aspects some of the steps that make starting exercise easier, (b) following a promotion message, having opinion leaders (i.e., fitness instructors or advisors) incorporate and present the coping strategies necessary for planning exercise to increase involvement in the face-to-face delivery of the message to a target layperson. In longer-term smoking-cessation or weight-loss programs with change-maintenance follow-ups, multiple methods (i.e., both behavior-change and social-persuasion messages) have been used to promote and maintain behavior. It seems probable that a similar approach could be attempted in order to promote and maintain exercise in the life-styles of different target groups of people.

Third, given the first and second suggestions, and considering that regular exercise and its associated behavioral/physiological/psychological outcomes represent a complex promotion and maintenance problem, it is unlikely that promotion efforts will be easy. Short-term, Band-Aid™ attempts at promotion are not solutions and underestimate the multifaceted complexity of the determinants of exercise behavior that characterize the exercise cycle.

Fourth, the cost-effectiveness of any promotion effort must be weighed against the target group's goal for exercise (see Perkins & Epstein, 1988). The expense of any promotion effort, both financial and human, must be balanced against what the individual desires and what promotion experts/ researchers think is good for the person. Promotion efforts that treat the individual as a passive lump of clay to the molded to a standard program of exercise just for reliable physiological outcomes are doomed to failure.

This chapter has been an attempt to summarize and suggest psychological methods of fitness promotion for exercise initiation and maintenance. In general, the overall theme has been to take a systematic approach that includes the use of theory to develop promotion strategies. This approach requires evidence to determine its success or failure, and thus, promotion can only advance with an interplay of associated research and practice. It is hoped that the target problems and needs identified in this chapter will promote much-needed research in both the behavioral-management and the mass-change areas in the future.

## REFERENCES

Ajzen, I. (1985). From intentions to actions: A theory of planned behavior. In J. Kuhl & Beckman (Eds.), *Action control from cognition to behavior*. Heidelberg, Germany: Springer.

Ajzen, I., & Fishbein, M. (1980). *Understanding attitudes and predicting social behavior*. Englewood Cliffs, NJ: Prentice-Hall.

Ajzen, I., & Madden, T. J. (1986). Prediction of goal directed behavior: Attitudes, intentions, and perceived behavioral control. *Journal of Experimental Social Psychology, 22*, 453–474.

Bandura, A. (1977). Self-efficacy: Toward a unifying theory of behavioral change. *Psychological Review, 84*, 191–215.

Bandura, A. (1986). *Social foundations of thought and action: A social cognitive theory*. Englewood Cliffs, NJ: Prentice-Hall.

Bandura, A. (1991). Self-efficacy mechanism in physiobiological activation and health-promoting behavior. In J. Madden IV (Ed.), *Neurobiology of learning, emotion and affect* (pp. 229–269), New York, NY: Raven Press.

Baun, W. B., & Bernacki, E. J. (1988). Who are corporate exercisers and what motivates them? In R. K. Dishman (Ed.), *Exercise adherence: Its impact on public health* (pp. 321–348). Champaign, IL: Human Kinetics.

Becker, M. H. (1976). Sociobehavioral determinants of compliance. In D. L. Sachett & R. B. Haynes (Eds.), *Compliance with therapeutic regimens* (pp. 40–50). Baltimore: Johns Hopkins University Press.

Brawley, L. R., & Horne, T. E. (1987). *Prediction of fitness class adherence: The use of attitudinal models*. (Report Project No. 8606-4042-2042. Ottawa, Canada: Canadian Fitness and Lifestyle Research Institute.

Brawley, L. R., & Horne, T. E. (1988). *Refining attitude–behavior models to predict adherence in normal and socially-supportive conditions* (Parts I & II; Report Project No. 8706-4042-2099. Ottawa: Canadian Fitness and Lifestyle Research Institute.

Brawley, L. R., Rodgers, W. M., & Horne, T. E. (1990). *Evaluating fitness promotion messages: A social cognition approach.* Research Report, Ontario Ministry of Tourism and Recreation, Toronto, June.

Canada Fitness Survey (1983). *Fitness and lifestyle in Canada.* Ottawa, Canada: Fitness and Amateur Sport, Government of Canada.

Desharnais, R., Bouillon, J., & Godin, G. (1986). Self-efficacy and outcome expectations as determinants of exercise adherence. *Psychological Reports, 59,* 1157–1159.

Dishman, R. K. (1988). *Exercise adherence: Its impact on public health.* Champaign, IL: Human Kinetics.

Dzewaltowski, D. A. (1989). Toward a model of exercise motivation. *Journal of Sport and Exercise Psychology, 11,* 251–269.

Dzewaltowski, D. A., Noble, J. M., & Shaw, J. M. (1990). Physical activity participation: Social cognitive theory versus the theories of reasoned action and planned behavior. *Journal of Sport and Exercise Psychology, 12,* 388–405.

Epstein, L. H., & Masek, B. J. (1978). Behavioral control of medicine compliance. *Journal of Applied Behavioral Analysis, 11,* 1–9.

Epstein, L. H., Wing, R. R., Thompson, J. K., & Griffin, W. (1980). Attendance and fitness in aerobics exercise. *Behavior Modification, 4,* 465–479.

Erling, J., & Oldridge, N. B. (1985). Effect of a spousal-support program on compliance with cardiac rehabilitation. *Medicine and Science in Sports and Exercise, 17,* 284.

Ewart, C. K., Taylor, B., Reese, L. B., & DeBusk, R. F. (1983). Effects of early postmyocardial infarction exercise testing on self-perception and subsequent physical activity. *American Journal of Cardiology, 51,* 1076–1080.

Fishbein, M., & Ajzen, I. (1975). *Belief, attitude, intention, and behavior: An introduction to theory and research.* Reading, MA: Addison-Wesley.

Godin, G., & Gionet, N. J. (1991). Determinants of an intention to exercise of an electric power commission's employees. *Ergonomics, 34,* 1221–1230.

Godin, G., & Shephard, R. J. (1990). Use of behavioural models in exercise promotion. *Sports Medicine, 10,* 103–121.

Godin, G., Valois, P., Shephard, R. J., & Desharnais, R. (1987). Prediction of leisure-time behavior: A path analysis (LISREL V) model. *Journal of Behavioral Medicine, 10,* 145–158.

Gould, D. (1987). Understanding attrition in children's sport. In D. Gould & M. Weiss (Eds.), *Advances in pædiatric sport sciences: Behavioral issues,* (pp. 61–85). Champaign, IL: Human Kinetics.

Horne, T. E. (1991, October). *Predictors of participation and on participation in moderate physical activity by rural Alberta homemakers.* Paper presented at the annual meeting of the Canadian Society for Psychomotor Learning and Sport Psychology, London, Ontario.

Hoyt, M. F., & Janis, I. L. (1975). Increasing adherence to a stressful decision via a motivational balance-sheet procedure: A field experiment. *Journal of Personality and Social Psychology, 35,* 833–839.

Jackson, J. J. (1979). Promoting physical recreation in social systems. *Recreation Research Review, 6,* 66–69.

Keefe, F. J., & Blumenthal, J. A. (1980). The life fitness program: A behavioral approach to making exercise a habit. *Journal of Behavior Therapy and Experimental Psychiatry, 11,* 31–34.

King, A. C., & Frederiksen, L. W. (1984). Low-cost strategies for increasing exercise behavior: Relapse preparation training and social support. *Behavior Modification, 8,* 3–21.

Kirschenbaum, D. S. (1992). Elements of effective weight control programs: Implications for exercise and sport psychology. *Journal of Applied Sport Psychology, 4,* 77–93.

Knapp, D. N. (1988). Behavioural management techniques and exercise promotion. In R. K. Dishman (Ed.), *Exercise adherence: Its impact on public health* (pp. 203–236). Champaign, IL: Human Kinetics.

Lau, R. R., Hartman, K. A., & Ware, J. E., Jr. (1986). Health as a value: Methodological and theoretical considerations. *Health Psychology, 5,* 25–43.

Maddux, J. E., Norton, L. W., & Stoltenberg, C. D. (1986). Self-efficacy expectancy, outcome expectancy, and outcome value: Relative effects on behavioral intentions. *Journal of Personality and Social Psychology, 51,* 783–789.

Marlatt, G. A. (1985). Relapse prevention: Theoretical rationale and overview of the model. In G. A. Marlatt & J. R. Gordon (Eds.), *Relapse prevention: Maintenance strategies in the treatment of addictive behaviors.* New York: Guilford Press.

Marlatt, G. A., & Gordon, J. R. (Eds.). (1985). *Relapse prevention: Maintenance strategies in the treatment of addictive behaviors* (pp. 3–70). New York: Guilford Press.

Marlatt, G. A., & Kaplan, B. E. (1972). Self-initiated attempts to change behavior: A study of New Year's resolutions. *Psychological Reports, 30,* 123–131.

Martin, J. E., Dubbert, P. M., Katell, A. D., Thompson, J. K., Raczynski, J. R., Lake, M., Smith, P. O., Webster, J. S., Sikora, T., & Choen, R. E. (1984). Behavioral control of exercise in sedentary adults: Studies 1 through 6. *Journal of Consulting and Clinical Psychology, 52,* 795–811.

Matarazzo, J. D. (1980). Behavioral health and behavioral medicine: Frontiers for a new health psychology. *American Psychologist, 35,* 807–817.

McAuley, E. (1991). Efficacy, attributional and affective responses to exercise participation. *Journal of Sport and Exercise Psychology, 13,* 382–393.

McAuley, E. (1992). The role of efficacy cognitions in the prediction of exercise behavior of middle-aged adults. *Journal of Behavioral Medicine, 15,* 65–68.

McAuley, E., & Jacobson, L. (1991). Self-efficacy and exercise participation in sedentary adult females. *American Journal of Health Promotion, 5,* 185–191.

McAuley, E., & Rowney, T. (1990). Exercise behavior and intentions: The mediating role of self-efficacy cognitions. In L. VanderVelden & J. H. Humphrey (Eds.), *Psychology and sociology of sport* (Vol. 2, pp. 3–15). New York: AMS and Press.

Meichenbaum, D., & Turk, D. C. (1987). *Facilitating treatment adherence: A practitioner's guidebook.* New York: Plenum Press.

Meyer, D., Leventhal, H., & Gutmann, M. (1985). Common sense model of illness: The example of hypertension. *Health Psychology, 4,* 115–135.

Miller Brewing Company. (1983). *The Miller Lite report on American attitudes toward sports.* Milwaukee, WI: Author.

Morgan, W. P., & Goldston, S. E. (Eds.). *Exercise and mental health.* New York: Hemisphere.

Morgan, W. P., & O'Connor, P. J. (1988). Exercise and mental health. In R. K. Dishman (Ed.), *Exercise adherence: Its impact on public health* (pp. 91–122). Champaign, IL: Human Kinetics.

Mummery, W. K., & Wankel, L. M. (1991, October). *Contribution of indirect behavioral and control beliefs to the prediction of physical activity intention in the Canadian population.* Paper presented at the annual meeting of the Canadian Society for Psychomotor Learning and Sport Psychology, London, Ontario.

Nelson, R. O., Haynes, S. C., Spong, R. T., Jarratt, R. B., & McKnight, D. L. (1983). Self-reinforcement: Appealing misnomer or effective mechanism? *Behavior Research and Therapy, 21,* 557–566.

Olson, J. M., & Zanna, M. P. (1981). *Promoting physical activity: A social psychological perspective.* Toronto, Canada: Report to the Ministry of Culture and Recreation.

Olson, J. M., & Zanna, M. P. (1987). Understanding and promoting exercise: A social psychological perspective. *Canadian Journal of Public Health, 78,* 1–7.

Perkins, K. A., & Epstein, L. H. (1988). Methodology in exercise adherence research. In R. K. Dishman (Ed.), *Exercise adherence: Its impact on public health* (pp. 399–416). Champaign, IL: Human Kinetics.

Perri, M., Nezu, A., McAllister, D., Gange, J., Jordan, R., & McAdoo, W. (1988). Effects of four maintenance programs on the long-term management of obesity. *Journal of Consulting and Clinical Psychology, 56,* 529–534.

Petty, R. E., & Cacioppo, J. T. (1981). *Attitudes and persuasion: Classic and contemporary approaches.* Dubuque, IA: W. C. Brown.

Petty, R. E., & Cacioppo, J. T. (1986). The elaboration likelihood model of persuasion. In L. Berkowitz (Ed.), *Advances in experimental social psychology* (Vol. 19, pp. 123–205). New York: Academic Press.

Poag-DuCharme, K. A., & Brawley, L. R. (1991a, October). *The goal dynamics of fitness classes: A preliminary analysis.* Paper presented at the annual meeting of the Canadian Society for Psychomotor Learning and Sport Psychology. London, Ontario.

Poag-DuCharme, K. A., & Brawley, L. R. (1991b, October). *The relationship of self-efficacy and social support to exercise intentions in the aged.* Paper presented at the annual meeting of the Canadian Society for Psychomotor Learning and Sport Psychology. London, Ontario.

Powell, K. E. (1988). Habitual exercise and public health: An epidemiological view. In R. K. Dishman (Ed.), *Exercise adherence: Its impact on public health* (pp. 15–40). Champaign, IL: Human Kinetics.

Powell, K. E., Spain, K. G., Christenson, G. M., & Mollenkamp, M. P. (1986). The status of the 1990 objectives for physical fitness and exercise. *Public Health Reports, 101,* 15–21.

Rejeski, W. J. (1992). Research in exercise motivation: A critique of theoretical directions. In G. C. Roberts (Ed.), *Motivation in sport and exercise* (pp. 129–157). Champaign, IL: Human Kinetics.

Riddle, P. K. (1980). Attitudes, beliefs, behavioral intentions and behaviors of men and women toward regular jogging. *Research Quarterly for Exercise and Sport, 51,* 663–674.

Rimer, B., & Glassman, B. (1984). How do persuasive health messages work? A health education field study. *Health Education Quarterly, 11,* 31–321.

Rodgers, W. M., & Brawley, L. R. (1991a). The role of outcome expectancies in participation motivation. *Journal of Sport and Exercise Psychology, 13,* 411–427.

Rodgers, W. M., & Brawley, L. R. (1991b, June). *The role of outcome and self-efficacy expectancies in motivating initiation of physical activity.* Paper presented at the annual meeting of the North American Society for the Psychology of Sport and Physical Activity, Monterey, CA.

Rodgers, W., Brawley, L. R., Horne, T. E., & Cargoe, S. (1990, May). *Fitness promotion by videotape: A social-cognitive analysis.* Paper presented at the annual meeting of the North American Society for the Psychology of Sport and Physical Activity, Houston, TX.

Rodgers, W., Horne, T. E., & Brawley, L. R. (1989, June). *Evaluating fitness messages promoting involvement: Effects on attitudes and behavioural intentions.* Paper presented at the annual meeting of the North American Society for the Psychology of Sport and Physical Activity. Kent State, OH.

Sallis, J. F., Haskell, W. L., Fortmann, S. P., Vranizan, M. S., Taylor, C. B., & Solomon, D. S. (1986). Predictors of adoption and maintenance of physical activity in a community sample. *Preventative Medicine, 15,* 331–341.

Sallis, J. F., & Hovell, M. F. (1990). Determinants of exercise behavior. In K. B. Pandolf & J. O. Holloszy (Eds.), *Exercise and sport sciences reviews* (Vol. 18, pp. 307–330). Baltimore: Williams & Wilkins.

Schifter, D. E., & Ajzen, I. (1985). Intention, perceived control, and weight loss: An application of the theory of planned behavior. *Journal of Personality and Social Psychology, 49,* 843–851.

Sherif, M. & Sherif, C. W. (1969). *Social psychology.* New York, NY: Harper & Row.

Sonstroem, R. J. (1988). Psychological models. In R. K. Dishman (Ed.), *Exercise adherence: Its impact on public health* (pp. 125–154). Champaign, IL: Human Kinetics.

Stevens, T., & Craig, C. L. (1990). *The well-being of Canadians: Highlights of the 1988 Campbell's survey.* Ottawa, Canada: The Canadian Fitness and Lifestyle Research Institute.

Strecher, V. J., DeVillis, B. M., Becker, M. H., & Rosenstock, I. M. (1986). The role of self-efficacy in achieving health behavior change. *Health Education Quarterly, 13,* 73–81.

Wankel, L. M. (1987). Enhancing motivation for involvement in voluntary exercise programs. In M. L. Maehr & D. A. Kleiber (Eds.), *Recent advances in motivation and achievement: Vol 5. Enhancing motivation (pp. 239–286).* Greenwich, CT: JAI Press.

Wankel, L. M. (1988). Exercise adherence and leisure activity: Patterns of involvement and interventions to facilitate regular activity. In R. K. Dishman (Ed.), *Exercise adherence: Its impact on public health* (pp. 369–396). Champaign, IL: Human Kinetics.

Wankel, L. M. (1991, October). *Understanding and predicting physical activity involvement: The theory of planned behavior.* Symposium presented at the annual meeting of the Canadian Society for Psychomotor Learning and Sport Psychology, London, Ontario.

Wankel, L. M., Yardley, J. K., & Graham, J. (1985). The effects of motivational interventions upon the exercise adherence of high and low self-motivated adults. *Canadian Journal of Applied Sport Sciences, 10,* 147–156.

Weinstein, N. D. (1984). Why it won't happen to me: Perceptions of risk factors and susceptibility. *Health Psychology, 3,* 431–457.

# 11

# Developmental Aspects of Exercise Psychology

## THELMA S. HORN AND RANDAL P. CLAYTOR

During the 1980s, the issue of youth fitness became a popular topic of discussion. Interest in the fitness status of American children and the subsequent call for programs to increase their level of physical activity was based largely on research conducted with adults, which suggested that a regular program of physical activity would result in decreased risk for cardiovascular disease and an increased state of well-being (Paffenbarger & Hyde, 1984; Plante & Rodin, 1990). However, as several writers (e.g., Corbin, 1987; Seefeldt, 1984) have noted, the results of research conducted with adults cannot necessarily be applied to children. Because children differ both physically and psychologically from adults, it is certainly possible that their response to exercise training may be both quantitatively and qualitatively different than that of adults.

The purpose of this chapter is to review the available research and theory on the relationship between children's fitness and their physical and psychological health. In particular, this topic is approached from both a developmental and a multidisciplinary perspective. The chapter is divided into two parts. In the first part, the research conducted to assess the health and fitness status of American children is briefly reviewed. Then, in the second part, the potential relationship between exercise training and children's mental and psychological health is more extensively explored. Within each of these sections, limitations in the current research methodologies and paradigms are noted, and clear directions for future research are provided.

## HEALTH AND FITNESS STATUS OF CHILDREN

Within the past decade, considerable data have been collected in an attempt to assess the health and fitness status of children. Collectively, these data provide information relative to children's level of (a) fitness (e.g., strength, flexibility, aerobic endurance), (b) physical activity (i.e., frequency and intensity of daily activity patterns, and (c) health (e.g., cardiovascular risk indicators). In the following sections, the results of the research in each of these areas are summarized.

### Children's Fitness

Although the term *fitness* has been defined in a variety of ways, most traditional conceptions of fitness have incorporated the notion of fitness as a "functional or movement capacity" (i.e., the ability to carry out daily tasks with vigor and alertness) (Pate, 1988). Typical components of fitness included such competencies as power, agility, muscular strength, muscular endurance, cardiovascular endurance, flexibility, speed, balance, and coordination.

More recently, however, it has been argued that definitions or conceptualizations of fitness should be more closely linked to health outcomes (e.g., see Pate, 1988; Simons-Morton, Parcel, O'Hara, Blair, & Pate, 1988). Using this perspective, *fitness* is defined in terms of the traits or capacities that are associated with low risk of such diseases as hypertension, coronary heart disease (CHD), adult-onset diabetes, and a variety of musculoskeletal problems. Components of fitness included under this definition are limited to muscular strength, muscular endurance, cardiorespiratory endurance, low back/hamstring flexibility, and body composition. Due to the topical content of this chapter, the health-related conceptualization of fitness is used herein.

**Developmental Trends in Children's Fitness Levels.**  Within the past two decades, several large-scale population-based studies have been conducted to assess the fitness status of American children (e.g., American Alliance for Health, Physical Education, Recreation, and Dance [AAHPERD], 1975; Reiff, Dixon, Jacoby, Ye, Spain, & Hunsicker, 1986; Ross & Gilbert, 1985; Ross & Pate, 1987). In addition, a wide variety of other studies have been conducted by researchers interested in assessing more specific aspects of children's fitness (see reviews by Beunen & Malina, 1988; Krahenbuhl, Skinner, & Kohrt, 1985; Rowland, 1990; Simons-Morton, O'Hara, Simons-Morton, & Parcel, 1987; Thomas & French, 1985). Despite relatively major differences in study design, sampling procedures, and instrumentation, some fairly consistent results have been obtained concerning the health-related fitness levels of American children. However, as discussed later in this section, there also have been numerous criticisms concerning the reliability and validity of the conclusions made on the basis of this research.

When the available data on children's fitness are examined from a developmental perspective, it is clearly apparent that children's fitness scores vary as a function of both age and gender. In regard to *cardiorespiratory endurance performance, muscular strength,* and *muscular endurance,* for example, the available research shows that both boys and girls exhibit a fairly steady increase in performance capabilities across the childhood years. However, during the adolescent years (i.e., ages 12–18 years), the incremental curves for boys and girls diverge. That is, boys' scores continue to show some increase in all of these areas during the adolescent years, while girls' scores tend to level off or even decline. Thus, while there appear to be small gender differences in these performance areas during the childhood years, there are considerable differences during and after adolescence.

In regard to *aerobic capacity,* Krahenbuhl et al. (1985), who reviewed the available literature in this area, concluded that the maximal aerobic power ($\dot{V}O_2$ max) relative to body weight remains relatively stable for boys between the ages of 6 and 17 years. In contrast, girls' scores on such tests show a progressive decline over the same age range.

In the area of *flexibility,* the data from the National Children and Youth Fitness Studies (Ross & Gilbert, 1985; Ross & Pate, 1987) indicate that girls' scores show little change from ages 6 to 9 years but then steadily increase from ages 10 to 16 years. In comparison, boys' scores show little change from ages 6 to 9 years, a slight decrease from 10 to 12 years, and then an increase from 13 to 17 years. At all ages, girls' flexibility scores are somewhat higher than that of their male peers.

In regard to *body composition,* examination of body fat indices in children of various ages has shown that relative body fat in boys remains fairly stable (13–15%) from ages 6 to 10, but then increases by 2–3% between the ages of 10 and 13 years. With the increase in muscle mass that occurs in boys during the adolescent growth spurt, body fat again decreases by 2–3% between the ages of 13 and 18 years. In contrast, the percentage of body fat increases progressively in girls across the childhood years. By 10 years of age, girls evidence about a 20% body fat index. During the adolescent years, percentage of body fat increases again to about a 25–26% level. Thus, it is apparent that from early childhood on, girls show significantly higher body-fat scores than do their male peers.

In summary, the data obtained from the field and laboratory studies that have been conducted over the past 20 years indicate that both age and gender have a significant impact on children's fitness scores. Interestingly, the size of the gender effect appears to increase as a function of age (i.e., there are greater gender differences after the age of 10 years than before) (Smoll & Schutz, 1990; Thomas & French, 1985). Despite these significant age and gender effects, it is necessary to use considerable caution in the interpretation of these developmental trends.

First, although it is tempting to conclude that the age-related changes that are consistently observed in children's fitness scores are due to the normal growth and maturation process, many other factors actually may explain these findings. First, with age may come an increased motivation to score well on performance-based fitness tests. Such increased motivation may result because children's interest in and use of peer comparison as a means to evaluate their physical competence increases significantly between the ages of 8 and 14 years (Horn & Hasbrook, 1986; Horn & Weiss, 1991). Given that many field fitness tests are based on the peer-comparison process (i.e., use of percentiles, class/group standings), older children may be more motivated to perform well in order to demonstrate relative competence than would younger children who are less oriented to the use of peer comparison. Second, performance on fitness tests may be at least partially a function of practice and/or past experience. Thus, children's scores may improve with age because they are more experienced at taking such tests. Third, children's movement and/or motor patterns become considerably more efficient with age. It is possible, for example, that improved endurance performance with age (e.g., decreases in a 1-mile-run time) may be due to biomechanical improvements in running patterns rather than to actual aerobic capacity. Finally, as children (particularly boys) get older, the physical demands placed on those who participate in organized sport programs increase measurably. Although there are conflicting reports in the literature as to whether children (especially at the prepubertal stage) will show improvement in cardiorespiratory function and strength capacities in response to exercise training, many of these studies have been methodologically weak and thus have introduced a number of confounding factors (see reviews by Gallahue, 1989; Krahenbuhl et al., 1985; Rowland, 1990). However, the training studies that have been conducted in accord with recommended exercise training guidelines (i.e., in terms of intensity, duration, frequency, and mode of exercise) have shown that significant improvements in children's maximal aerobic power and in their strength capabilities can be made. Thus, the age-related increases in fitness test scores that have been reported, particularly in samples of male children, may actually be due to sports-associated training programs rather than to growth and maturation. In summary, then, we must be cautious in concluding that the increases in fitness scores that occur across the childhood years are due only to the physical growth and maturation process.

Similar concerns can be raised about the causes and correlates of the gender differences typically found in both field and laboratory-based data. Specifically, boys have been found to score higher than girls in tests of cardiorespiratory endurance and muscular strength and endurance. Girls, in contrast, show better flexibility scores and also have higher body-fat content. Although these gender differences are somewhat evident in childhood, the differences increase significantly at puberty (Smoll & Schutz, 1990; Thomas & French, 1985). Traditionally, such gender differences have been attributed to naturally occurring physiological differences between males and females. Although there appear to be very few anthropometric differences between prepubescent boys and girls, a number of such differences appear during late childhood or early adolescence and continue into adulthood (Hansman, 1970; Malina, 1984; Roche & Malina, 1983). Because the particular anthropometric variables in which males and females differ (e.g., percentage of body fat, muscle mass, limb length, body physique) are biomechanically and physiologically related to performance on tasks that require strength, power, and endurance, the physiologically based explanation for gender differences in physical performance may certainly be justified.

Recently, however, a few investigators have questioned the ability of these physiological factors to explain all or even a significant amount of the variation between boys and girls in their fitness or physical performance scores (e.g., Smoll & Schutz, 1990; Thomas & French, 1985). This caution is based on several pieces of evidence suggesting that other factors may be equally explanatory. First, because there are very few physiological differences between boys and girls prior to puberty (particularly before 10 years of age) (see review by Malina, 1984), there should be few, if any, performance differences. However, as noted in the earlier sections, both field and laboratory studies have indicated that at least some gender differences in performance are evident from early childhood on. Thus, as Rowland (1990) has concluded, "the physiological differences between males and females are smaller than the performance gap" (p. 77).

A more direct assessment of the extent to which anthropometric variables are predictive of physical performance outcomes has been attempted by Smoll and Schutz (1990) with a sample of 2142 Canadian physical education students in Grades 3, 7, and 11. The results of their study verified the previously reported finding that the percentage of variance in children's physical performance scores that can be attributed to gender increased dramatically from Grade 3 to Grade 11. Specifically, gender accounted for up to 23% of the performance variability at Grade 3 and between 34% and 72% of the variability at Grade 11. However, their analysis of the degree to which anthropometric variables (particularly percentage of body fat) contributed to these gender differences indicated that for some tasks (e.g., standing long jump, flexed arm hang, timed run), there was actually a decrease with age in the percentage of explained variance. These results led Smoll and Schutz to conclude that with increasing age, gender differences in performance may be proportionately more a function of socioenvironmental factors than of biological factors. The authors also noted that percentage of body fat may itself be very much affected by level of physical activity and exercise. Thus, the notion that gender differences in fitness levels are primarily or predominantly explained by naturally occurring biological differences is not supported.

It is apparent, then, that other factors must be contributing to gender differences in fitness performance. One factor that appears to be particularly important is the comparative level of physical activity and/or sport-related training that boys and girls engage in during the childhood and adolescent years. Eaton and Enns (1986) conducted a meta-analysis using 90 studies, which assessed the frequency and/or intensity of motor activity in boys and girls from the prenatal to the early adolescent years. A significant effect size was found, indicating that males were generally more active than females. However, these authors also found that the effect size increased considerably with the age of the child. Although significant gender differences in activity level were already present during early infancy (0–11 months), the effect sizes were larger for the older groups. Unfortunately, the authors could find only six prenatal studies that assessed gender differences in activity level. Although the effect size for this group of studies was not significant, the authors note that additional studies could result in a different finding.

Given that *level* of physical activity (both frequency and intensity) may have a significant impact on children's physical fitness, it certainly would not be surprising that girls, who—as a group—are more sedentary, would exhibit lower levels of fitness at all ages than their more active male peers. The most likely explanation for the more sedentary life-style of girls lies in the sex-role socialization process, which does not encourage the development of physical competence in females. Specifically, in our society, because competence in the physical domain is not seen to be as valuable for females as it is for males, girls may not receive the same social and environmental support for the development of physical competence as do boys. A number of studies have revealed support for such socioenvironmental hypotheses (see Boutilier & SanGiovanni, 1983).

The fact that socioenvironmental factors can explain a large portion of the variation between males and females in physical performance does not completely negate the contribution of biological factors. Obviously, there are significant size and body-composition differences in postpubertal males and females, and these differences certainly affect physical performance capabilities. However, as Thomas and French (1985) note, the negative sociocultural messages concerning the appropriateness of physical activity for females may result in an overestimation of true (i.e., biologically based) differences in motor- or physical-skill capacities.

Finally, it should also be noted that the preceding discussion, which focused solely on gender differences in performance, obscures the fact that there is also much variation within each gender in fitness performance scores. That is, although the data may show that males as a group will differ significantly from females as a group on any single physical performance or fitness index, this certainly does not imply that all girls are more flexible than or less cardiovascularly fit than all boys. Rather, there is considerable overlap, both pre- and postpuberty in the physical capabilities of males and females. Thus, as Rowland (1990) concludes, there are probably more similarities than differences in the fitness scores of boys and girls. Furthermore, it is also important to keep in mind that many factors other than gender have a relatively larger impact on physical proficiency. Thus, an overemphasis on gender contrasts can obscure more important determinants of children's physical fitness status.

**Limitations and Future Directions.**    Despite the amount of data collected in the past decade, the information obtained to date concerning children's fitness status has been criticized for a variety of limitations in regard to research design (e.g., lack of longitudinal studies) Beunen & Malina, 1988; Branta, Haubenstricker, & Seefeldt, 1984; Gallahue, 1989), assessment procedures (e.g., use of unreliable or invalid instrumentation, low interrater and/or intrarater reliability) (Rowland, 1990), and interpretation or evaluation of obtained data (i.e., use of normatively defined fitness standards and/or lack of validated criterion cutoff scores) (Looney & Plowman, 1990; Safrit, Baumgartner, Jackson & Stamm, 1980; Simons-Morton et al., 1988).

In addition to the foregoing problems, the research work to date has also been limited in terms of subject sampling (Duda & Allison, 1990; Thomas & French, 1985). Specifically, the subjects in the research studies cited in the previous section have been limited in terms of age (primarily 10–18 years), race (mostly white), and socioeconomic background (mostly middle class). In addition, many of the laboratory studies have used children who were volunteers and/or currently involved in a physical activity program (e.g., competitive athletic teams) (Simons-Morton et al., 1987). Even in the large-scale population-based data-collection projects, when children from a wide variety of socioeconomic, racial, and activity backgrounds are used, the data are not always analyzed to determine how and/or whether such socioenvironmental factors are related to fitness levels. Given the evidence suggesting that individuals from selected ethnic and socioeconomic backgrounds are more susceptible to some specific hypokinetic diseases and that physical activity levels, exercise behavior, and motor proficiency vary as a function of ethnic and/or socioeconomic background (see excellent review by Duda & Allison, 1990), it seems essential that future research should be conducted to examine children's fitness level as a function of such factors.

Many of the foregoing problems are compounded by the difficulties involved in obtaining valid and reliable fitness or physical-performance scores from children. Several writers (e.g., Clarke, 1986; Seefeldt, 1984) have detailed a number of problems researchers face when attempting to obtain such data: (a) the difficulty in motivating younger children, in particular, to exert a maximum performance effort; (b) the probability that the use of some mechanical-assessment devices (e.g., heart-rate monitors, mouthpieces) may distract the child's attention away from performance; (c) the possibility that immature movement patterns may inhibit the testing process (e.g., balance problems on a moving treadmill); and (d) ethical concerns related to the informed-assent process. These difficulties certainly provide some explanation for the limited amount of physiological research on children's performance capabilities. In addition, recognition of these problems suggests that some caution should be used in the interpretation of the data obtained to date.

Finally, extreme caution must be observed in attempting to interpret children's fitness scores relative to their health status. Although it is commonly believed that American children of today are unfit, that conclusion is presently unwarranted for at least two reasons. First, conclusive statements about the status of children's health-related fitness cannot currently be made because we do not yet know what level of fitness is essential for optimal health during the childhood and adolescent years. Most traditional interpretations of children's fitness levels are based on normative comparisons (e.g., percentile scores or standard scores). That is, the fitness levels of individual children or groups of children are evaluated as to how their scores compare to that of their age-group peers. Although such normative comparisons may be useful for some purposes, they provide virtually no information concerning the health status of individual children. For example, a child who scores at the thirtieth percentile for his or her age group on the 1-mile-run test may still be at a sufficient level of fitness for optimal health benefits even though he or she may be called "less cardiovascularly fit" than the majority of his or her peers. Thus, we cannot use such normative data to speculate about children's health status.

A second, and perhaps more crucial, point with regard to the interpretation of children's fitness scores is that a link between fitness and health has not been established definitively yet. In fact, as some researchers (e.g., Meredith, 1988; Powell, Thompson, Caspersen, & Kendrick, 1987; Simons-Morton et al., 1988) have noted, studies conducted with adult subjects have clearly shown that it is *physical activity* rather than *physical fitness* that is associated with positive health benefits. That is, adults who are physically active appear to be at reduced risk for developing a variety of health problems (e.g., heart disease, diabetes, osteoporosis, some forms of cancer). In contrast, a strong association between fitness status and health has not been established. Thus, an individual whose fitness scores are high but who is physically inactive may not necessarily be at reduced risk for selected health problems. Although comparable research work with children has not been conducted, the research with adults suggests that we should be less concerned with children's scores on fitness tests than with their level of physical activity. It is for these reasons, in combination with initial research indicating that there may be little carryover from childhood to adulthood in health-related aspects of fitness, that a number of writers (e.g., Sallis & McKenzie, 1991; Simons-Morton et al., 1987) have suggested that the emphasis in children's physical-activity programs should be on physical activity rather than on physical-fitness status. That is, children should be encouraged to participate in and to enjoy some form of moderate to vigorous physical activity rather than to achieve some preestablished level of fitness. Such a recommendation seems appropriate considering the current lack of definitive and valid information concerning optimal levels of fitness during the childhood and adolescent years.

Given the number and severity of the criticisms concerning our current knowledge of children's fitness levels, it is obvious that considerably more research is needed before we will have an adequate understanding of children's fitness levels and how such levels relate to their physical health. The next two sections review the research that has been conducted to examine children's physical-activity patterns and their cardiovascular health.

## Children's Physical-Activity Levels

Recent reports have indicated that anywhere from 7.6 to 20% of American adults ages 18–65 years regularly participate in forms of physical activity that can be characterized as moderate to vigorous in nature and that an additional 40% of adults are sedentary (Caspersen, Christenson, & Pollard, 1986; Stephens, Jacobs, & White, 1985). Comparable attempts to assess the activity level of children have been hindered by the difficulty encountered in measuring the intensity, frequency, and duration of children's daily activity (Klesges & Klesges, 1987; Saris, 1986). The three types of instruments most typically employed by researchers in this area of study have included self-report assessments (e.g., diaries, activity-recall questionnaires), observational measures (i.e., data collected by external observers), and mechanical or electronic monitors (e.g., portable heart-rate monitors, motion sensors).

Unfortunately, each of these measurement techniques has limitations, particularly with regard to assessment of physical-activity levels in children (see critiques by Klesges & Klesges, 1987; Noland, Danner, Dewalt, McFadden, & Kotchen, 1990; Saris, 1986). Thus, no one system of measurement has yet been demonstrated to be the most valid. However, recent advancements in the sophistication of the instrumentation (Noland et al., 1990; O'Hara, Baranowski, Simons-Morton, Wilson, & Parcel, 1989; Puhl, Greaves, Hoyt, & Baranowski, 1990) may ultimately result in more reliable and accurate data concerning children's activity levels.

Despite these measurement problems, a number of research studies have been conducted in an attempt to describe the amount of physical activity children exhibit either in physical education classes or in more unstructured settings such as recess time, or after-school free play. The results of these studies are briefly summarized in the following paragraphs.

**Physical Education Activity Levels.** The NCYFS population studies conducted in the 1980s (Ross, Dotson, Gilbert, & Katz, 1985; Ross, Pate, Corbin, Deply, & Gold, 1987) showed that the majority of school-aged children across the country are enrolled in physical-education classes. However, only about a third of these students take physical education on a daily basis, and participation rates vary markedly by grade. In addition, most of the activities constituting the physical-education classes were found to be oriented toward sports and games rather than toward fitness and/or lifelong physical activities (e.g., Ross et al., 1985).

Recently, several observational studies have been conducted to examine more closely the amount of physical activity children get in physical-education classes (e.g., Parcel, Simons-Morton, O'Hara, Baranowski, Kolbe, & Bee, 1987; Placek, Silverman, Shute, Dodds & Rife, 1982). The combined results of these studies show that children spend very little class time engaged in moderate to vigorous physical activity. In fact, a large portion of the class time is devoted to management and organizational activities. In addition, Klausen, Rasmussen, and Schibye (1986) noted that there was extreme variation in activity level among children in the same class. Thus, even if the class as a whole is involved in a moderate to vigorous physical activity, not all children may be participating at that level.

In general, then, the results of these studies show that children are not engaged in vigorous physical activity for significant portions of their physical-education class time. In response to this observation, however, it must be pointed out that the development of fitness levels in children is not the only objective of school-based physical-education programs. Rather, physical educators must also be concerned with teaching children both the fundamental motor skills (catching, throwing, kicking) and the more activity-specific skills needed for successful participation in a variety of sports and physical activities (e.g., tennis, golf, racquetball) (Corbin, 1987; Haywood, 1991; Seefeldt & Vogel, 1987). In addition, most physical-education curriculums specify other social, cognitive, and affective objectives. Thus, the amount of class time that physical-education teachers can allocate specifically to fitness-related activities must necessarily be limited to a relatively small portion of the total available. Of course, as Haywood, in particular, has pointed out, physical-education instructional activities can be structured in such a way that both skill-related and fitness objectives are simultaneously accomplished. Thus, it may not be so much what physical-education teachers teach as how they teach it that may need to be changed. Nevertheless, as Corbin has suggested, it may well be that physical education should not be considered the only unit responsible for the development of fitness and/or physical activity in children.

**Unstructured Activity Level.** A variety of studies have also been conducted to examine children's physical activity patterns in more unstructured situations (e.g., Andersen, Ilmarinen, Rutenfrantz, Ottmann, Berndt, Kylian, & Ruppel, 1984; Gilliam, Freedson, Greenen, & Shahraray, 1981; Kemper, Dekker, Ootjers, Post, Ritmeester, Snel, Splinter, Essen, & Verschuur, 1985; Sallis, Patterson, McKenzie, & Nader, 1988; Simons-Morton, O'Hara, Parcel, Huang, Baranowski, & Wilson, 1990). Although these studies certainly have varied considerably in methodology, research design, sample size, subject age, and gender, they have generally all reported the consistent finding that children do not voluntarily participate in a significant amount of regular vigorous physical activity during unstructured play or leisure time periods. Furthermore, the results of these studies suggest that activity level declines as a function of age. That is, it appears that children in the early elementary years spend more time per day in vigorous physical activity than do children in later childhood. Other studies have shown that there is a particularly significant decline in the level of vigorous physical activity for both boys and girls during adolescence (12–18 years) (e.g., Andersen et al., 1984; Kemper et al., 1985).

There is also at least initial evidence to show that girls spend significantly less time in vigorous physical activity at all age levels than do their male peers (Andersen et al., 1984; Gilliam et al., 1981; Kemper et al., 1985; Ross & Gilbert, 1985). Again, however, based on the effect sizes calculated by Eaton and Enns (1986), using 90 independent studies, it is most likely that gender differences in level of physical activity increase as a function of age. In an interesting follow-up study, Eaton and Yu (1989) found that the comparably earlier maturation rates of girls can explain some of the gender differences in activity level. However, significant differences between boys and girls in level of activity remained even when maturational level was statistically controlled. Thus, Eaton and Yu conclude that maturity is only one of several mechanisms that explain the degree of sex differences in activity level.

As noted earlier, the results of these studies must be examined with some caution, due to the difficulty in obtaining a valid and reliable indicator of the frequency and intensity of activity level in children. Nevertheless, the available data suggest that children are not as active as it is perhaps commonly believed. Furthermore, the significant age and gender differences in activity level suggest the need to examine further the correlates and causes of interindividual variation in children's activity patterns. An interesting example of this type of research is illustrated in a recent study conducted by Sallis and associates (Sallis et al., 1988), who used multiple regression analyses to estimate the relative effects of a variety of familial variables (e.g., family cardiovascular disease risk, parents' activity level) on the activity level of preschool children. Continued research in this area will certainly result in the identification of additional physiological, anthropometric, psychological, and socioenvironmental variables that can explain variations among individual children in regard to participation in vigorous physical activity (see more extensive development of this argument by Duda & Allison, 1990). Of course, as noted earlier in regard to children's fitness levels, further research is also necessary to determine how much physical activity is necessary for optimal health benefits. Although present data support the idea that children are not very physically active, the implications of such results for health purposes are largely still unknown. However, based on comparable research with adults (see reviews by Meredith, 1988; Powell et al., 1987; Simons-Morton et al., 1988), it appears that physical activity may be more relevant to health than is physical fitness. Thus, the fact that children, as a group, are relatively inactive and that activity levels decline with age should be of greater concern to us than their scores on relevant fitness tests.

## Children's Health

The demonstrated link between exercise and cardiovascular health in adults stimulated comparable research with children to determine their health status relative to the development of CHD. Because several comprehensive reviews of these studies have been written about this topic recently (e.g., Despres, Bouchard, & Malina, 1990; Gilliam & MacConnie, 1984; Montoye, 1986), the results are only briefly summarized here.

In general, the results of research with children have supported the notion that children exhibit the same health-risk factors as adults. Specifically, several investigators have shown that significant numbers of children between the ages of 7 and 17 years exhibit such risk factors as obesity, hypertension, hyperlipidemia, and diabetes (Gilliam, Katch, Thorland, & Weltman, 1977; Lauer, Connor, Leaverton, Reiter, & Clarke, 1975; Wilmore & McNamara, 1974). In addition, selected risk factors have even been detected in preschoolers (Hunter, Wolf, Sklov, Webber, Watson, & Berenson, 1982; Lundberg, 1983). Furthermore, postmortem studies conducted with children (Strong, Eggen & Oalmann, 1972; Strong & McGill, 1969) and young adults (Enos, Beyer, & Holmes, 1955; McNamara, Molot, Stremple, & Cutting, 1971; Newman, Freedman, Voors, Gard, Srinivasan, Cresanta, Williamson, Webber, & Berenson, 1986) have suggested that the atherosclerotic process (i.e., the deposit of fat along the arterial walls) has already begun during the early years of life.

Although we do not yet have conclusive long-term research to show that the presence of risk factors during childhood is significantly predictive of incidence and/or severity of CHD in adulthood, a few tracking studies have been completed. The results of these studies show that there is at least some stability across the childhood, adolescent, and young adult years in regard to the presence of risk factors (see reviews by Cresanta, Hyg, Burke, Downey, Freedman, & Berenson, 1986, and Despres et al., 1990).

In summary, the research in this area indicates that certain risk factors are present in childhood and that such factors appear to be at least relatively stable into early adulthood. Such information certainly should lead to the hypothesis that interventions conducted with children who exhibit high-risk health profiles would reduce these children's vulnerability and that such interventions should begin as early as possible.

As noted in the introduction to this chapter, interest among practitioners, as well as researchers, in children's fitness was stimulated to a great extent by research conducted with adults showing that participation in a regular program of moderate to vigorous physical activity results in (a) decreased risk for a number of cardiovascular-related diseases and (b) increased mental well-being. The next section of this chapter describes the much smaller amount of research that has been conducted to examine the effects of exercise training on children's mental health.

## EXERCISE TRAINING AND CHILDREN'S MENTAL HEALTH

Researchers who have empirically tested the relationship between physical activity and mental health in children have focused primarily on self-esteem and, to a lesser extent, on such related psychological constructs as locus of control, anxiety, and depression. More recently, there has also been some interest in examining the effects of exercise training on children's reactivity to stress. The research in each of these two areas of study is discussed separately in the following two sections.

### Self-Esteem and Related Constructs

Although there has been some confusion in the past concerning the use of such related terms as self-esteem, self-worth, self-concept, self-efficacy, and perceived competence, a consensus definition of these terms has been achieved in recent years (e.g., Fox, 1988; Sonstroem, 1984). Specifically, *self-*

*concept* is the term that is now used to describe an individual's overall awareness of the self in terms of physical attributes, personal characteristics, social identities, and/or behaviors (e.g., "I am a female," "I am an athlete," "I am introverted"). In contrast, *self-esteem* refers to the individual's evaluation of or affective reaction to these attributes or characteristics. In other words, while *self-concept* can be defined as the individual's perception of self, *self-esteem* can be defined as the value the individual places on those self-perceptions (i.e., degree of satisfaction with what he or she is).

A variety of other self-related constructs have also been used by researchers in their attempts to examine the relationship between physical activity and self-perceptions. These constructs include self-efficacy, self-confidence, and perceived competence. Typically, these constructs are used to represent more specific components or dimensions of self-esteem and are usually employed to measure children's perceptions of the self and/or personal ability in regard to particular achievement domains or performance contexts. As discussed later in this chapter, these constructs represent more specific subdomains of the global self-esteem construct and are thus subsumed under the more general term, *self-esteem*.

As noted earlier, most of the research that has been conducted to examine the relationship between physical activity and psychological well-being in children has focused on self-esteem. This may be due to the fact that self-esteem is one of the more accessible psychological constructs to measure. Also, self-esteem appears to be a primary antecedent or director of behavior and thus may be one of the most important psychological constructs to study. Three reviews (Gruber, 1986; Sonstroem, 1982, 1984) of the research on exercise and self-esteem have been published. Because Sonstroem's reviews have focused primarily on research with adults, while Gruber's review is limited to exercise and self-esteem in children, only the results of Gruber's analysis are discussed in this section.

Gruber (1986) began by identifying 27 controlled experimental studies, which were conducted to examine the relationship between children's participation in some form of physical activity and subsequent changes in their self-esteem and/or related personality dimensions. Using meta-analytic statistical procedures to collate the results across studies, Gruber found a significant overall effect size indicating that participation in a physical-activity program does have a measurable impact on children's self-esteem.

In addition to this main effect, Gruber (1986) also examined the extent to which several other factors might mediate the overall relationship between physical activity and self-esteem. The first of these subanalyses indicated that participation in physical activity has a relatively greater impact on the self-esteem of what Gruber called "handicapped" children than on "nonhandicapped" children. Children who were classified in this analysis as being "handicapped" included those who were emotionally disturbed, trainable and educable mentally retarded, economically disadvantaged, and perceptually handicapped. As Gruber notes, these results are probably due to the relatively lower self-esteem scores evidenced by "handicapped" children prior to participation in a physical-activity program. Thus, as in other areas of research, the greatest gain to be found in intervention programs is evident in those who are lowest in the variable that is targeted for improvement.

Another secondary analysis conducted by Gruber (1986) showed that the greatest gain in self-esteem occurred when the physical-activity training programs consisted of physical fitness and/or aerobic types of activities rather than sport or dance skill or perceptual-motor activities. As Gruber speculates, the relatively greater psychological benefits to be gained from an aerobic or fitness program may be due to the fact that individual progress in such programs is more directly and visibly evident than in other sport- or movement-activity programs. Thus, the child's perception of competence or success may be facilitated to a greater degree. Further discussion concerning the role of perceived success in the psychological adaptation process is provided at the end of this section.

Although the research conducted to date has certainly provided some interesting information concerning the effects of exercise and physical activity on self-esteem in children, recent advances in self-concept theory and measurement suggest exciting new directions for research in this area. From a theoretical perspective, for example, a number of writers (e.g., Harter, 1983; Shavelson, Hubner, & Stanton, 1976) have argued that self-concept and/or self-esteem should be conceptualized as a multidimensional construct rather than a unidimensional one. Traditionally, self-esteem was perceived to be unidimensional (see Figure 11.1a), measured by assessing the individual's evaluation of the self across a wide variety of general and specific life situations. These individual evaluations were then summed to provide a composite score representing the individual's global or overall level of self-esteem.

Within the past decade, this singular conceptualization of self-esteem has given way to a multidimensional approach, which postulates that an individual can have very different perceptions or judgments of the self, depending on the particular domain (e.g., social, cognitive, physical) in which the self is being evaluated. Although the various domain-specific self-perceptions do contribute to an overall or global self-esteem (see Figure 11.1b), this global construct is more than just the sum of the individual parts and is thus assessed independently from its parts (e.g., Harter, 1985).

A related but somewhat different way to view self-esteem is from a hierarchical perspective (Shavelson et al., 1976) (see Figure 11.1c). This approach also postulates the existence of a global or overall self-esteem construct that is linked to self-perceptions in a number of subdomains (e.g., physical, cognitive, social). In addition, however, a series of hierarchical sublevels are added, suggesting that each subdomain can be compartmen-

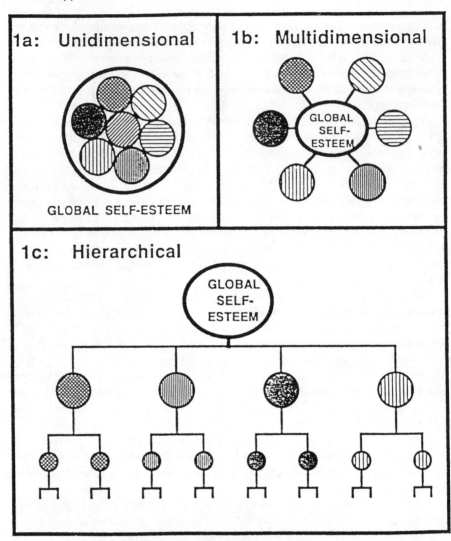

**Figure 11.1.** Three models of self-esteem structure. From "The Physical Self-perception Profile: Development and Preliminary Validation" by Kenneth R. Fox and Charles B. Corbin, 1989, *Journal of Sport and Exercise Psychology, 11*(4), p. 409. Copyright 1989 by Human Kinetics Publishers, Inc. Reprinted by permission.

talized into increasingly more specific components. An individual's academic self-esteem, for example, can be further divided into perceptions of ability in specific subject areas (e.g., English, math). In the physical domain, Fox and Corbin's (1989) initial work with college students has shown that the physical domain self-perceptions can be further divided into four subdomains, comprising perceived sports competence, perceived bodily attractiveness, perceived physical strength and muscular development, and perceived level of physical conditioning and exercise (see Figure 11.2). Based on the hierarchical notion of self-esteem, it could be hypothesized that each of these four subdomains can be further differentiated. The perceived sports competence subdomain, for example, could be broken down into specific sports (e.g., basketball, baseball, gymnastics) or sport groups (individual sports vs. team sports).

From a developmental perspective, researchers (e.g., Harter, 1988; Marsh & Shavelson, 1985) have found that children as young as 4 years exhibit differentiation in their perceptions of the self (i.e., they can judge themselves differently, depending on the domain). However, the number of domains increase with age. Harter's self-perception scale for children ages 8–12 years includes 5 subscales. In contrast, the adolescent version includes 8 subscales, and the adult version comprises 11. Interestingly, Harter and Pike (1984), in a separate study, found that the self-judgments of children between the ages of 4 and 7 years were differentiated along only two dimensions. Specifically, the cognitive and physical competence judgments loaded together, and items relating to social acceptance and behavioral conduct formed the second dimension. Thus, it certainly appears that an individual's propensity to form a multidimensional assessment of the self increases as a function of age.

In regard to the hierarchical model of self-esteem, Marsh and his colleagues (e.g., Marsh, Byrne, & Shavelson, 1988; Marsh & Holmes, 1990) have

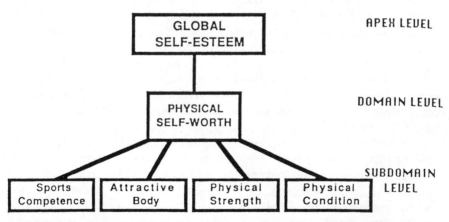

**Figure 11.2.** Hypothesized three-tier hierarchical organization of self-perceptions. From "The Physical Self-perception Profile: Development and Preliminary Validation" by K. R. Fox and C. B. Corbin, 1989, *Journal of Sport and Exercise Psychology, 11*(4), p. 414. Copyright 1989 by Human Kinetics Publishers, Inc. Reprinted by permission.

recently used a variety of statistical techniques to provide empirical support for this model. More specific to the physical domain, Fox and Corbin's (1989) psychometric work with college students has also resulted in support for at least a three-tier hierarchical structure (see Figure 11.2). However, as Fox and Corbin (1989) and Marsh and Holmes (1990) caution, the particular hierarchical dimensions and subdimensions within both the academic and physical domains may not yet have been adequately specified. Nevertheless, these initial results suggest that self-esteem cannot be investigated adequately without assuming a multidimensional approach.

Application of these multidimensional theoretical models to the field of exercise psychology would lead to the hypothesis that an exercise training program would have greatest impact on the subcomponents or components of self-esteem that are most directly related to the goals of that training program. Specifically, a weight-training program may have significant impact on the participants' perceptions of physical appearance and body image. Although these domain-specific self-constructs are perhaps more subject to change than is global self-esteem, ultimately, of course, increases in the individual's domain-specific self-esteem can also positively influence global self-esteem. This effect on global self-esteem will most probably occur if the exercise training program is of sufficient intensity and/or duration. For example, in the sports domain, a child who experiences success in her first competitive softball season may show an increase in perceived softball competence. However, continued (i.e., sustained) success in softball may result in increased physical self-esteem and perhaps ultimately in increased global self-esteem. From a measurement perspective, then, it is important that researchers who are testing the psychological effects of an exercise program on children measure global self-esteem, physical self-esteem, and the more domain-specific subcomponents of the physical construct. Otherwise, the potential effects of the exercise training may not be adequately assessed.

Empirical support for this multidimensionally based hypothesis in the physical domain has been found in a few recent studies. First, in two group-comparison studies, Marsh and Jackson (1986; Jackson & Marsh, 1986) found that female athletes had significantly higher physical self-concepts than did nonathletes. In contrast, group differences on other domain-specific measures of self-concept were either much smaller or nonsignificant. Similar results were obtained by Fox and Corbin (1989) in a study conducted with college students. Their correlational analyses showed that the type of sport or physical activity in which individuals were active was significantly related to their scores on the various subscales. High scores on the perceived strength subscale, for example, were significantly correlated with weight training. Correspondingly, participation in ball-sport activities was more highly related to the sport competence subscale. In a more training-oriented study, Marsh and Peart (1988) found that eighth-grade girls (ages 11–14 years) who participated in a 6-week, relatively noncompetitive cardiovascular aerobics training program showed significant improvement in physical ability self-concept and a lower but still significant increase in the physical appearance self-concept. No training effect was found for the other domain-specific measures of self-concept or for general self-concept. In addition, no changes in any of the self-concept dimensions were found in a comparable group of control subjects. The combined results of these studies provide support for the multidimensional model of self-esteem and for the differential impact of the various exercise or sport training programs on individual self-esteem subdomains.

One other recent advance in self-esteem theory may have relevance for sport and exercise psychology researchers. Specifically, several theorists (e.g., Harter, 1988; Rosenberg, 1982) have suggested that individuals may vary in the degree of importance they place on certain aspects of the self-esteem structure. One child, for example, may place greater importance on athletic sport competence while her or his peer may place greater emphasis on perceived body attractiveness. Such interindividual variation in the relevance or importance of the various subdomains may have a significant impact on the child's global self-esteem.

For example, the child who places great emphasis on sport competence but who is generally unsuccessful in this area will have lower physical and global self-esteem than her or his peer who is equally unsuccessful in sports but who values it less highly. In the fitness area, then, a child who participates successfully in an exercise training program (i.e., experiences a training-induced increase in fitness) but who does not value competence in this domain will probably not show an increase in physical self-esteem as a function of the training program. In contrast, a child who highly values physical strength, conditioning, and exercise but who perceives low competence in these areas may show very significant improvement in physical self-esteem after successful participation in a training program.

Harter's (1988) life span analysis of the causes and correlates of self-esteem has shown clear support for this model. Specifically, her work with individuals ranging in age from 8 to 50 years showed that correspondence between *perceived* competence in a particular subdomain (e.g., athletic competence) and the *importance* that individuals assigned to that subdomain was a very significant predictor of global self-esteem. That is, individuals who perceived themselves to be incompetent in a domain they also deemed to be very important were significantly more apt to have low global self-esteem than individuals whose perceptions of incompetence in a specific domain were combined with low ratings of importance in that same domain. It is for these reasons that the recent psychometric work conducted by Fox and Corbin (1989) for the purpose of developing a physical self-perception profile has included an accompanying instrument to measure the perceived importance of the various subscales. This importance construct may be necessary for researchers to take into consideration when investigating the psychological effects of exercise training on children.

As noted earlier, much less work has been conducted with children to assess the impact of exercise training on psychological constructs other than self-esteem or self-concept. The few studies that have been conducted have shown positive effects. Duke, Johnson, and Nowicki (1977), for example, found a significant increase in internal locus of control in children who participated in an 8-week sport fitness camp. Similarly, Holloway, Beuter, and Duda (1988), who conducted a 12-week training program for increasing strength in adolescent females, showed that significant increases could be obtained in subjects' self-efficacy concerning their strength competence. These situationally specific positive training effects also generalized, however, to confidence and self-efficacy in other areas of life and were reflected in an increase in the more general measure of perceived physical ability. The authors explain this generalized effect by suggesting that because females in our society tend to be low in actual and perceived strength capabilities, they may show comparably greater increases in perceived competence as a result of intensive training.

In a somewhat unusual study conducted with 24 children, Alpert, Field, Goldstein, and Perry (1990) found that the positive psychological benefits of a cardiovascular fitness program can be extended to preschoolers. These researchers pre- and posttested children (ages 3–5 years) on a variety of physical tasks (e.g., submaximal aerobic exercise test, agility test) and on a general self-esteem scale. Following an 8-week cardiovascular aerobics program, the 12 trained children showed significant increases in self-esteem from pre- to posttraining, while a comparable set of children who had been assigned to a playground control group showed no change in self-esteem. The significant increase in global self-esteem found in this study may have been due to the lack of differentiation in the self-perceptions of children in this age group. This, of course, suggests that the less differentiated global self-esteem of children at younger ages may be more open to change than it is for older children who show increased differentiation.

Although research with adults has shown that participation in an exercise training program can result in decreased levels of anxiety and depression (see recent review by Plante & Rodin, 1990), little research with children has been conducted in either of these areas. One study (MacMahon & Gross, 1988) did find that participation in a 3-month aerobic exercise program was effective in both increasing self-concept and decreasing depression levels in 32 incarcerated adolescent males ages 14–18 years. In discussing these results, the authors suggest that these subjects, the majority of whom exhibited at least a mild level of depression at the pretraining time, may have been particularly likely to benefit from such an intervention program. Similar results were found in a laboratory training study conducted with undergraduate male and female subjects in our lab (Horn,

Claytor, & Phelps, 1991). Specifically, significant decreases in trait anxiety and significant increases in internal locus of control were found after subjects participated in an intensive 10-week aerobic training program. However, such positive psychological changes were found only in subjects who scored above the trait anxiety population mean before the training program began. The results of these studies, which are consistent with those obtained by Gruber (1986) in his meta-analysis of the self-esteem literature, suggest that exercise training may have the greatest psychological impact on those individuals who exhibit what may be defined as "at risk" psychological profiles prior to the training program.

In summary, the research that has been conducted to examine the effects of exercise training on children's mental health has supported the hypothesis that participation in a physical activity program can result in increased self-esteem and an internal locus of control and decreased anxiety and depression. In particular, the research suggests that such positive psychological adaptation will be most likely to occur in subjects who are at greatest risk psychologically.

It is important to keep in mind that these results are based on what is really a minimal amount of research. Furthermore, much of the research that has been conducted to date has suffered from theoretical, methodological, and measurement problems (see Plante & Rodin, 1990, and Sonstroem, 1984, for a more detailed discussion). From a theoretical and/or measurement perspective, very few studies have assumed a multidimensional approach to the measurement of self-esteem. Thus, the effects of physical training may not have been assessed accurately. In addition, serious methodological problems are evident, in that many studies have not (a) included control groups and/or have not used random assignment of subjects to groups, (b) quantified the training program or the subjects' responses to it, (c) specified the type of training used in the program (e.g., aerobic, anaerobic), (d) controlled for between-subject differences in initial or pretraining fitness levels, or (e) assessed the stability of any psychological changes through the use of follow-up assessment procedures.

Given the theoretical and methodological problems identified in the preceding paragraph, it is obvious that there remains a need for well-conducted and well-controlled studies in this area. In addition, future research is certainly needed to address questions concerning how and/or why psychological adaptation can occur as a result of exercise training. More specifically, do changes in psychological health result from increased fitness (i.e., actual physiological adaptations) or from mere participation in a physical activity program? As several writers and researchers (e.g., King, Taylor, Haskell, & DeBusk, 1989; Plante & Rodin, 1990; Sonstroem, 1984) have recently noted, the changes in psychological health that have been seen in adult subjects who participated in an exercise training program appear to have resulted from *perceived* as opposed to *actual* changes in fitness. That is, it may not be necessary for individuals to obtain an actual fitness change in order for them to benefit psychologically from an exercise program. Thus, it has been speculated that the positive psychological changes are not due to exercise-induced physiological changes but to such things as an increased sense of mastery, perception of personal control, or personal self-efficacy. This is certainly an interesting question to consider and one that will need to be addressed in future research work with both children and adults.

## Reactivity to Stress

In recent years, there has been considerable interest in the exercise psychology literature concerning the notion that exercise training might have a positive effect on individuals' reactivity to environmental stress. The research work that has been conducted to test this hypothesis with adult subjects has revealed equivocal findings (see Salazar et al., Chapter 5, this volume). In the following pages of this chapter, the research on children's reactivity patterns is examined. This review begins with an examination of the factors that affect the strength and intensity of children's reactivity to environmental and/or laboratory stressors and then ends with a discussion concerning the viability of exercise training as a mediator of such reactivity patterns.

Considerable research evidence indicates that children, just like adults, experience an increase in physiological and emotional arousal as a result of exposure to various environmental stressors (see comprehensive reviews by Beidel, 1989, and Jemerin & Boyce, 1990). Specifically, heightened neuroendocrine activity, increased cardiovascular responses, and accompanying emotional arousal have been observed in children subjected to a variety of stressful conditions (e.g., public speaking, academic examinations, laboratory stress protocols, dental examinations).

In establishing that stress-induced reactivity does exist in children, however, most researchers have also noted that there is considerable variability among children in their reactivity patterns (i.e., there is interindividual variability in the onset, intensity, and/or length of the stress response) (Beidel, 1989; Jemerin & Boyce, 1990; Murphy, Alpert, Willey, & Somes, 1988). Furthermore, there appears to be a relatively small subset of children within any given population of children who respond to stressful environmental conditions with exaggerated or comparatively high physiological and/or emotional reactivity. This type of exaggerated pattern is sometimes referred to as a "hyperreactive pattern." Based on a review of the cardiovascular reactivity research, Jemerin and Boyce (1990) estimated that 15–20% of primary school children fit such a hyperreactive profile. Finally, there is some, albeit limited, evidence to suggest that children's reactivity patterns (i.e., the strength and intensity of the individual response to stressors) are relatively stable across the preschool, childhood, and adolescent years (Matthews, Rakaczky, Stoney, & Manuck, 1987; Sallis, Patterson, McKenzie, Buono, Atkins, & Nader, 1989). These results suggest that the way in which an individual child responds to stress may represent a relatively stable individual difference variable (i.e., generalizable over time and across stressors). If this is the case, then children who are identified as hyperreactors during early childhood may maintain such a pattern throughout succeeding developmental stages.

Most researchers and writers consider such a hyperreactive pattern to be potentially negative for several reasons. First, high levels of arousal can result in impaired physical and cognitive performance (e.g., Beuter, Duda, & Widule, 1989; Sarason, 1980; Weinberg, 1978). Second, high anxiety has also been associated with a number of negative behavioral responses, such as withdrawal from challenge situations, lack of persistence following failure, and decrements in use of appropriate problem-solving and attentional strategies (Dweck & Leggett, 1988; Wine, 1980). However, the greatest concern in regard to hyperreactivity in children is the potential impact such a pattern may have on their health. As Jemerin and Boyce (1990) point out in their review of the literature, children and young adults who are highly reactive and/or who exhibit an overactive behavioral pattern (e.g., aggressiveness) have been found to be more susceptible to illness and injury (Bijur, Stewart-Brown, & Butler, 1986; Dembroski, MacDougall, Slaats, Eliot, & Buell, 1981; Horwitz, Morgenstern, DiPietro, & Morrison, 1988). Similarly, initial research has tied a hyperreactive pattern to the development of such health problems as hypertension and cardiovascular disease (Borghi, Costa, Boschi, Mussi, & Ambrosioni, 1986; Falkner, Onesti, & Hamstra, 1981).

As noted earlier, it is apparent that there is considerable variation among children in their reactivity to environmental stress. Given such diversity, a number of research studies have been conducted in recent years in an attempt to identify the factors that can explain such interindividual variation in reactivity. The factors that have been identified to date can be separated into three categories: demographic variables, psychological characteristics, and socioenvironmental influences. Each of these categories are briefly discussed in the following section.

**Factors Associated with Reactivity Patterns in Children.**    From a demographic perspective, researchers have identified a number of variables (e.g., age, gender, race, parental history of hypertension), which appear to affect children's reactivity to stress. To assess the impact of age on stress reactivity, several researchers have conducted cross-sectional laboratory research studies in order to compare the intensity of the stress response across children and adults of varying ages. The combined results of these studies show some age-related differences in reactivity. Specifically, adults exhibit greater increases in systolic blood pressure during stress situations than do children (Matthews & Stoney, 1988; Palmer, Ziegler, & Lake, 1978). However, adults also show reduced heart-rate response in comparison to children (Gintner, Hollandsworth, & Intrieri, 1986; Palmer et al., 1978). In addition, Matthews and Stoney (1988) demonstrated that among children ages 7–18 years, increased age was related to smaller heart-rate responses to stress. Thus, relatively consistent support has been found for the notion that aging reduces the magnitude of the heart-rate response to behavioral stress but enhances the systolic-blood-pressure responses.

Based on epidemiological research indicating that there are some differences between men and women in risk for CHD, a number of researchers have begun testing the hypothesis that such sex-differential risk is due to sex differences in physiological responses to stress. In a recent meta-analysis of this research, Stoney and colleagues (Stoney, Davis, & Matthews, 1987) found that adult males do exhibit both significantly higher systolic-blood-pressure responses and urinary epinephrine levels in response to stress than do adult females. In addition, there was some evidence that females showed greater heart-rate reactivity than did their male peers. No significant effects were found for diastolic blood pressure or for urinary norepinephrine or cortisol. Thus, Stoney and colleagues concluded that there is some support for the hypothesis that men show greater physiological reactivity to acute behavioral stress than do women. However, these authors also note that many other factors (e.g., type of stressor, task demand, behavioral characteristics) may mediate the link between an individual's gender and her or his level of reactivity to stress. In addition, recent research (e.g., Kaplan, Whitsett, & Robinson, 1990) has shown that the psychophysiological patterns of adult (premenopausal) women do vary significantly as a function of the menstrual cycle. Such cyclical variation in female subjects may have served as a confounding factor in previous gender-difference studies. Thus, the degree to which men and women differ in reactivity and the reasons for such differences has not yet been assessed adequately.

The data regarding sex differences in reactivity during the childhood years are also somewhat equivocal. Although two studies did find that boys exhibited greater increases in systolic blood pressure than did girls (Murphy et al., 1988; Schmidt, Thierse, & Eschweiler, 1986), other studies have shown no differences in blood-pressure response (e.g., Matthews & Stoney, 1988). However, Matthews and Stoney provide initial evidence to suggest that the presence or absence of sex differences may depend on the age of the subjects. Specifically, these researchers found no gender differences in the reactivity responses of elementary- and middle-school-aged children but did find significant differences in systolic blood-pressure reactivity in their high-school-aged subjects during some specific tasks. Matthews and Stoney suggest that this gender-by-age interaction effect could be due to the sex-differential hormonal changes that occur in children during the early adolescent years. However, as Matthews and Stoney also note, the gender differences in reactivity could also be a function of task type. In their study, for example, women and girls showed greater increases in heart rate during a serial subtraction (arithmetic) task than did their male peers. However, no sex differences were found in two other tasks (i.e., mirror-image tracing and an isometric handgrip task.)

The intriguing finding that sex differences in reactivity may not occur until the adolescent years is consistent with research in the developmental psychology literature showing that sex differences in achievement cognitions and related constructs either begin during the adolescent years or are significantly enhanced during this time period (Maccoby & Jacklin, 1974; Parsons, 1981). Thus, the finding that sex differences in reactivity may begin in adolescence appears to be part of an overall developmental pattern that may be either biologically or environmentally determined. As Matthews and Stoney (1988) note, however, the fact that sex constitutes one risk factor for CHD, especially coronary artery disease, provides clear justification for continued research to determine the factors related to the age-by-gender interaction effect in regard to reactivity.

Another demographic variable that appears to be related to degree of reactivity is parental history of hypertension. A number of research studies have been conducted to examine whether children whose parents are hypertensive will show greater reactivity to stressors than will children who do not have a parental history of hypertension. Recently, Fredrickson and Matthews (1990) conducted a meta-analysis using the available studies in this area. Their results clearly indicated that normotensive offspring of hypertensive parents did exhibit moderately larger and more reliable blood-pressure and heart-rate responses to stressors than did normotensive individuals whose parents were not hypertensive. Interestingly, from a developmental perspective, their results also showed that the observed group differences in reactivity were more pronounced in older samples of subjects (i.e., offspring who were 20 years or older) than in the younger samples (i.e., offspring who were aged 19 or younger). Overall, however, parental history of hypertension does appear to be one factor that affects children's reactivity patterns.

Based on observed epidemiological differences between African-American and European-American individuals in their rate and severity of hypertension (Anderson, 1989), a few researchers have begun investigating race as a factor that may affect children's reactivity to stress. The results of these studies provide some evidence that African-American children exhibit greater increases in blood pressure in response to stressors than do European-American children (e.g., Murphy, Alpert, Moes, & Somes, 1986; Murphy, Alpert, Willey, & Somes, 1988). Although some researchers have attributed observed racial differences in reactivity to selected physiological factors (e.g., plasma renin levels and sodium excretion), others have cited possible sociocultural explanations (see comprehensive review by Anderson, 1989). Armstead, Lawler, Gorden, Cross and Gibbons (1989), for example, have found that African-American college students who were exposed to racist scenarios exhibited significantly greater increases in blood pressure than they did when exposed to anger-provoking but not racist scenarios. Based on these results, Armstead et al. have suggested that African-American adults may be significantly more apt to develop hypertension because of the cumulative effects of daily exposure to racism. In addition, Anderson (1989) has identified a variety of other sociocultural factors that may mediate the relationship between race and stress-induced reactivity. Thus, although the research to date has identified race as *one* factor that affects reactivity to stress, the etiology of such racial differences are as yet undetermined. Clearly, however, as Anderson concludes, future researchers in this area should probably be directed toward an examination of the interaction of sociocultural and biological factors in determining patterns of reactivity. In addition, an examination of the interindividual variability within the designated racial groups may also yield as much or more information than the comparison of reactivity patterns across racial groups. Thus, this remains an interesting and potentially informative area of research.

In addition to demographic factors, research evidence has been accumulated to suggest that certain *psychological* characteristics or traits affect children's reactivity patterns. Specifically, research reported in the developmental-psychology and sport-psychology literatures has indicated that such psychological characteristics as high trait anxiety, low self-esteem, and low self-efficacy have all been associated with heightened cardiovascular, emotional, and/or behavioral reactivity to stressful conditions (e.g., Beidel, 1989; Scanlan & Lewthwaite, 1984; Yan Lan & Gill, 1984). Similarly, Engebretson, Matthews, and Scheier (1989) have demonstrated that styles of anger expression were important determinants of systolic blood-pressure responses in college-aged male subjects, particularly when subjects were not allowed to use their preferred modes of expressing anger. The literature of the Type A behavior pattern also reveals a significant association between this behavior pattern and exaggerated heart-rate and blood-pressure responses in children who are exposed to challenging laboratory procedures (Brown & Tanner, 1988; Lawler, Allen, Critcher, & Standard, 1981; Lundberg, 1983; Schmidt et al., 1986). In addition, McCann and Matthews (1988) have found a significant link between adolescents' potential for hostility and their blood-pressure responses to behavioral stressors. As these researchers suggest, given recent research suggesting that hostility may be a more significant risk factor for CHD than the more global Type A measure, further research to examine the link between hostility and psychophysiological reactivity in children is warranted.

Finally, a series of studies by Kagan and his associates (e.g., Kagan, Reznick, Clarke, Snidman, & Garcia-Coll, 1984; Kagan, Reznick, & Snidman, 1987) have pointed out an interesting association between an inhibited behavioral pattern (i.e., extreme cautiousness, shyness, and/or behavioral withdrawal) and degree of reactivity when exposed to unfamiliar and/or challenging conditions. In particular, Kagan et al. (1987) showed that children who were identified via behavioral observation during the second or third year of life as behaviorally inhibited tended to maintain this pattern through their sixth year of life. In addition, exposing these children and a comparable group of uninhibited children (characterized by fearless and outgoing temperament) to unfamiliar and/or mildly challenging laboratory conditions resulted in significant group differences in reactivity. Specifically, the inhibited children showed significantly greater physiological (e.g., heart rate, pupillary dilation) and neuroendocrine (e.g., salivary levels of cortisol, urinary levels of norepinephrine) reactivity to these laboratory stressors than did the uninhibited children. Given the longitudinal nature of this data-collection project and the variety of measures used to assess reactivity, the obtained results provide strong support for the notion that children with certain psychological profiles are more apt to exhibit a hyperreactive response to stress than are children who do not have such profiles.

A third category of variables that may affect children's reactivity patterns includes those that can be grouped under the general heading of *sociocultural* or *environmental factors*. Although there has been relatively little work completed in this area, initial results suggest that children's reactivity patterns are linked to a number of family environment factors. Woodall and Matthews (1989) found, for example, that male children raised in families who scored low on positive affiliation (i.e., lack of cohesive, expressive, and/or supportive family relationships) and high in authoritarianism (i.e., high levels of structure, control, and restrictiveness) exhibited greater increases in heart-rate reactivity in response to a laboratory stress protocol than did boys raised in families who did not show such patterns. Similar relationships have been found by researchers who have examined the etiology of test anxiety in children (see reviews by Dusek, 1980, and Krohne, 1980). Krohne (1980) specifically identified four parental childrearing patterns that appear to play a central role in developing high trait anxiety in children: (1) high frequencies of negative reinforcement, (2) high intensity of negative reinforcement, (3) inconsistency in regard to performance and/ or behavioral feedback, and (4) a restrictive emotional environment. Although the results of these studies show only that there is an associative relationship between family environment factors and children's reactivity patterns, a more interesting issue for future researchers is to test whether the link is actually causal in nature. That is, do these, and perhaps other, parental behaviors actually cause children to develop a hyperreactive pattern, or do they both reflect another common factor, which may be biological or environmental? In addition, there are quite probably many other more wide-ranging sociocultural or environmental variables that could also be implicated in regard to the development of high reactivity in children. Thus, research in this area is just beginning.

The combined results of the research presented in this section show that the variation among children in their reactivity to environmental stress can be attributed, at least in part, to a variety of demographic, psychological, and/or socioenvironmental factors. Certainly, this is not an inclusive list, as there quite probably are many factors or even categories of factors (e.g., physiological) that are also associated with reactivity patterns in children. Thus, future research efforts should be directed toward the identification of such additional factors and/or the examination of the interrelationships among the various factors. Such information is of particular value because it may provide some insight concerning the causes and correlates of a hyperreactive stress pattern. Ultimately, such research work would allow us to develop a profile that characterizes children who show high reactivity to environmental stressors.

Given the potentially negative health consequences that may be associated with a hyperreactive stress pattern, some researchers have recently begun focusing their attention on possible intervention strategies. An aerobic-exercise training program has been proposed as one of these possible intervention strategies. The potential relationship between exercise training and modification of children's reactivity responses is examined in the next section.

**Exercise Training and Stress Reactivity in Children.** Within the past decade, a number of studies have been conducted to test the hypothesis that exercise training moderates individuals' psychophysiological reactivity to a variety of laboratory stressors. Unfortunately, for purposes of this chapter, this research has been limited to adult subjects. To our knowledge, no empirical, laboratory-based training studies have yet been conducted with subjects under the age of 18 years. A few researchers, however, have examined the relationship between children's exercise activity and their reactivity to stress using a more field-based approach. Brown and his colleagues (Brown & Lawton, 1986; Brown & Siegel, 1988) have demonstrated, for example, that adolescents who reported that they exercised on a regular basis experienced fewer physical illnesses under conditions of high life stress (e.g., parental separation, change in residence, negative interactions with adults or peers, social exclusion) than did their less physically active peers. Thus, exercise appears to buffer or temper the potentially negative impact of naturally occurring but stressful life events on children's physical and mental health. Although the results of these studies do provide some support for the hypothesis that exercise training can modulate children's reactivity to stress, the methodological procedures used in these field-based studies do not allow as direct a test of the exercise–reactivity relationship as do the more well-controlled laboratory studies.

Undoubtedly, the dearth of laboratory studies to assess the relationship between children's physical activity and their stress reactivity can be attributed, at least in part, to the difficulties involved in conducting such studies with children. Nevertheless, as the research reviewed in the preceding section clearly shows, children do exhibit a measurable increase in physiological and emotional arousal as a result of exposure to various environmental stressors. Furthermore, there appears to be a subset of children who respond to stressful conditions with exaggerated reactivity. Thus, research to examine the relationship between exercise training and reactivity in children would certainly seem to be warranted. However, such research must be carefully designed and conducted if an adequate assessment of this relationship is to be obtained. In the following paragraphs, we offer four specific recommendations concerning future research studies. These recommendations are based on the foregoing review of the literature on reactivity patterns in children and on recently published reviews and critiques of the research in this area (see, for example, Chodzko-Zajko, 1991; Claytor, 1991; Pickering & Gerin, 1990; Plante & Rodin, 1990; Sothmann, Hart, & Horn, 1991).

The first and most obvious recommendation is that future research studies must be methodologically well designed and conducted. Specifically, based on a review of the research conducted to date with adult subjects, the following measurement and experimental design issues appear to be the most important:

1. Use of training studies rather than—or in addition to—cross-sectional studies

2. Employment of appropriate control groups

3. Use of accurate and valid instrumentation to measure subjects' pre- and posttraining fitness levels

4. Use of stress protocols that are of sufficient intensity and/or duration to allow the emergence of potential differences between trained and untrained subjects

5. Use of exercise training protocols that are sufficiently rigorous to result in a significant increase in subjects' actual and perceived fitness levels

6. Careful consideration and specification of the type of stimulus used to elicit a stress response (e.g., physical vs. behavioral stressors; active vs. passive coping demands; novel vs. familiar tasks) because the effects of exercise training may vary as a function of the type of stressor used

Our second recommendation is that future researchers should assume a multidimensional approach in measuring children's stress responses. A review of the available literature on stress reactivity clearly shows that there is considerable disparity across studies in the measures that individual researchers have used to assess reactivity in their subjects. Some investigators, for example, use cardiovascular indicators (e.g., heart rate, blood pressure), while others have chosen to use neuroendocrine indices (e.g., plasma levels of epinephrine, norepinephrine, cortisol). In addition, from a more psychological perspective, reactivity has also been measured using a variety of emotional indicators (i.e., through use of self-report questionnaires). Unfortunately, the scores obtained from the various measurement systems do not appear to be highly correlated (Kagan et al., 1987; Murphy et al., 1988; Nesse, Curtis, Thyer, McCann, Huber-Smith, & Knopf, 1985). Thus, as Murphy et al. note, the various measures cannot really be considered to be equivalent indices of reactivity. Because we do not know at this point which particular index will provide the most valid measure of reactivity in children, the most prudent strategy may be to employ a set of indices that represent as many of the assessment domains as possible. Based on comparable research with adults, it certainly appears that exercise training may have an impact on some reactivity indices but not on others (e.g., Claytor, 1991). Thus, considerably more information concerning the effect of exercise training on children's reactivity can be obtained when a more multidimensional measurement approach is used.

Consistent with the theme of this chapter, our third recommendation is that future research on reactivity in children must be conducted from a developmental perspective. Such an approach is necessary because children change in both quantitative and qualitative ways as they mature. In the self-esteem literature, for example, our review of the research showed that self-esteem scores change qualitatively as a function of age (i.e., maturation is associated with increased differentiation). Similarly, there also appear to be age and age-by-gender changes in regard to reactivity patterns. Given such age-dependent response patterns, it would be inappropriate for an individual researcher who is conducting a study with a sample of children ranging in age from 8 to 18 years to analyze the results as a composite across ages. As the literature reviewed in this chapter would clearly suggest, the statistical results may differ for 8-year-olds as compared to 14-year-olds. Thus, a developmental approach must be used in collecting and analyzing data.

Finally, as we have noted a number of times throughout this chapter, it does appear as if participation in an exercise training program may be most beneficial for those children who are psychologically at risk. Applying this same maxim to the stress-reactivity area would lead to the hypothesis that a significant exercise-induced change in children's reactivity patterns would be most likely to occur in those children who are hyperreactors prior to the training period. From a related perspective, Sothmann et al. (1991), who recently reviewed the available literature on exercise and plasma catecholamine reactivity in adult subjects, identified several other, more physiologically based, subject characteristics that may affect the relationship between exercise and reactivity to stress. Whether these characteristics will also apply to children is, of course, currently unknown. Nevertheless, it is our belief that future research should carefully investigate the possibility that exercise training will have the largest (or perhaps the only significant) effect on those children who are hyperreactors before the training.

## SUMMARY

As stated in the introductory section, our purpose in writing this chapter was to review the available research and theory on the relationship between children's fitness and their physical and psychological health. In particular, we chose to approach this topic from both a multidimensional and a developmental perspective. Thus, our review emphasized the changing relationships that may occur with regard to the link between physical activity and health across the childhood and adolescent years.

Although our review of the available research revealed some interesting results concerning children's health and fitness, we also discovered that there is still much work to be accomplished. In regard to children's fitness, for example, although we have a fair amount of data concerning children's performance on relevant fitness tests, we have virtually no information concerning how or even whether such performance capacities relate to their physical health. Based on comparable research with adults, we can speculate, at this point, that children's physical activity patterns may be more important for health purposes than their actual fitness status. However, the research conducted to date on children's physical activity levels clearly indicates that they do not spend significant amounts of time per day in activities that are moderate to vigorous in nature. Furthermore, physical activity levels appear to decline with age, and there is a particularly significant drop during the adolescent years. Based on these research results, it is our recommendation that future research should be directed toward an examination of the factors that affect children's physical activity levels. This recommendation is based on the fact that there is considerable variation among individual children in activity level, and the information regarding the factors that are associated with an inactive life-style could be used to design more effective physical-activity programs.

In the second part of this chapter, we reviewed the research that has been conducted, to test whether participation in an exercise training program can have measurable effects on children's mental health. Although much of this research has been plagued by methodological and theoretical flaws, the work that has been completed clearly indicates that physical activity participation can have a very beneficial effect on several aspects of children's psychological health, including their self-esteem, locus of control, and depression levels. Comparable research to assess the relationship between exercise training and children's reactivity to stress has not yet been conducted, but a review of the literature in this area indicates that such research is warranted.

As we noted several times throughout this chapter, future research on the physical-activity–health link should be methodologically well designed and conducted. Furthermore, children's pretraining psychological status should be taken into consideration, as it appears that children who are psychologically at risk may benefit most from an exercise training program. Certainly, the possibility exists that exercise intervention programs conducted during the childhood or adolescent years will have a particularly significant effect on individuals' physical and psychological health. However, considerably more research is necessary before this possibility can be stated with greater assurance.

## REFERENCES

Alpert, B., Field, T., Goldstein, S., & Perry, S. (1990). Aerobics enhances cardiovascular fitness and agility in preschoolers. *Health Psychology, 9,* 48–56.

American Alliance for Health, Physical Education, Recreation, and Dance (AAHPERD) (1975). *AAHPERD Youth Fitness Test manual.* Reston, VA: AAHPERD.

Anderson, N. B. (1989). Racial differences in stress-induced cardiovascular reactivity and hypertension: Current status and substantive issues. *Psychological Bulletin, 105,* 89–105.

Anderson, K. L., Ilmarinen, M., Rutenfrantz, J., Ottmann, W., Berndt, I., Kylian, H., & Ruppel, M. (1984). Leisure time sport activities and maximal aerobic power during late adolescence. *European Journal of Applied Physiology, 52,* 431–436.

Armstead, C. A., Lawler, K. A., Gorden, G., Cross, J., & Gibbons, J. (1989). Relationship of racial stressors to blood pressure responses and anger expression in black college students. *Health Psychology, 8,* 541–556.

Beidel, D. C. (1989). Assessing anxious emotion: A review of psychophysiological assessment in children. *Clinical Psychology Review, 9,* 717–736.

Beunen, G., & Malina, R. M. (1988). Growth and physical performance relative to the timing of the adolescent spurt. In K. B. Pandolf (Ed.), *Exercise and sport sciences reviews* (Vol. 16), pp. 503–540). New York: Macmillan.

Beuter, A., Duda, J. L., & Widule, C. J. (1989). The effect of arousal on joint kinematics and kinetics in children. *Research Quarterly for Exercise and Sport, 60,* 109–116.

Bijur, P. E., Stewart-Brown, S., & Butler, N. (1986). Child behavior and accidental injury in 11,966 preschool children. *American Journal of Diseases in Children, 140,* 487–492.

Borghi, C., Costa, F. V., Boschi, S., Mussi, A., & Ambrosioni, E. (1986). Predictors of stable hypertension in young borderline subjects: A five-year follow-up study. *Journal of Cardiovascular Pharmacology, 8* (Suppl. 5), S138–S141.

Boutilier, M. A., & SanGiovanni, L. (1983). *The sporting woman.* Champaign, IL: Human Kinetics.

Branta, C., Haubenstricker, J., & Seefeldt, V. (1984). Age changes in motor skills during childhood and adolescence. In R. L. Terjung (Ed.), *Exercise and sport sciences reviews* (Vol. 12), pp. 467–520). Lexington, MA: D. C. Heath.

Brown, J. D., & Lawton, M. (1986). Stress and well-being in adolescence: The moderating role of physical exercise. *Journal of Human Stress, 12,* 125–131.

Brown, J. D., & Siegel, J. M. (1988). Exercise as a buffer of life stress: A prospective study of adolescent health. *Health Psychology, 7,* 341–353.

Brown, M. S., & Tanner, C. (1988). Type A behavior and cardiovascular responsivity in preschoolers. *Nursing Research, 37,* 152–191.

Caspersen, C. J., Christenson, G. M., & Pollard, R. A. (1986). Status of the 1990 physical fitness and exercise objectives—Evidence from NHIS 1985. *Public Health Reports, 101,* 587–592.

Chodzko-Zajko, W. J. (1991). Physical fitness, cognitive performance, and aging. *Medicine and Science in Sports and Exercise, 23,* 868–872.

Clarke, D. H. (1986). Children and the research process. In G. A. Stull (Ed.), *Effects of physical activity on children* (pp. 9–13). Champaign, IL: Human Kinetics.

Claytor, R. P. (1991). Stress reactivity: Hemodynamic adjustments in trained and untrained humans. *Medicine and Science in Sports and Exercise, 23,* 873–881.

Corbin, C. B. (1987). Youth fitness, exercise and health: There is much to be done. *Research Quarterly for Exercise and Sport, 58,* 308–314.

Cresanta, J. L., Hyg, M. S., Burke, G. L., Downey, A. M., Freedman, D. S. & Berenson, G. S. (1986). Prevention of atherosclerosis in childhood. *Pediatric Clinics of North America, 33,* 835–858.

Dembroski, T. M., MacDougall, J. M., Slaats, S., Eliot, R. S., & Buell, J. C. (1981). Challenge-induced cardiovascular response as a predictor of minor illnesses. *Journal of Human Stress, 7,* 2–5.

Despres, J. P., Bouchard, C., & Malina, R. (1990). Physical activity and coronary heart disease risk factors during childhood and adolescence. In K. B. Pandolf & J. O. Holloszy (Eds.), *Exercise and sport sciences reviews* (Vol. 18), pp. 243–262). Baltimore: Williams and Wilkins.

Duda, J. L., & Allison, M. T. (1990). Cross-cultural analysis in exercise and sport psychology: A void in the field. *Journal of Sport and Exercise Psychology, 12,* 114–131.

Duke, M., Johnson, T. C., & Nowicki, S. (1977). Effects of sports fitness camp experience on locus of control orientation in children 6–14. *Research Quarterly, 48,* 280–283.

Dusek, J. B. (1980). The development of test anxiety in children. In I. G. Sarason (Ed.), *Test anxiety: Theory, research, and applications* (pp. 87–110). Hillsdale, NJ: Erlbaum.

Dweck, C. S., & Leggett, E. L. (1988). A social-cognitive approach to motivation and personality. *Psychological Review, 95,* 256–273.

Eaton, W. O., & Enns, L. R. (1986). Sex differences in human motor activity level. *Psychological Bulletin, 100,* 19–28.

Eaton, W. O., & Yu, A. P. (1989). Are sex differences in child motor activity level a function of sex differences in maturational status? *Child Development, 60,* 1005–1011.

Engebretson, T. O., Matthews, K. A., & Scheier, M. F. (1989). Relations between anger expression and cardiovascular reactivity: Reconciling inconsistent findings through a matching hypothesis. *Journal of Personality and Social Psychology, 57,* 513–521.

Enos, W. J., Beyer, J. C., & Holmes, F. H. (1955). Pathogenesis of coronary disease in American soldiers killed in Korea. *Journal of the American Medical Association, 158,* 912–914.

Falkner, B., Onesti, G., & Hamstra, B. (1981). Stress response characteristics of adolescents with high genetic risk for essential hypertension: A five-year follow-up. *Clinical and Experimental Hypertension, 3,* 583–591.

Fox, K. R. (1988). The self-esteem complex and youth fitness. *Quest, 40,* 230–246.

Fox, K. R., & Corbin, C. B. (1989). The Physical Self-perception Profile: Development and preliminary validation. *Journal of Sport and Exercise Psychology, 11,* 408–430.

Fredrickson, M., & Matthews, K. A. (1990). Cardiovascular responses to behavioral stress and hypertension: A meta-analytic review. *Annals of Behavioral Medicine, 12,* 30–39.

Gallahue, D. L. (1989). *Understanding motor development: Infants, children, adolescents.* Indianapolis, IN: Benchmark Press.

Gilliam, T. B., Freedson, P. S., Geenen, D. L., & Shahraray, B. (1981). Physical activity patterns determined by heart rate monitoring in 6–7 year old children. *Medicine and Science in Sports and Exercise, 13,* 65–67.

Gilliam, T. B., Katch, V. L., Thorland, W. G., & Weltman, A. W. (1977). Prevalence of coronary heart disease risk factors in active children, 7 to 12 years of age. *Medicine and Science in Sports and Exercise, 9,* 21–25.

Gilliam, T. B., & MacConnie, S. E. (1984). Coronary heart disease risk in children and their physical activity patterns. In R. A. Boileau (Ed.), *Advances in pediatric sport sciences* (Vol. 1, pp. 171–187). Champaign, IL: Human Kinetics.

Gintner, G. G., Hollandsworth, J. G., & Intrieri, R. C. (1986). Age differences in cardiovascular reactivity under active coping conditions. *Psychophysiology, 23,* 113–120.

Gruber, J. J. (1986). Physical activity and self-esteem development in children: A meta-analysis. In G. A. Stull & H. M. Eckert (Eds.), *Effects of physical activity on children.* Champaign, IL: Human Kinetics.

Hansman, C. (1970). Anthropometry and related data. In R. W. McCammon (Ed.), *Human growth and development* (pp. 101–154). Springfield, IL: Thomas.

Harter, S. (1983). Developmental perspectives on the self-system. In E. M. Hetherington (Ed.), *Handbook of child psychology: Vol. 4. Socialization, personality, and social development* (pp. 275–385). New York: Wiley.

Harter, S. (1985). *Manual for the Self-perception Profile for Children.* Unpublished manuscript, University of Denver, Department of Psychology.

Harter, S. (1988). Causes, correlates, and the functional role of global self-worth: A lifespan perspective. In J. Kolligian & R. Sternberg (Eds.), *Perceptions of competence and incompetence across the lifespan.* New Haven, CT: Yale University Press.

Harter, S., & Pike, R. (1984). The pictorial perceived competence scale for young children. *Child Development, 55,* 1969–1982.

Haywood, K. (1991). The role of physical education in the development of active lifestyles. *Research Quarterly for Exercise and Sport, 62,* 151–156.

Holloway, J. B., Beuter, A., & Duda, J. L. (1988). Self-efficacy and training for strength in adolescent girls. *Journal of Applied Social Psychology, 18,* 699–719.

Horn, T. S., Claytor, R. P., & Phelps, D. (1991, June). *The effect of pre-training psychological status on psychological adaptation to an exercise training program.* Paper presented at the North American Society for the Psychology of Sport and Physical Activity, Asilomar, CA.

Horn, T. S., & Hasbrook, C. A. (1986). Informational components influencing children's perceptions of their physical competence. In M. R. Weiss & D. Gould (Eds.), *The Olympic Scientific Congress Proceedings: Vol. 10. Sport for children and youths* (pp. 81–88). Champaign, IL: Human Kinetics.

Horn, T. S., & Weiss, M. R. (1991). A developmental analysis of children's self-ability judgments in the physical domain. *Pediatric Exercise Science, 3,* 310–326.

Horwitz, S. M., Morgenstern, H., DiPietro, L., & Morrison, C. L. (1988). Determinants of pediatric injuries. *American Journal of Diseases in Children, 142,* 605–611.

Hunter, S. M., Wolf, T. M., Sklov, M. C., Webber, L. S., Watson, R. M., & Berenson, G. S. (1982). Type A coronary-prone behavior pattern and cardiovascular risk factor variables in children and adolescents: The Bogalusa heart study. *Journal of Chronic Disease, 35,* 613–621.

Jackson, S. A., & Marsh, H. W. (1986). Athletic or antisocial: The female sport experience. *Journal of Sport Psychology, 8,* 196–211.

Jemerin, J. M., & Boyce, W. T. (1990). Psychobiological differences in childhood stress response: II. Cardiovascular markers of vulnerability. *Journal of Developmental and Behavioral Pediatrics, 11,* 140–150.

Kagan, J., Reznick, J. S., Clarke, C. Snidman, N., & Garcia-Coll, C. (1984). Behavioral inhibition to the unfamiliar. *Child Development, 55,* 2212–2225.

Kagan, J., Reznick, J. S., & Snidman, N. (1987). The physiology and psychology of behavioral inhibition in children. *Child Development, 58,* 1459–1473.

Kaplan, B. J., Whitsett, S. F., & Robinson, J. W. (1990). Menstrual cycle phase is a potential confound in psychophysiology research. *Psychophysiology, 27,* 445–450.

Kemper, H. C. G., Dekker, H., Ootjers, G., Post, B., Ritmeester, J. W., Snel, J., Splinter, P., Essen, L. S., & Verschuur, R. (1985). The problems of analyzing longitudinal data from the study, "Growth and health of teenagers." In R. A. Binkhorst, H. C. G. Kemper, & W. H. M. Saris (Eds.), *Children and exercise* (Vol. 9, pp. 233–251). Champaign, IL: Human Kinetics.

King, A. C., Taylor, C. B., Haskell, W. L., & DeBusk, R. F. (1989). Influence of regular aerobic exercise on psychological health: A randomized controlled trial of healthy middle-aged adults. *Health Psychology, 8,* 305–324.

Klausen, K., Rasmussen, B., & Schibye, B. (1986). Evaluation of the physical activity of school children during a physical education lesson. In J. Rutenfrantz, R., Morellin, & F. Klimt (Eds.), *Children and exercise* (Vol. 12, pp. 93–101). Champaign, IL: Human Kinetics.

Klesges, L. M., & Klesges, R. C. (1987). The assessment of children's physical activity: A comparison of methods. *Medicine and Science in Sports and Exercise, 19,* 511–517.

Krahenbuhl, G. S., Skinner, J. S., & Kohrt, W. M. (1985). Developmental aspects of maximal aerobic power in children. In R. L. Terjung (Ed.), *Exercise and sport sciences reviews* (Vol. 13, pp. 503–538). New York: Macmillan.

Krohne, H. W. (1980). Parental child-rearing behavior and the development of anxiety and coping strategies in children. In I. G. Sarason & C. D. Spielberger (Eds.), *Stress and anxiety* (Vol. 7). Washington, DC: Hemisphere.

Lauer, R. M., Connor, W. E., Leaverton, P. E., Reiter, M. A., & Clarke, W. R. (1975). Coronary heart disease risk factors in school children: The Muscatine study. *The Journal of Pediatrics, 86*, 697–706.

Lawler, K. A., Allen, M. T., Critcher, E. C., & Standard, B. A. (1981). The relationship of physiological responses to the coronary-prone behavior pattern in children. *Journal of Behavioral Medicine, 4*, 203–216.

Looney, M. A., & Plowman, S. A. (1990). Passing rates of American children and youth on the FITNESSGRAM criterion-referenced physical fitness standards. *Research Quarterly for Exercise and Sport, 61*, 215–223.

Lundberg, U. (1983). Note on Type A behavior and cardiovascular responses to challenge in 3–6 year old children. *Journal of Psychosomatic Research, 27*, 39–42.

Maccoby, E. E., & Jacklin, C. N. (1974). *The psychology of sex differences.* Stanford, CA: Stanford University Press.

MacMahon, J. R., & Gross, R. T. (1988). Physical and psychological effects of aerobic exercise in delinquent adolescent males. *American Journal of Diseases in Children, 142*, 1361–1366.

Malina, R. (1984). Physical growth and maturation. In J. R. Thomas (Ed.), *Motor development during childhood and adolescence* (pp. 2–26). Minneapolis, MN: Burgess.

Marsh, H. W., Byrne, B. M., & Shavelson, R. J. (1988). A multifaceted academic self-concept: Its hierarchical structure and its relation to academic achievement. *Journal of Educational Psychology, 80*, 366–380.

Marsh, H. W., & Holmes, I. W. M. (1990). Multidimensional self-concepts: Construct validation of responses by children. *American Educational Research Journal, 27*, 89–117.

Marsh, H. W., & Jackson, S. A. (1986). Multidimensional self-concepts, masculinity and femininity as a function of women's involvement in athletics. *Sex Roles, 15*, 391–415.

Marsh, H. W., & Peart, N. D. (1988). Competitive and cooperative physical fitness training programs for girls: Effects on physical fitness and multidimensional self-concepts. *Journal of Sport and Exercise Psychology, 10*, 390–407.

Marsh, H. W., & Shavelson, R. J. (1985). Self-concept: Its multifaceted, hierarchical structure. *Educational Psychologist, 20*, 107–125.

Matthews, K. A., Takaczky, C. J., Stoney, C. M., & Manuck, S. B. (1987). Are cardiovascular responses to behavioral stressors a stable individual difference variable in childhood. *Psychophysiology, 24*, 464–473.

Matthews, K. A., & Stoney, C. M. (1988). Influences of sex and age on cardiovascular responses during stress. *Psychosomatic Medicine, 50*, 46–56.

McCann, B. S., & Matthews, K. A. (1988). Influences of potential for hostility, Type A behavior, and parental history of hypertension on adolescents' cardiovascular responses during stress. *Psychophysiology, 25*, 503–511.

McNamara, J. J., Molot, M. A., Stremple, J. F., & Cutting, R. T. (1971). Coronary artery disease in combat casualties in Vietnam. *Journal of the American Medical Association, 216,* 1185–1186.

Meredith, M. D. (1988). Activity or fitness: Is the process or the product more important for public health? *Quest, 40,* 180–186.

Montoye, H. J. (1986). Physical activity, physical fitness, and heart disease risk factors in children. In G. A. Stull & H. M. Eckert (Eds.), *Effects of physical activity on children* (pp. 127–152). Champaign, IL: Human Kinetics.

Murphy, J. K., Alpert, B. S., Moes, D., & Somes, G. (1986). Race and cardiovascular reactivity: A neglected relationship. *Hypertension, 8,* 1075–1083.

Murphy, J. K., Alpert, B. S., Willey, E. S., & Somes, G. W. (1988). Cardiovascular reactivity to psychological stress in healthy children. *Psychophysiology, 25,* 144–152.

Nesse, R. M., Curtis, G. C., Thyer, B. A., McCann, D. S., Huber-Smith, M., & Knopf, R. F. (1985). Endocrine and cardiovascular responses during phobic anxiety. *Psychosomatic Medicine, 47,* 320–332.

Newman, W. P., Freedman, D., Voors, A. W., Gard, P. D., Srinivasan, S. R., Cresanta, J. L., Williamson, G. D., Webber, L. S., & Berenson, G. S. (1986). Relation of serum lipoprotein levels and systolic blood pressure to early atherosclerosis. *New England Journal of Medicine, 314,* 138–144.

Noland, M., Danner, F., Dewalt, K., McFadden, M., & Kotchen, J. M. (1990). The measurement of physical activity in young children. *Research Quarterly for Exercise and Sport, 61,* 146–153.

O'Hara, N. M., Baranowski, T., Simons-Morton, B. G., Wilson, B. S., & Parcel, G. S. (1989). Validity of the observation of children's physical activity. *Research Quarterly for Exercise and Sport, 60,* 42–47.

Paffenbarger, R. S., Jr., & Hyde, R. T. (1984). Exercise in the prevention of coronary heart disease. *Preventive Medicine, 13,* 3–22.

Palmer, G. J., Ziegler, M. G., & Lake, C. R. (1978). Response of norepinephrine and blood pressure to stress increases with age. *Journal of Gerontology, 33,* 482–487.

Parcel, G. S., Simons-Morton, B. G., O'Hara, N. M., Caranowski, T., Kolbe, L. J., & Bee, D. E. (1987). School promotion of healthful diet and exercise behavior: An integration of organizational change and social learning theory interventions. *Journal of School Health, 57,* 150–156.

Parsons, J. (1981). Attributions, learned helplessness, and sex differences in achievement. In S. R. Yussen (Ed.), *The development of achievement.* New York: Academic Press.

Pate, R. R. (1988). The evolving definition of physical fitness. *Quest, 40,* 174–179.

Pickering, T. G., & Gerin, W. (1990). Cardiovascular reactivity in the laboratory and the role of behavioral factors in hypertension: A critical review. *Annals of Behavioral Medicine, 12,* 3–16.

Placek, J., Silverman, S., Shute, S., Dodds, P., & Rife, F. (1982). Academic learning time (ALT-PE) in a traditional elementary physical education setting: A descriptive analysis. *Journal of Curriculum and Instruction, 17,* 41–47.

Plante, T. G., & Rodin, J. (1990). Physical fitness and enhanced psychological health. *Current Psychology: Research and Reviews, 9,* 3–24.

Powell, K. E., Thompson, P. D., Caspersen, C. J., & Kendrick, J. S. (1987). Physical activity and the incidence of coronary heart disease. *Annual Review of Public Health, 8,* 253–287.

Puhl, J., Greaves, K., Hoyt, M., & Baranowski, T. (1990). Children's Activity Rating Scale (CARS): Description and calibration. *Research Quarterly for Exercise and Sport, 61,* 26–36.

Reiff, G. G., Dixon, W. R., Jacoby, D., Ye, G. X., Spain, C. G., & Hunsicker, P. A. (1986). *The President's Council on Physical Fitness and Sports national school population fitness study.* Ann Arbor, MI: University of Michigan.

Roche, A. F., & Malina, R. M. (Eds.) (1983). *Manual of physical status and performance in childhood* (Vol. 1). New York: Plenum.

Rosenberg, M. (1982). Psychological selectivity in self-esteem formation. In M. Rosenberg & H. B. Kaplan (Eds.), *Social psychology of the self-concept* (pp. 535–545). Arlington Heights, IL: Harlan Davidson.

Ross, J. G., Dotson, C. O., Gilbert, G. G., & Katz, S. J. (1985). What are kids doing in school physical education? *Journal of Physical Education, Recreation, and Dance, 56,* 73–76.

Ross, J. G., & Gilbert, G. G. (1985). The National Children and Youth Fitness Study: A summary of findings. *Journal of Physical Education, Recreation, and Dance, 56,* 45–50.

Ross, J. G., & Pate, R. R. (1987). The National Children and Youth Fitness Study II: A summary of findings. *Journal of Physical Education, Recreation, and Dance, 58,* 51–56.

Ross, J. G., Pate, R. R., Corbin, C. B., Deply, L. A., & Gold, R. S. (1987). What is going on in the elementary physical education program? *Journal of Physical Education, Recreation, and Dance, 58,* 78–84.

Rowland, T. (1990). *Exercise and children's health.* Champaign, IL: Human Kinetics.

Safrit, M. J., Baumgartner, T. A., Jackson, A. S., & Stamm, C. L. (1980). Issues in setting motor performance standards. *Quest, 32,* 152–162.

Sallis, J. F., & McKenzie, T. R. (1991). Physical education's role in public health. *Research Quarterly for Exercise and Sport, 62,* 124–137.

Sallis, J. F., Patterson, T. L., McKenzie, T. L., Buono, M. J., Atkins, C. J., & Nader, P. R. (1989). Stability of systolic blood pressure reactivity to exercise in young children. *Journal of Developmental and Behavioral Pediatrics, 10,* 38–43.

Sallis, J. F., Patterson, T. L., McKenzie, T. L., & Nader, P. R. (1988). Family variables and physical activity in preschool children. *Journal of Developmental and Behavioral Pediatrics, 9,* 57–61.

Sarason, I. G. (Ed.). (1980). *Test anxiety: Theory, research, and applications.* Hillsdale, NJ: Erlbaum.

Saris, W. H. M. (1986). Habitual physical activity in children: Methodology and findings in health and disease. *Medicine and Science in Sports and Exercise, 18,* 253–263.

Scanlan, T. K., & Lewthwaite, R. (1984). Social psychological aspects of competition for male youth sport participants: I. Predictors of competitive stress. *Journal of Sport Psychology, 6,* 208–226.

Schmidt, T. H., Thierse, H., & Eschweiler, J. (1986). Behavioral correlates of cardio-vascular reactivity in school children. In T. H. Schmidt, T. M. Dembroski, & G. Blumchen (Eds.), *Biological and psychological factors in cardiovascular disease* (pp. 187–227). New York: Springer-Verlag.

Seefeldt, V. (1984). Physical fitness in preschool and elementary school-aged chil-dren. *Journal of Physical Education, Recreation, and Dance, 10,* 33–37,40.

Seefeldt, V., & Vogel, P. (1987). Children and fitness: A public health perspective— A response. *Research Quarterly for Exercise and Sport, 58,* 331–333.

Shavelson, R. J., Hubner, J. J., & Stanton, G. C. (1976). Self-concept: Validation of construct interpretations. *Review of Educational Research, 46,* 407–441.

Simons-Morton, B. G., O'Hara, N. M., Parcel, G. S., Huang, I. W., Baranowski, T., & Wilson, B. (1990). Children's frequency of participation in moderate to vigorous physical activities. *Research Quarterly for Exercise and Sport, 61,* 307–314.

Simons-Morton, B. G., O'Hara, N. M., Simons-Morton, D. G., & Parcel, G. S. (1987). Children and fitness: A public health perspective. *Research Quarterly for Exercise and Sport, 58,* 295–302.

Simons-Morton, B. G., Parcel, G. S., O'Hara, N. M., Blair, S. N., & Pate, R. R. (1988). Health-related physical fitness in childhood: Status and recommendations. *An-nual Review of Public Health, 9,* 403–425.

Smoll, F. L., & Schutz, R. W. (1990). Quantifying gender differences in physical performance: A developmental perspective. *Developmental Psychology, 26,* 360–369.

Sonstroem, R. J. (1982). Exercise and self-esteem: Recommendations for expository research. *Quest, 33,* 124–139.

Sonstroem, R. J. (1984). Exercise and self-esteem. In R. L. Terjung (Ed.), *Exercise and sport sciences reviews* (pp. 123–155). Lexington, MA: D. C. Heath.

Sothmann, M. S., Hart, B. A., & Horn, T. S. (1991). Plasma catecholamine response to acute psychological stress in humans: Relation to aerobic fitness and exercise training. *Medicine and Science in Sports and Exercise, 23,* 860–867.

Stephens, T., Jacobs, D. R., Jr., & White, C. C. (1985). A descriptive epidemiology of leisure time physical activity. *Public Health Reports, 100,* 147–158.

Stoney, C. M., Davis, M. C., & Matthews, K. A. (1987). Sex differences in physiologi-cal responses to stress and in coronary heart disease: A causal link? *Psycho-physiology, 24,* 127–131.

Strong, J. P., Eggen, D. A., & Oalmann, M. C. (1972). The natural history, geographic pathology and epidemiology of atherosclerosis. In R. W. Wissler & J. C. Geer (Eds.), *The pathogenesis of atherosclerosis* (pp. 20–40). Baltimore: Williams and Wilkins.

Strong, J. P., & McGill, H. C. (1969). The pediatric aspects of atherosclerosis. *Journal of Atherosclerosis Research, 9,* 251–265.

Thomas, J. R., & French, K. E. (1985). Gender differences across age in motor performance: A meta-analysis. *Psychological Bulletin, 98,* 260–282.

Weinberg, R. S. (1978). The effects of success and failure on the patterning to neuromuscular energy. *Journal of Motor Behavior, 10,* 53–61.

Wilmore, J. H., & McNamara, J. J. (1974). Prevalence of coronary heart disease risk factors in boys, 8 to 12 years of age. *The Journal of Pediatrics, 84,* 527–533.

Wine, J. D. (1980). Cognitive-attentional theory of test anxiety. In I. G. Sarason (Ed.), *Test anxiety: Theory, research, and applications*. Hillsdale, NJ: Erlbaum.

Woodall, K. L., & Matthews, K. A. (1989). Familial environment associated with Type A behaviors and psychophysiological responses to stress in children. *Health Psychology, 8,* 403–426.

Yan Lan, L., & Gill, D. L. (1984). The relationships among self-efficacy, stress responses, and a cognitive feedback manipulation. *Journal of Sport Psychology, 6,* 227–238.

# 12

# A Cognitive Perspective on the Stress-Reducing Effects of Physical Exercise

**BONITA C. LONG**

## OVERVIEW

Within the clinical practice of health psychology and behavioral medicine, exercise has become a popularly recommended stress-management treatment often viewed as an adjunct to psychotherapy (Burks & Keeley, 1989). Although most stress-management programs include training in relaxation, self-monitoring methods, and cognitive strategies (Hillenberg & DiLorenzo, 1987; Woolfolk & Lehrer, 1984), a comprehensive theoretical rationale that accounts for their efficacy is lacking. An approach that may provide a rationale for the efficacy of exercise as a treatment for stress is the study of cognitive processes—a dominant trend in much of psychology (Cantor, 1990; Turk & Salovey, 1985). Thus, the purpose of this chapter is to describe an integrative cognitive framework for understanding stress and coping processes and to provide a rationale for considering exercise as both a preventive coping resource and a responsive coping behavior. In addition, I examine cognitive constructs (e.g., self-schemata, possible selves, self-efficacy) that relate to the stress-appraisal process so that the effects of exercise on stress are clarified. Finally, recommendations are made for both research and practice.

## PHYSICAL EXERCISE AND STRESS

Aerobic or physical fitness is a biologically defined characteristic that has frequently been associated with a lower incidence of coronary heart disease and is hypothesized to be related to coping with stress or illness (for recent reviews, see Paffenbarger, 1988; Powell, Thompson, Caspersen, & Kendrick, 1987; Sedgwick, Taplin, Davidson, & Thomas, 1984). The results of a meta-analysis of aerobic fitness and reactivity to psychosocial stress, conducted by Crews and Landers (1987), indicated that people who are fit respond to psychosocial stress in a hyporeactive way. However, Van Doornen, de Geus, and Orlebeke (1988) question the prediction that fit people are hyporeactive to stress and claim that this hypothesis is based on a questionable analogy between physiological responses to aerobic exercise and responses to psychological stress. Despite criticism of the physiological explanation for the effects of exercise on stress, research indicates that high levels of aerobic fitness and regular exercise habits are related to lower anxiety, less emotionality, and less depression (e.g., Doan & Sherman, 1987; Eysenck, Nias, & Cox, 1982; Hughes, 1984; Long, 1984). Thus, as Van Doornen et al. (1988) and others (Dienstbier, 1989; Long, 1983) suggest, psychological processes may well explain the effectiveness of exercise as a stress-management treatment, especially because not all aerobically fit or exercising individuals appear to benefit psychologically from exercise. For example, data from exercise programs for stressed adults indicate that highly aerobically fit individuals, compared with less-fit individuals, do not show greater stress reductions (Long, 1983; Moses, Steptoe, Mathews, & Edwards, 1989). In addition, anxiety reduction and long-term maintenance of anxiety reduction is not found for all exercising individuals (Long, 1985; Long & Haney, 1988b; Steptoe, 1989).

## STRESS AND COPING THEORY

For a model of stress to be useful in guiding treatment of any sort, it must reflect the multidimensional, dynamic, and complex nature of stress. Two models of stress have been criticized for their lack of recognition of the role of cognition in the stress process: (1) stimulus models, which focus on precipitating factors such as life events; and (2) response models, which emphasize physiological reactivity. Recent models emphasize the role of appraisal in determining arousal and are referred to as "transactional models." According to Lazarus and Folkman's (1984) transactional model, stress occurs when an individual appraises a situation as one in which she or he is unable to cope adequately when confronted with specific valued and significant demands.

*Coping* is defined as "constantly changing cognitive and behavioral efforts to manage specific external and/or internal demands that are appraised as taxing or exceeding the resources of the person" (Lazarus & Folkman, 1984, p. 141). Coping is viewed as the process of responding to a specific stressful situation. Two distinct functions of coping were initially defined by the Ways of Coping Checklist developed by Folkman and Lazarus (1980). Managing or altering the problem causing the distress is considered a problem-focused coping function, and regulating the emotional response to the problem is considered an emotion-focused coping function. Both types of coping include efforts to manage stress, regardless of outcome, and previous investigations show that people generally use both forms of coping in virtually every type of stressful encounter (Folkman & Lazarus, 1980, 1985). See Figure 12.1 for an illustration of these relations.

Lazarus and Folkman (1984) postulate that antecedent conditions, such as beliefs about oneself and recognition of personal *resources for coping* (e.g., self-esteem and energy), moderate the stress process because they interact with other conditions to produce both short-term and long-term outcomes such as health and well-being. Thus, Lazarus and Folkman recognize the role of self-esteem, energy, and stamina—resources that people draw upon in order to cope. Additionally, Matheny, Aycock, Pugh, Curlette, and Cannella (1986) further develop the concept of coping resources by defining them as conditions or attributes that either (a) decrease the likelihood that demands will be perceived as stressors or (b) increase the effectiveness of coping behaviors. These resources serve a preventive function and are essential elements of the stress and coping process. Matheny et al. label them "preventive coping" resources.

*Coping behaviors*, on the other hand, are actions taken to deal with encountered stressors (a problem-focused coping function) or one's reaction to them (an emotion-focused coping function). Coping behaviors mediate the stress response because they are generated in the stressful encounter and are hypothesized to change the relationship between the antecedent state and the outcome (e.g., morale, health, well-being) of the stressful situation (Folkman & Lazarus, 1988).

Cognitive appraisal is of central importance to this transactional model of stress and is defined as an evaluative or judgmental process through which the individual judges the significance of a transaction with the envi-

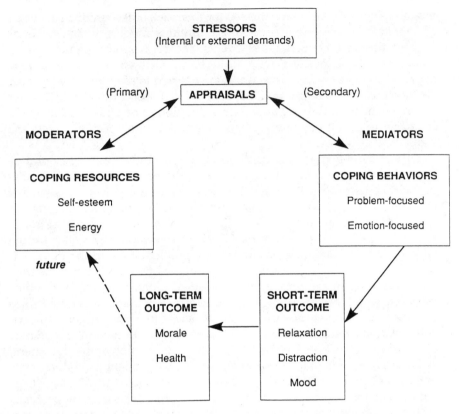

**Figure 12.1.** Cycle of stress and coping—the mediating and moderating effects of coping during the stress process.

ronment. *Primary appraisal* follows from the recognition that the situation is important and potentially taxing (i.e., appraisals of challenge, threat, or harm–loss). Secondary appraisal is a judgment about the options for coping, including the extent to which (a) the outcome is amenable to change and (b) appropriate coping resources are available. Secondary appraisal may cause revisions of the primary appraisal. The product of this appraisal process is the event's implicit meaning for that individual. "For example, the loss of a job might mean, to one individual, a threat that can be handled, to a second person, a threat with which one cannot cope, and a chance to demonstrate one's worth to a third" (Thompson & Janigian, 1988, p. 262).

## COGNITIVE THEORY: SELF-SCHEMA

Whereas appraisal is construed as a judgmental process, human judgment, in turn, is affected by the integration of both situational information and acquired knowledge—two fundamentally contrasting elements (Brewin, 1989). In familiar situations, as compared with novel events, acquired knowledge results in automatic processing, which draws on theoretical structures such as internal models, schemata, and associative networks. *Schemata* are cognitive structures of organized prior knowledge, abstracted from specific experiences, which act as guides for the processing of information and the retrieval of stored information (Fiske & Taylor, 1984).

According to Safran, Segal, Hill, and Whiffen (1990) cognitive schema theories have much to offer in terms of understanding the efficacy of diverse treatment programs because these constructs help us understand the way in which individuals create representations of their experiences and how these representations influence their subsequent behaviors. One particular type of structure has been the focus of extensive research effort and is of particular relevance to the stress process: the *self-schema*, which is conceptually similar to the term *self-concept*. The self-schema is typically described as an organization of information about who one perceives oneself to be and about who one perceives that others want one to be, as stored in long-term memory. Self-schemata are cognitive structures that are derived from past experience and that involve generalizations about the self that are focused on aspects of the self regarded by the individual as important (Markus, 1977). For example, given a performance situation, a self-schema would be a knowledge structure that summarizes information about the self that relates to the performance domain. Research in a variety of domains (e.g., Type A personality, exercise, body weight) has demonstrated that self-schemata affect the processing of information about both the self and others (Kendzierski, 1988, 1990; Markus, Hamill, & Sentis, 1987; Strube et al., 1986).

Cognitive schemata not only help us to make sense of the enormous array of information confronting us, but also lead us to formulate various errors or biases in our information processing. An example is the process of confirmatory hypothesis testing—that is, individuals tend to seek information that is consistent with their previously existing schemata (Snyder & Swann, 1978). People are also more likely to remember information that is consistent with existing schemata (Snyder & Uranowitz, 1978) and to maintain schemata well beyond what is supported by current information (Slusher & Anderson, 1989). In general, research indicates that people are likely to both recall and attend to information that is consistent with self-schemata, as compared to information that is not (see review by Schrauger, 1982).

Self-schemata may contain images of specific events that have taken place, as well as memories of expressive motor and autonomic responses to those events (Safran et al., 1990). Potential selfhoods include social categories, roles, particular personal features, attributes, and habits. These self-schemata are similar in structure to the type of emotion schemata described by Leventhal (1984)—that is, expectations about people or things (e.g., "people are threatening and harmful"), beliefs about the self (e.g., "I am incompetent"), and expectations about how one must behave to avoid threats to self (e.g., "I must avoid threatening situations"). As defined by Markus (1977), individuals are schematic in regard to a particular attribute when they consider that attribute to be either extremely self-descriptive or extremely nondescriptive, and when the attribute is considered to be important to self-image. For example, exercise as an attribute would be self-descriptive for an avid exerciser, whereas exercise would be nondescriptive as an attribute for someone who is a nonexerciser (see Kendzierski, 1990). These beliefs and expectations are implicit in the generalized representation of the self. In summary, *self-schemata* are multifaceted structures that subsume many self-representations—positive and negative; present, past, and future.

## Possible Selves

Cognitive behavioral theorists have distinguished between core and peripheral cognitive structures (Arnkoff, 1980; Guidano & Liotti, 1983; Mahoney, 1985), with *core cognitive structures* considered to be fundamental assumptions about the way the individual construes the self and the world. Although self-schemata have been described as core structures (Safran, 1990), that subset of self-schemata that contain representations of future selves may be particularly central to a transactional model of stress and coping. As James (1910) postulated, an awareness of one's potential is the most significant component of the self.

The term *possible selves* has been used to describe subcomponents of self-schemata that include conceptions of the future, both hoped for and feared (Markus & Nurius, 1987). Possible selves that are hoped for (positive possible selves) might include the powerful or leader self, the slim and fit self, the revered and esteemed self. Negative possible selves may include one's fears and anxieties such as visions of being a failure and unwanted, or the undervalued and unrecognized self. Possible selves are the cognitive manifestations of "enduring goals, aspirations, motives, fears, and threats" (Markus & Nurius, 1987, p. 158). Oyserman and Markus (1990) suggest that possible selves are subsets of personalized goals, outcomes, or expectancies. "It is the sense of one's self in a desired end-state—me with an exciting job or me with a happy family—that organizes and energizes actions in the pursuit of the end-state" (Oyserman & Markus, 1990, p. 113). Similarly, negative possible selves may also be motivational in developing action to avoid or prevent feared outcomes. Thus, possible selves are conceived to be generalizations about future selves, derived from past experience, which provide organization and direction—motivation for action.

In order to explain possible selves, Markus and Nurius (1986; Nurius & Markus, 1986) suggest that the self should be conceived as a set of self-conceptions that are a "continually active, changing array of available self-knowledge" (p. 957). The working self-schema is a subset of one's complete set of self-conceptions—the set that is active at any one time. For example, "when an individual experiences a defeat, rejection, or a lapse in will power, the working self-schema may be configured with conceptions of negative possibilities" (Markus & Nurius, 1987, p. 164). In other instances, the working self-schema may contain largely positive possibilities.

Thoughts and images of what is possible may provide an opportunity for the individual to construct a self that is an alternative to the present one. Individuals who cannot instantiate future selves may be trapped in an unchangeable course of action. However, if alternative conceptions of the self, which are vivid and well-elaborated, can be brought into the working self-schema, then they may enable the individual to decrease both threats to self-esteem and maladaptive actions.

So far, there is a paucity of research on the effects of self-schemata on behavior, despite their hypothesized properties. However, recent research has provided some evidence that self-schemata and possible selves predict behaviors such as exercising and delinquency (Kendzierski, 1990; Oyserman & Markus, 1990). Furthermore, Oyserman and Markus hypothesized and provided some support for the notion that motivation is greatest when an individual has a balance of both negative (feared) and positive (desired) possible selves. However, more research is warranted before drawing this conclusion. In summary, possible self structures are a link between general beliefs about oneself and any given action or performance.

## Self-Efficacy

Possible selves are conceived as the self-relevant internal structures that give rise to generalized feelings of self-efficacy (Bandura, 1986), competence (Harter, 1985), and internal locus of control (Lefcourt, 1976). Self-efficacy, the self-evaluative process regarding a stimulus domain, has been given a large amount of explanatory power in social-learning theory (Gecas, 1989; Turk & Salovey, 1985). Although self-efficacy and possible selves are conceptually distinct, little or no research has examined their discriminant validity. According to Bandura (1977), self-efficacy is the conviction that one can carry out the behavior required to produce a desired outcome. Outcome expectancy, however, is a person's expectation that a given behavior will lead to a certain outcome. Thus, an individual may have a high outcome expectancy but may not believe that he or she is capable of performing the given behavior. The strength of individuals' beliefs in their efficacy is likely to determine not only the inferences that they make about their behavior, but also whether and how they attempt to try to cope with a difficult situation (Bandura, 1977; Turk & Salovey, 1985). For example, an individual who perceives himself or herself as inefficacious may consider difficulties as being much greater than they are in reality and may also avoid situations believed to be beyond their capabilities. Thus, individuals' beliefs about their efficacy (i.e., a component of possible selves) influence their thought processes, emotional reactions, and behaviors during both anticipatory and actual transactions (e.g., Bandura, Reese, & Adams, 1982; Barling & Abel, 1983; O'Leary, 1985).

Self-efficacy will also influence both how much effort people exert and how long people persist when confronted with aversive circumstances (Bandura, 1977). People who have strong misgivings about their capabilities (i.e., negative self-schema, low efficacy expectations) reduce their efforts or give up, whereas those who have a strong sense of competence (i.e., positive self-schemata, high efficacy expectations) are likely to persist (Turk, 1979; Turk & Salovey, 1985). Because competencies are often achieved through continued effort (Bandura, 1977), factors that contribute to giving up may restrict opportunities to experience events that might lead to enhanced perceptions of self-efficacy.

Turk and Salovey (1985) summarized this process by suggesting that people who judge themselves to be inefficacious may not only exaggerate the severity of threats but may also worry about problems that rarely occur. Subsequently, they experience high levels of distress, which, in turn, heighten their thoughts of personal inefficacy and contribute to their mal-adaptive behaviors. High distress levels may result in attention to difficulties rather than to information that might reduce the threat. Thus, the maladaptive behavior may substantiate the individual's self-perceptions as being inadequate, helpless, or weak (a negative self-schema). This confirmation may increase avoidance of problematic situations (increase emotion-focused coping) or reduce task-relevant efforts (decrease problem-focused coping), thereby creating a self-defeating cycle (Turk & Salovey, 1985).

### Stress, Coping, and Cognitive Theories: An Integration

Cognitive appraisal, the central construct in the transactional model of stress, involves processing two types of information: acquired knowledge (e.g., self-schema) and situational information. Thus, appraisals are based on self-schemata, particularly possible selves that are instantiated or brought into focus (e.g., "I can be an A student"; "I can run for an hour"), and on the situational demands (e.g., "I only have 2 days to write the report"; "I've only trained for 4 weeks"). For example, when an individual is confronted with a demanding situation, the individual finds meaning in the event through appraisals of the situation (e.g., challenge, harm–loss, or threat) based on previously acquired knowledge (e.g., self-schema) and the situational requirements.

Specific components of self-schemata are particularly important influences on motivation and coping behavior. These components are an individual's feared and expected possible selves and self-efficacy expectancies. Markus and Nurius (1986) claim that possible selves provide the link between self-schemata and motivation. Choosing among competing behaviors or actions, and pursuing chosen actions depend on one's set of possible selves; thus, possible selves may affect both the appraisal process and the coping strategies. For example, a positive possible self of "me, the energetic teacher" will affect both the appraisal of a demanding, energy-draining, teaching task, and the initiation and persistence of coping behavior used to deal with these demands.

Furthermore, an individual who is unable to cognitively counter fears or threats in a believable self-relevant way through instantiating a positive possible self may be unable to respond to a stressor with adequate coping behaviors. Thus positive self-efficacious possible selves are construed as preventive coping resources because they may affect the appraisal process (decrease appraisals of threat or harm–loss), thereby moderating the stress-outcome relationship. Furthermore, they may enhance the effectiveness of coping behaviors. Research indicates that self-efficacy is associated with greater likelihood of initiation and greater persistence of task-related behaviors (Feltz, 1988; Stumpf, Brief, & Hartman, 1987), specifically with problem-focused coping strategies (Fleishman, 1984; Folkman, Lazarus, Dunkel-Schetter, DeLongis, & Gruen, 1986; Long, 1989).

The integration of cognitive-schema theory and the transactional model of stress provides a backdrop to examine the efficacy of exercise as a treatment program. See Figure 12.2 for an illustration of these relationships.

## EXERCISE: COPING AND COGNITIVE PROCESSES

### Exercise as a Coping Behavior

Exercise may fulfill at least two different functions of coping—both as an emotion-focused strategy and as a preventive coping resource. Thus, both primary and secondary appraisals of potentially stressful events may be affected by exercise behaviors.

**Exercise as an Emotion-Focused Coping Response.** Exercise as an emotion-focused function is examined first because the most obvious influence of exercise on the stress process, and the most researched, is as a means of inducing relaxation (deVries, 1976), changing mood (Morgan, 1976), and providing a psychological distraction (Bahrke & Morgan, 1978). When confronted with a distressing situation, individuals may exercise to distract themselves from the situation, to induce physical relaxation, or to enhance their mood. Physical exercise is considered an emotion-focused coping strategy because, in this case, exercise fulfills the function of regulating emotional and physiological reactions to the stressor event. Thus, exercise is a mediator of the stress–outcome process (see Figure 12.2).

There is no conclusive evidence suggesting that in order for exercise to be an effective emotion-focused coping strategy, exercise must produce a physical conditioning effect (i.e., increase aerobic capacity). It appears that the exercise experience need only be physically relaxing, psychologically distracting, or mood enhancing, and that it reduce either the emotional or the physiological reaction to a stressor. Yet characteristics of exercise (e.g., type, intensity, and duration) necessary to provide emotional regulation probably vary from individual to individual. There is some suggestion from research that exercise that (a) involves large-muscle groups (e.g., jogging, cycling, swimming), (b) is sustained for 20–30 minutes, and (c) is of a

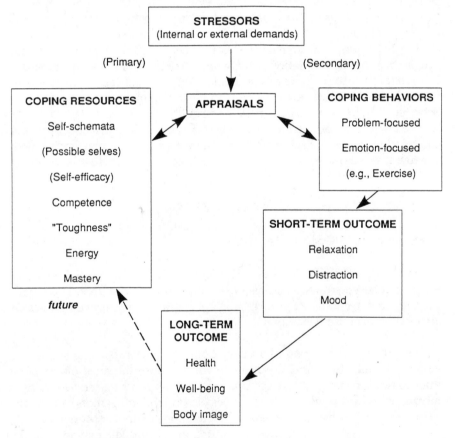

**Figure 12.2.** Cycle of stress and coping—the effects of cognitive processes and exercise on the stress process.

moderate intensity will provide an emotion-focused coping function (Morgan, 1976; Moses et al., 1989).

The mediating effects of exercise on outcome can be related to both short-term and long-term outcomes. The short-term effects include immediate reductions in emotional or physiological reactions, whereas long-term effects occur if exercise is maintained regularly. The result is enhanced cardiovascular health, with the concomitant increase in physiological stamina and energy. In addition, exercise may serve as a means of weight control and muscle development/definition, resulting in a body shape that is socially sanctioned and thus contributes to a positive body image.

**Exercise as a Resource for Preventive Coping: Self-Schemata, Possible Selves, and Self-Efficacy.**   In order to determine whether exercise affects the primary appraisal process—that is, serves as a preventive coping resource that affects appraisals of the challenge, threat, or harm–loss of situations—it is necessary to examine how exercise affects self-schemata and in particular, possible selves and self-efficacy.

Experiences associated with the exercise habits of an individual constitute the content of the self-schema stored in long-term memory. The self-schema may consist of many pieces of information derived from exercise history, including expressive motor and autonomic responses to exercise. Particularly important are elements that contribute to a positive possible self. As a result of exercising, the self-schema may contain many positive self-conceptions—for example, "I am fit, competent, and goal directed." Negative self-conceptions may also be formed—for example, "I'll get fat, and I'll be unattractive if I do not continue exercising." An individual who has an exercise schema that is instantiated in future situations is better able to process information with regard to the contents of the exercise schema, and thus to appraise situations differently than an individual lacking such a self-schema.

There are several ways in which physical exercise may contribute to an internal or external demand being appraised as less threatening or harmful. Individuals who experience mood changes or muscular relaxation through exercise may have confidence that the negative affect and physiological arousal accompanying a distressing event can be modified; that is, they have the acquired knowledge that exercising will help them feel better, and this has become part of their self-schemata. Much research has supported the notion that perceived control over emotional reactions is effective in reducing stress (Wallston, Wallston, Smith, & Dobbins, 1987). Thus, for persons who exercise, a stressor may be appraised as less threatening or harmful, compared with nonexercisers who may not have readily available means of reducing body tension or of enhancing mood. In this case, the effects of exercise do not depend on exercise inducing a physiological conditioning effect, but rather depend on whether the individuals have had positive experiences with exercise in the past and can anticipate similar results in the future (i.e., they have formed and can draw on positive possible selves).

With regard to the self-efficacy component of self-schemata, it has been proposed that individuals who master a difficult exercise task enhance self-efficacy for strenuous or difficult tasks, and that this appraisal generalizes (Dienstbier, 1989; Long, 1984, 1985; Long & Haney, 1988a, 1988b). Thus, individuals who have maintained exercise programs may well have developed components of self-schemata that are positive regarding self-efficacy or competence (Hughes, 1984). If their acquired knowledge from regular exercise was stored in long-term memory as self-schemata relating to mastery, control, and self-regulation, then they will have positive schemata as resources when confronted with potentially stressful situations, provided the situation is not too novel.

Documented consequences of chronic physical activity include enhanced self-esteem, self-efficacy, health, stamina, and energy (Doan & Sherman, 1987; Hughes, 1984; Ossip-Klein et al., 1989; Sonstroem, 1988)—all are important components of self-schemata. These consequences result because exercisers may respond favorably to actual or perceived improvements in fitness (Hughes, 1984), and exercise may provide a series of graded-mastery experiences that enhance self-efficacy, improve self-concept, and increase the probability of coping behavior (Bandura, 1977; Beck, Rush, Shaw, & Emery, 1979). Dienstbier (1989) suggests that the arousal and energy obtained from exercising contributes to secondary appraisals of coping potential. Dienstbier provides evidence that what may be called a "tough" physiological pattern dominated by pituitary–adrenal–cortical arousal is empirically linked with challenge and positive emotions; and when this toughening is achieved, the energy needed to cope in challenge–stress situations is readily available. Furthermore, individuals who become aware of this energy are likely to appraise coping as manageable. "With such appraisals, subjects enter a positive spiral involving physiology (energy and an awareness of it) and positive appraisal, for the awareness that one can cope with the situation and an expectation of success should result in the arousal pattern associated with toughening" (Dienstbier, 1989, p. 93).

There is some empirical support indicating that personal resources such as self-esteem, stamina, and energy are associated with greater problem-focused coping (Fleishman, 1984), and that greater problem-focused coping is associated with less anxiety and greater well-being (Folkman et al., 1986; Long, 1989). Thus, exercise may increase coping effectiveness by increasing the use of problem-focused coping as a result of instantiating positive possible selves and providing readily available stores of energy.

In summary, exercise as a preventive coping resource is a component of both the primary appraisal process (a judgment regarding the extent to which the situation is important and potentially taxing) and the secondary appraisal process (a judgment about the options for coping, the extent to which the outcome is amenable to change, and whether appropriate coping behaviors or resources are available). However, Lazarus and Folkman (1984) claim that appraisals are interactive and reciprocal processes; thus, both primary and secondary appraisals interact with one another and should not be considered to be independent processes.

## Implications for Research and Practice

An integration of cognitive-schema theory and stress theory helps us understand the role of self in the stress and coping process, and it provides the basis for the development of effective stress-management interventions. Despite the fact that far less research exists on how to change self-schemata than on describing their effects, several implications for the use of exercise as a stress treatment are apparent. Both short-term and long-term effects must be considered. Short-term effects relate to the emotion-focused function of exercise and are valuable means of coping with stress, particularly when there is little or no control over the stressor (Suls & Fletcher, 1985). It may also be helpful in conjunction with problem-focused strategies. Folkman et al. (1986) found evidence that dealing with one's reactions to a stressful event is associated with greater use of problem-focused coping. They speculated that some forms of emotion-focused coping may facilitate problem solving.

Dienstbier (1989), however, argues that therapists should not implement relaxation therapies for stressed individuals but rather should use what he calls "toughening" procedures. He provides support for the notion that exercise training builds toughness that is relevant to either physical or mental challenge–threat situations. Dienstbier suggests that a program of aerobic exercise is an acceptable toughening experience and that even modest training programs should have an impact on toughening. However, within a transactional model of stress and coping, exercise can be both a means of relaxation and an energizer. Furthermore, emotion-focused coping strategies (e.g., progressive muscle relaxation, meditation, biofeedback) are widely used and accepted, and there is evidence for the utility of emotion-focused coping for short-term low-control situations (Suls & Fletcher, 1985). Emotion-focused coping is also an important element in most major theoretical formulations of stress (e.g., Janis's emotional-drive theory, 1958; Leventhal & Johnson's self-regulation theory, 1983; and Lazarus and Folkman's cognitive-appraisal model, 1984).

Gurin and Brim's (1984) review of how change occurs in adulthood points to several means of enhancing self-efficacy that related to the exercise experience. For example, there is evidence that success changes efficacy more when feedback is tied to performance, when success if obviously due to the succeeder's skills, when success occurs in varied circumstances, and when performance implies improvement rather than a leveling off (Bandura, 1977). Furthermore, efficacy is positively affected by events (a) that our culture construes as resulting from individual motivation, and (b) that occur in a situation seen by others, who reaffirm the individual's role in the outcome. Thus, an exercise program may provide success feedback for an activity (a) that is culturally sanctioned and public, (b) that is construed to be due to the exerciser's motivation and skill, (c) that can be performed in many circumstances, and (d) that at least initially shows performance improvements rather than performance plateaus.

Relationships between group members and the exercise leader are important, too. The exercise leader who values and accepts participants even when they do not meet their exercise goals thereby disconfirms the exerciser's belief that he or she must always be perfect in order to maintain the esteem of important others. Thus, similar to the *client–therapist relationship*, the exercise leader provides an opportunity for "generating perturbations in extant, maladaptive cognitive schemata and restructuring them into a more functional processing system" (Carson, 1982, p. 78).

However, hoped-for possibilities (positive possible selves) may be easily threatened or undermined, and unless they are vividly elaborated, deliberately invoked, and reaffirmed, they may easily be lost from the working self-concept (Markus & Nurius, 1987). By exercising regularly, an individual's self-schema of mastery is frequently reinforced, particularly if the exercise program contains graded increments of difficulty. Thus, the exerciser's environment is modified so that it is reinforcing, and alternative views of self are frequently activated to enhance their strength (see cognitive therapies such as Beck et al., 1979; McMullin & Giles, 1985). Goldfried (1980) argues that a major objective in therapy is for the therapist to intervene in a way that creates new, adaptive, and noncharacteristic behaviors from the client. Consequently, the challenge is to create well-elaborated (vivid) possible selves through an exercise program that overtly emphasizes an alternative view of the self (e.g., "I am competent; I can regulate my emotional stress reaction"). Furthermore, the exercise leader can enhance this process by making more overt the relationship between exercise activity and self-concept. Because individuals often exercise with others (friends, family members), the social environment may also provide reinforcement for exercise accomplishments. The result is an increased chance of instantiating a positive possible self in response to familiar but trying situations. Thus, for individuals for whom exercising becomes an enduringly salient aspect of the self, exercise may contribute to an alternative self-schema.

Although not yet documented empirically, exercise probably relates most directly to one's sense of competence, and therefore, exercise may be more effective for individuals who have deficits in their sense of efficacy—a fundamental and core component of one's sense of self (Bandura, 1986; Gecas, 1989). Research should explore changes in self-schemata, possible selves, and self-efficacy as a result of exercise programs. Some beginning work has been done regarding exercise schemata and exercise behaviors (Kendzierski, 1988, 1990). However, there is a need (a) to examine exercise as a stress-management treatment in light of transactional theories of stress and coping that address emotion- and problem-focused coping strategies, as well as preventive coping resources, and (b) to determine the relative effects of exercise on self-schemata, possible selves, and self-efficacy.

## ACKNOWLEDGMENTS

I would like to thank Sara Comish and Beth Haverkamp for their thoughtful comments on an earlier version of this paper.

## REFERENCES

Arnkoff, D. (1980). Psychotherapy from the perspective of cognitive therapy. In M. Mahoney (Ed.), *Psychotherapy process: Current issues and future directions* (pp. 339–362). New York: Plenum Press.

Bahrke, M. S., & Morgan, W. P. (1978). Anxiety reduction following exercise and meditation. *Cognitive Therapy and Research, 2*, 323–333.

Bandura, A. (1977). Self-efficacy: Toward a unifying theory of behavioral change. *Psychological Review, 84*, 191–215.

Bandura, A. (1986). *Social foundations of thought and action: A social cognitive theory.* Englewood Cliffs, NJ: Prentice-Hall.

Bandura, A., Reese, L., & Adams, N. E. (1982). Microanalysis of action and fear arousal as a function of differential levels of perceived self-efficacy. *Journal of Personality and Social Psychology, 43*, 5–21.

Barling, J., & Abel, M. (1983). Self-efficacy beliefs and performance. *Cognitive Therapy and Research, 7*, 265–272.

Beck, A. T., Rush, A. H., Shaw, B. F., & Emery, G. (1979). *Cognitive therapy of depression.* New York: Guilford Press.

Brewin, C. R. (1989). Cognitive change processes in psychotherapy. *Psychological Review, 96*, 379–394.

Burks, R., & Keeley, S. (1989). Exercise and diet therapy: Psychotherapists' beliefs and practices. *Professional Psychology: Research and Practice, 20*, 62–64.

Cantor, N. (1990). From thought to behavior: "Having" and "doing" in the study of personality and cognition. *American Psychologist, 45*, 735–750.

Carson, R. C. (1982). Self-fulfilling prophecy, maladaptive behavior, and psychotherapy. In J. C. Anchin & D. J. Kiesler (Eds.), *Handbook of interpersonal psychotherapy* (pp. 64–77). New York: Pergamon Press.

Crews, D. J., & Landers, D. M. (1987). A meta-analytic review of aerobic fitness and reactivity to psychosocial stressors. *Medicine Science in Sports and Exercise, 19*, S114–S120.

deVries, H. A. (1976). Immediate and long-term effects of exercise upon resting muscle action potential. *Journal of Sports Medicine and Physical Fitness, 8,* 1–11.

Dienstbier, R. A. (1989). Arousal and physiological toughness: Implications for mental and physical health. *Psychological Review, 96,* 84–100.

Doan, R. E., & Sherman, A. (1987). The therapeutic effect of physical fitness on measures of personality: A literature review. *Journal of Counseling and Development, 66,* 28–36.

Eysenck, H. J., Nias, D. K., & Cox, D. N. (1982). Sport and personality. *Advances in Behavior Research and Therapy, 4,* 1–56.

Feltz, D. L. (1988). Gender differences in the causal elements of self-efficacy on a high avoidance motor task. *Journal of Sport and Exercise Psychology, 10,* 151–166.

Fiske, S. T., & Taylor, S. E. (1984). *Social cognition.* New York: Random House.

Fleishman, J. A. (1984). Personality characteristics and coping patterns. *Journal of Health and Social Behavior, 37,* 229–244.

Folkman, S., & Lazarus, R. (1980). An analysis of coping in a middle-aged community sample. *Journal of Health and Social Behavior, 21,* 219–239.

Folkman, S., & Lazarus, R. (1985). If it changes it must be a process: Study of emotion and coping during three stages of a college examination. *Journal of Personality and Social Psychology, 48,* 159–170.

Folkman, S., & Lazarus, R. (1988). The relationship between coping and emotion: Implication for theory and research. *Social Science Medicine, 36,* 309–317.

Folkman, S., Lazarus, R., Dunkel-Schetter, C., DeLongis, A., & Gruen, R. (1986). Dynamics of a stressful encounter: Cognitive appraisal, coping, and encounter outcomes. *Journal of Personality and Social Psychology, 5,* 992–1003.

Gecas, V. (1989). The social psychology of self-efficacy. *Annual Review of Sociology, 15,* 291–316.

Goldfried, M. R. (1980). Toward a delineation of therapeutic change principles. *American Psychologist, 35,* 991–999.

Guidano, V. F., & Liotti, G. (1983). *Cognitive processes and emotional disorders.* New York: Guilford Press.

Gurin, P., & Brim, O. G., Jr. (1984). Change in self in adulthood: The example of sense of control. In P. Baltes & O. G. Brim (Eds.), *Life span development and behavior* (Vol. 6, pp. 281–334). San Diego, CA: Academic Press.

Harter, S. (1985). Competence as a dimension of self-evaluation. In R. L. Leahy (Ed.), *The development of the self* (pp. 55–121). San Diego, CA: Academic Press.

Hillenberg, J. B., & DiLorenzo, T. M. (1987). Stress management training in health psychology practice: Critical clinical issues. *Professional Psychology: Research and Practice, 18,* 402–404.

Hughes, J. R. (1984). Psychological effects of habitual aerobic exercise: A critical review. *Preventive Medicine, 13,* 66–78.

James, W. (1910). *Psychology: The briefer course.* New York: Holt.

Janis, I. L. (1958). *Psychological stress.* New York: Wiley.

Kendzierski, D. (1988). Self-schemata and exercise. *Basic and Applied Social Psychology, 9,* 45–59.

Kendzierski, D. (1990). Exercise self-schemata: Cognitive and behavioral correlates. *Health Psychology, 9,* 69–82.

Lazarus, R., & Folkman, S. (1984). *Stress, appraisal and coping.* New York: Springer.

Lefcourt, H. M. (1976). *Locus of control: Current trends in theory and research.* Hillsdale, NJ: Erlbaum.

Leventhal, H. (1984). A perceptual-motor theory of emotion. In L. Berkowitz (Ed.), *Advances in experimental and social psychology* (Vol. 17, pp. 117–182). New York: Academic Press.

Leventhal, H., & Johnson, J. E. (1983). Laboratory and field experimentation: Development of a theory of self-regulation. In P. J. Wooldridge, M. H. Schmitt, J. K. Skipper, Jr., & R. C. Leonard (Eds.), *Behavioral science and nursing theory* (pp. 189–262). St. Louis: C. V. Mosby.

Long, B. C. (1983). Aerobic conditioning and stress reduction: Participation or conditioning? *Human Movement Science, 2,* 171–183.

Long, B. C. (1984). Aerobic conditioning and stress inoculation: A comparison of stress management interventions. *Cognitive Therapy and Research, 8,* 517–547.

Long, B. C. (1985). Stress management interventions: A 15-month follow-up of aerobic conditioning and stress inoculation training. *Cognitive Therapy and Research, 9,* 471–478.

Long, B. C. (1989). Sex-role orientation, coping strategies, and self-efficacy of women in traditional and nontraditional occupations. *Psychology of Women Quarterly, 13,* 307–324.

Long, B. C., & Haney, C. J. (1988a). Coping strategies for working women: Aerobic exercise and relaxation interventions. *Behavior Therapy, 19,* 75–83.

Long, B. C., & Haney, C. J. (1988b). Long-term follow-up of stressed working women: A comparison of aerobic exercise and progressive relaxation. *Journal of Sport and Exercise Psychology, 10,* 461–470.

Mahoney, M. J. (1985). Psychotherapy and human change processes. In M. H. Mahoney & A. Freeman (Eds.), *Cognition and psychotherapy* (pp. 3–48). New York: Plenum Press.

Markus, H. (1977). Self-schemata and processing information about the self. *Journal of Personality and Social Psychology, 35,* 63–78.

Markus, H., Hamill, R., & Sentis, K. P. (1987). Thinking fat: Self-schemas for body weight and the processing of weight relevant information. *Journal of Applied Social Psychology, 17,* 50–71.

Markus, H., & Nurius, P. S. (1986). Possible selves. *American Psychologist, 41,* 954–969.

Markus, H., & Nurius, P. (1987). Possible selves: The interface between motivation and the self-concept. In K. Yardley & T. Honess (Eds.), *Self and identity: Psychosocial perspectives* (pp. 157–172). New York: Wiley.

Matheny, K. B., Aycock, D. W., Pugh, J. L., Curlette, W., & Cannella, K. A. S. (1986). Stress coping: A qualitative synthesis with implications for treatment. *The Counseling Psychologist, 14,* 499–549.

McMullin, R. E., & Giles, T. R. (1985). *A cognitive-behavior therapy: A restructuring approach.* New York: Grune & Stratton.

Morgan, W. P. (1976). Psychological consequences of vigorous physical activity and sport. *Annals of the New York Academy of Sciences, 301,* 15–30.

Moses, J., Steptoe, A., Mathews, A., & Edwards, S. (1989). The effects of exercise training on mental well-being in the normal population: A controlled trial. *Journal of Psychosomatic Research, 33,* 47–61.

Nurius, P. S., & Markus, H. (1986). *The working self-concept: Contextual variability within a stable system.* Unpublished manuscript, University of Michigan.

O'Leary, A. (1985). Self-efficacy and health. *Behavior Research and Therapy, 23,* 437–451.

Ossip-Klein, D., Doyne, E., Bowman, E., Osborn, K., McDougall-Wilson, I., & Neimeyer, R. (1989). Effects of running or weight lifting on self-concept in clinically depressed women. *Journal of Consulting and Clinical Psychology, 57,* 158–161.

Oyserman, D., & Markus, H. R. (1990). Possible selves and delinquency. *Journal of Personality and Social Psychology, 59,* 112–125.

Paffenbarger, R. S. (1988). Contributions of epidemiology to exercise science and cardiovascular health. *Medicine Science in Sports and Exercise, 20,* 426–438.

Powell, K. E., Thompson, P. D., Caspersen, C. J., & Kendrick, J. S. (1987). Physical activity and the incidence of coronary heart disease. *Annual Review in Public Health, 8,* 253–287.

Safran, J. D. (1990). Towards a refinement of cognitive therapy in light of interpersonal therapy: I. Theory. *Clinical Psychology Review, 10,* 87–105.

Safran, J. D., Segal, Z. V., Hill, C., & Whiffen, W. (1990). Refining strategies for research on self-presentations in emotional disorders. *Cognitive Therapy and Research, 14,* 143–160.

Schrauger, J. S. (1982). Selection and processing of self-evaluative information: Experimental evidence and clinical implications. In G. Weary & H. Mirels (Eds.), *Integration of clinical and social psychology* (pp. 128–153). New York: Oxford University Press.

Sedgwick, A. W., Taplin, R. E., Davidson, A. H., & Thomas, D. W. (1984). Relationships between physical fitness and risk factors for coronary heart disease in men and women. *Australian/New Zealand Journal of Medicine, 14,* 208–214.

Slusher, M. P., & Anderson, C. A. (1989). Belief perseverance and self-defeating behavior. In R. Curtis (Ed.), *Self-defeating behaviors: Experimental research, clinical impressions, and practical implications* (pp. 11–40). New York: Plenum Press.

Snyder, M., & Swann, W. B. (1978). Hypothesis testing processes in social interaction. *Journal of Personality and Social Psychology, 36,* 1202–1212.

Snyder, M., & Uranowitz, S. W. (1978). Reconstructing the past: Some cognitive consequences of person perception. *Journal of Personality and Social Psychology, 36,* 941–950.

Sonstroem, R. J. (1988). Psychological models. In R. K. Dishman (Ed.), *Exercise adherence: Its impact on public health* (pp. 125–153). Champaign, IL: Human Kinetics.

Steptoe, A. (1989). Coping and psychophysiological reactions. *Advances in Behavioral Research and Therapy, 11,* 259–270.

Stumpf, S. A., Brief, A. P., & Hartman, K. (1987). Self-expectations and coping with career related events. *Journal of Vocational Behavior, 31,* 91–108.

Strube, M. J., Berry, J. M., Lott, C. L., Fogelman, R., Steinhart, G., Moergen, S, & Davison, L. (1986). Self-schematic representation of the Type A and B behavior patterns. *Journal of Personality and Social Psychology, 51,* 170–180.

Suls, J., & Fletcher, B. (1985). The relative efficacy of avoidant and nonavoidant coping strategies. *Health Psychology, 4,* 249–288.

Thompson, S. C., & Janigian, A. S. (1988). Life schemes: A framework for understanding the search for meaning. *Journal of Social and Clinical Psychology, 7,* 260–280.

Turk, D. C. (1979). Factors influencing the adaptive process with chronic illness. In I. G. Sarason & C. D. Spielberger (Eds.), *Stress and anxiety* (Vol. 6). Washington, DC: Hemisphere.

Turk, D. C., & Salovey, P. (1985). Cognitive structures, cognitive processes, and cognitive-behavior modification: I. Clinical issues. *Cognitive Therapy and Research, 9,* 1–17.

Van Doornen, L. J. P., De Geus, J. C. N., & Orlebeke, J. F. (1988). Aerobic fitness and the physiological stress response: A critical evaluation. *Social Science and Medicine, 26,* 303–307.

Wallston, K. A., Wallston, B. S., Smith, S., & Dobbins, C. (1987). Perceived control and health. *Current Psychological Research and Reviews, 6,* 5–25.

Woolfolk, R. L., & Lehrer, P. M. (Eds.). (1984). *Principles and practice of stress management.* New York: Guilford Press.

# 13

# Aerobic Exercise in Prevention and Treatment of Psychopathology

**THOMAS G. PLANTE**

An inordinate amount of attention has been focused on the myriad emotional and physical benefits attributed to a program of exercise. Exercise is popularly perceived as an elixir for improved self-esteem, mood, stability, and stamina. Exercise has been championed by a society eager to embrace self-improvement, spawning a billion-dollar business in the fitness boom of the 1970s and 1980s. Yet despite thousands of popular-press articles extolling the virtues of exercise, professional literature in the field of exercise psychology has been neither as prolific nor as conclusive. Scientifically researched questions remain, despite the current of popular belief: Does exercise enhance mood, reduce stress, and lend itself as an effective treatment for emotional disorders? This chapter attempts to summarize the current body of professional literature in the field and to clarify the actual, mythical, and as-yet incompletely tested notions regarding the effects of exercise on psychological functioning.

A great deal of attention has been given to the role of physical fitness and aerobic exercise in the prevention and treatment of psychopathology. Exercise has been used to decrease symptoms associated with *major affective disorders* such as major depression and bipolar illness, *anxiety disorders* such as generalized anxiety disorder and panic disorder, and as an adjunct treatment for *thought disorders* such as schizophrenia. Exercise also has been used as an adjunctive treatment for persons with mental retardation, autism, and the emotional turbulence associated with adolescence. Furthermore, exercise has been used to enhance psychological functioning and well-being among people who are mildly to moderately stressed but do not meet any diagnostic criteria for a psychiatric disorder. Many authors have reported that participation in a regular aerobic exercise program among the nonpsychiatric population may actually prevent future psychiatric symptoms and disorders.

The purpose of this chapter is to present and discuss the research evidence concerning the use of aerobic exercise in the prevention and treatment of psychopathology. It is hoped that an understanding of the potential preventive aspects of exercise in psychiatric disturbances is enhanced by examining how exercise influences psychological variables such as psychological well-being, mood, anxiety, depression, personality variables, and cognition. This is followed by an exploration of the use of exercise as a treatment intervention approach with an array of significant psychiatric disturbances, such as affective, thought, and substance abuse disorders.

## CURRENT STATE OF THE PROFESSIONAL AND POPULAR LITERATURE

Well over 1000 articles have been published in scientific journals regarding the psychological and psychiatric effects of exercise (Hughes, 1984; Plante & Rodin, 1990). In preparation for this chapter, more than 250 published articles were located in the professional literature since 1980 alone. The number of articles and reports published in popular magazines on this topic is staggering. Curiously, while the professional literature focuses on the use of exercise in treating significant physical and emotional problems, the popular press focuses on enhancing physical and emotional functioning among the general population. The vast majority of popular magazine articles that focus on the psychological benefits of regular exercise highlight its tension- and stress-reducing effects, while the majority of professional articles focus on the use of exercise for treating a wide range of psychiatric disorders.

A number of articles reviewing the exercise and psychopathology literature have been published (e.g., Biddle & Fox, 1989; Browman, 1981; Doan & Scherman, 1987; Folkins & Sime, 1981; Hales & Travis, 1987; Hughes, 1984; Ledwidge, 1980; MacMahon, 1990; Martinsen, 1989; Mobily, 1982; North, McCullagh, & Tran, 1990; Oberman, 1984; Phelps, 1987; Plante & Rodin, 1990; Raglin, 1990; Ransford, 1982; Rippe, Ward, Porcari & Freedson, 1988; Sachs, 1982; Simons, McGowan, Epstein, Kupfer, & Robertson, 1985a; Sonstroem, 1984; Taylor, Sallis, & Neddle, 1985; Tomporowski & Ellis, 1986). Most of these reviews, however, have focused on narrow, very specific aspects of the connection between exercise and psychopathology or on specific populations. For example, some of these reviews have highlighted the role of exercise in treating anxiety and/or depressive disorders (e.g., Hales & Travis, 1987; Ledwidge, 1980; Martinsen, 1989; North et al., 1990; Ransford, 1982; Simons et al., 1985a). Others have examined only aerobic exercise (e.g., Hughes, 1984; Sachs, 1982), while some have examined the role of exercise on self-esteem (Sonstroem, 1984) or on personality functioning (Doan & Scherman, 1987). Others have examined the role of exercise on nonpsychiatric populations (e.g., Plante & Rodin, 1990).

The last comprehensive review of the exercise and mental health literature was the 1981 article by Folkins and Sime, which appeared in the *American Psychologist*. This excellent and often-cited review examined the literature on the effects of exercise on cognition, perception, work behavior, sleep, social behavior, affect, personality, and self-concept. These authors concluded that exercise leads to improved mood, self-concept, and work behavior, as well as improved cognitive functioning during and immediately following exercise. The authors also concluded that except for self-concept, personality is not affected by improvements in physical fitness.

Plante and Rodin (1990) recently updated the Folkins and Sime (1981) article by reviewing the professional literature on exercise and psychological functioning published since 1980. This review found that exercise improves mood and psychological well-being (especially immediately following exercise), self-concept, and self-esteem, but it has little affect on personality functioning. In addition, Plante and Rodin (1990) found that exercise is likely to decrease mild anxiety, depression, and stress, and it may improve some work-relevant behaviors. They report that research concerning cognition and physiological stress responsivity is currently somewhat unclear. The conclusions provided by the review by Plante and Rodin (1990) support many of those of Folkins and Sime (1981) based on an earlier group of studies.

## AEROBIC EXERCISE IN THE PREVENTION OF PSYCHOPATHOLOGY

As mentioned earlier, exercise may prevent some types of psychiatric disturbances by decreasing many of the symptoms associated with a number of psychiatric disorders. For example, many studies have examined the role of exercise in altering *psychological variables* such as perceived well-being and mood, anxiety, stress, and depression, *personality factors* such as Type A behavior pattern and self-esteem, and *cognitive processes* such as attention, concentration, memory, and confusion. If exercise improves these psychological states, then exercise may act as a buffer against many psychiatric problems such as anxiety and depressive disorders. In this section, we examine the role of exercise in altering psychological well-being and mood; personality, especially self-concept; and cognitive processes. A review of the results of this research is presented in Table 13.1.

**TABLE 13.1  EXERCISE IN THE PREVENTION AND TREATMENT OF PSYCHOPATHOLOGY: SUMMARY OF RESEARCH FINDINGS**

| Psychological variable | Research results |
| --- | --- |
| Prevention | |
| Psychological well-being and mood | Improves functioning, especially immediately following workout |
| Personality | Little effect on trait measures |
| Type A behavior | Mixed, inconclusive |
| Locus of control | Mixed, inconclusive |
| Extroversion | Mixed, inconclusive |
| Self-concept | Improves |
| Cognition | Mixed, inconclusive; most compelling evidence among elderly population |
| Treatment | |
| Depression | Improves mild to moderate symptoms |
| Anxiety | Improves mild to moderate symptoms |
| Psychoses | Inconclusive, little effect on thought disorder |
| Alcoholism and other substance abuse | Inconclusive |
| Somatoform | Inconclusive |

## Psychological Well-Being and Mood

In seeking to understand the beneficial effects of exercise and how they are produced, it is important to consider separately the changes in mood and well-being immediately after an exercise workout and the longer-term benefits of maintaining an exercise regimen. A number of studies (e.g., Berger & Owen, 1983, 1988; Lichtman & Posner, 1983; Roth, 1989; Steptoe & Cox, 1988) have tested the short-term effects of exercise by examining the hypothesis that exercise improves mood and well-being immediately following an exercise workout. Other studies (e.g., Blumenthal, Williams, Needels, & Wallace, 1982b; Goldwater & Collins, 1985; Hayden & Allen, 1984; Hughes, Casal, & Leon, 1986; King, Taylor, Haskell, & DeBusk, 1989; Lobitz, Brammell, Stoll, & Niccoli, 1983; Lobstein, Mosbacher, & Ismail, 1983; Moses, Steptoe, Mathews, & Edwards, 1989; Sothmann, & Ismail, 1984) have focused on the longer-term benefits of exercise.

The majority of these studies report improvements in psychological well-being and/or mood among exercisers. Most studies failing to find associations between exercise and mood tend to have significant methodological flaws. Specifically, research supports the notion that moderate physical activity can improve mood states such as anxiety, depression, tension, and fatigue, as well as well-being, immediately following an exercise workout. However, high-intensity exercise might actually increase negative mood states such as tension and anxiety (Steptoe & Cox, 1988). While there is evidence that exercise improves general mood and well-being on a long-term basis, support for these long-term, cumulative effects is not as compelling as the recent research on the immediate effects of exercise on mood and well-being following a workout.

Curiously, one especially interesting study in this area (King et al., 1989) failed to find significant changes in depression, tension, well-being, or mood following a 6-month aerobic exercise program. These authors studied 120 middle-aged subjects who were randomly assigned to either a home-based aerobic exercise program or a control group. Although perceived fitness was associated with a decrease in tension following the exercise program, actual fitness (as measured by maximum volume of oxygen uptake, $\dot{V}O_2$ max) was not associated with any psychological improvements. This study raises the important question concerning the effects of perceived versus actual fitness on the psychological improvements associated with exercise.

The vast majority of studies examining the role of exercise on psychological well-being and mood support the notion that exercise will improve well-being and mood states such as anxiety, stress, depression, tension, and fatigue. The research focusing on the changes in these mood states immediately following an exercise workout is most compelling, while the research examining changes in these mood states following an extensive, more long-term exercise program are less clear and convincing. The notion that these benefits may primarily be due to perceived rather than actual improvements in physical fitness is an intriguing concept and an important question for future research.

## Personality and Self-Concept

A number of researchers have examined changes in personality and self-concept as a result of exercise conditioning. With so much attention on the relationship between the Type A behavior pattern and coronary disease, some recent studies have attempted to use exercise to change aspects of this problematic personality style. While many studies focused specifically on changes in Type A behavior (e.g., Lobitz et al, 1983; Roskies, Seraganian, Oseasohn, Hanley, Collu, Martin, & Smilga, 1986) or self-esteem/self-concept (Parent & Whall, 1984; Pauly, Palmer, Wright, Pfeiffer, 1982; Perri & Templer, 1985; Plummer & Koh, 1987; Tucker, 1982; Valliant & Asu, 1985), others studied more global personality functioning (e.g., Jasnoski & Holmes, 1981; Lobstein et al., 1983; Plante & Karpowitz, 1987).

**Type A Behavior Pattern.**    Research results examining changes in Type A behavior due to exercise have been mixed. For example, Roskies et al. (1986) examined 107 Type A males and randomly assigned them to either an aerobic exercise group, a cognitive-behavioral stress management group, or a weight-training group. All groups met for a 10-week period. Results indicated that the stress-management group, but not the aerobic exercise group, showed substantial reductions in Type A behavior, while the weight-training group showed some reduction. However, Lobitz et al. (1983) found reductions in Type A behavior among exercisers but not among subjects in their anxiety-management group. Unfortunately, both of these studies used a fairly short training program (i.e., 10 and 7 weeks, respectively), and neither reported follow-up results.

**Global Personality Functioning.**    A number of studies have examined changes in global personality functioning associated with exercise (e.g., Jasnoski & Holmes, 1981; Lobstein et al., 1983, Plante & Karpowitz, 1987). Unlike the earlier published research examining personality and exercise, many of the recent studies (Plante & Karpowitz, 1987; Roskies et al., 1986) failed to find significant associations between personality and exercise. This trend may reflect the fact that more and more people are exercising. While some specific kinds of individuals may have exercised on a regular basis a number of years ago, numerous people with all types of personality characteristics now exercise. Exercising reflects more of the norm than the exception. Therefore, research does not support the contention that exercise alone will significantly alter trait personality characteristics or styles.

**Self-Concept.**   The vast majority of studies examining improvements in self-concept and self-esteem associated with aerobic exercise are plagued with important methodological flaws, such as failing to use control groups, using numerous dependent measures with few subjects, and failing to randomly assign subjects to experimental and control conditions (e.g., Parent & Whall, 1984; Pauly et al., 1982; Perri & Templer, 1985; Plummer & Koh, 1987; Tucker, 1982; Valliant & Asu, 1985). Almost all of the studies examining self-concept or self-esteem report significant associations between these variables and exercise. For example, a number of these investigations revealed significant improvements in self-concept and/or self-esteem following an exercise program (Pauly et al., 1982; Perri & Templer, 1985; Tucker, 1982; Valliant & Asu, 1985), while others found that physically active subjects scored higher on self-concept and/or self-esteem than did sedentary subjects (Parent & Whall, 1984; Plummer & Koh, 1987).

**Summary.**   Research investigating the effects of exercise on personality functioning and self-concept consistently suggests that exercise improves self-concept, self-esteem, and self-assurance. Research also implies that exercise improves creative thinking. However, empirical evidence regarding the effects of exercise on Type A behavior, locus of control, extroversion, and other personality dimensions is inconclusive. Furthermore, research on personality characteristics that differentiate exercisers from nonexercisers is also contradictory and inconclusive. Unfortunately, the examination of the short- versus long-term, cumulative effects of exercise on personality and self-concept have not yet been explored adequately.

## Cognitive Processes

Many studies have examined the association between exercise and cognitive processes such as attention, concentration, and confusion. In fact, an extensive and excellent review on the effects of exercise on cognitive functioning has been published (Tomporowski & Ellis, 1986). Studies comparing the test performance of subjects differing in physical fitness during and after short-duration, moderately intense exercise (e.g., Sjoberg, 1980) generally support the view that cognitive functioning is facilitated by an increase in physical arousal. However, methodological shortcomings, as well as the use of cognitive tasks that are easily influenced by motivation, confound many of these studies. The effects of long-duration exercise are even less clear. For example, Tomporowski, Ellis, and Stevens (1987) studied subjects of low, moderate, and high fitness after each group had engaged in a strenuous run. No differential effects for any group, compared to a no-exercise control group, were found for performance on a memory task.

Much of the research examining the association between cognitive function and physical fitness focuses on the elderly. Spirduso (1980) reviewed this literature and concluded that a positive relationship exists between physical fitness and psychomotor speed (i.e., reaction time and movement time) among elderly subjects. However, Spirduso (1980) warned that the methodological problems in this area of research are troublesome. More-recent research has shown that aerobic fitness training improves cognitive and neuropsychological test performance among the elderly (Clarkson-Smith & Hartley, 1989; Dustman, Ruhling, Russell, Shearer, Bonekat, Shigeoka, Wood, & Bradford, 1984; Stones & Kozma, 1989). Furthermore, Blumenthal and Madden (1988) report that memory-search performance was positively correlated with aerobic fitness. However, unlike Dustman et al. (1984), Blumenthal and Madden failed to find an association between memory-search performance and changes in fitness associated with a 12-week exercise training program. Perhaps these differences could be attributed to the fact that Blumenthal and Madden used a fairly brief exercise program (12 weeks) and examined only memory-search performance, while Dustman et al. (1984) used a 48-week exercise program and examined a wide range of neuropsychological functioning.

Current data has failed to provide clear and convincing support for the notion that physical exercise improves cognitive functioning. However, some research suggests that physical fitness may improve cognitive functioning among elderly subjects. Tomporowski and Ellis (1986) suggest that this research has been plagued by methodological problems, as well as the fact that most studies in this area were conducted in a piecemeal fashion, with little emphasis on theory-based parametric approaches.

## AEROBIC EXERCISE IN THE TREATMENT OF PSYCHOPATHOLOGY

Exercise has been utilized as a treatment approach for a wide variety of psychiatric disorders and disturbances. The most common disorders treated with exercise include depressive and anxiety disorders. However, exercise has also been used in the treatment of psychoses such as schizophrenia, of alcohol and other substance abuse, and of somatoform disorders. Furthermore, exercise has been used in the treatment of many organic disorders, such as autism and mental retardation. In fact, a multicontributor book has been published (Sachs & Buffone, 1984) that specifically uses running as an adjunct treatment for a wide variety of these psychiatric disturbances.

In this section, we examine the role that exercise has played in the treatment of psychiatric disturbances and survey the literature using exercise as a treatment approach for depression, anxiety, psychosis (such as schizophrenia), alcohol and other substance abuse, and somatoform disorders. A review of the results of this research is presented in Table 13.1.

## Depression

Numerous studies have used some form of exercise to treat clinically depressed adult, adolescent, and child patients (e.g., Conroy, Smith & Felthous, 1982; Doyne et al., 1987; Greist, Klein, Eischens, Gurman, & Morgan, 1979; Kavanagh, Shephard, Tuck, & Oureshi, 1977; Klein, Greist, Gurman, Neimeyer, Lesser, Bushnell, & Smith, 1985; Martinsen, Medhus, & Sandvik, 1985; Martinsen, Strand, Paulsson, & Kaggestad, 1989c). Adequate research has not been conducted with patients experiencing bipolar disorders or depression with psychotic features. The vast majority of studies examining the role of exercise in treating depression suggests that exercise will improve mild to moderate depressive symptoms among clinically depressed patients. However, methodological problems are often prominent in this research area. Furthermore, a few recent research studies have questioned the role of an aerobic requirement for treatment effects. For example, Doyne et al. (1987) demonstrated that anaerobic exercise (such as weight lifting) may be just as effective in treating depression as aerobic exercise (such as running). Martinsen et al. (1985, 1989c) also found that aerobic effects were not required to achieve an antidepressant effect in their depressed subjects.

## Anxiety

Although a number of authors have used exercise to treat patients with anxiety disorders, some researchers have noticed that exercise may induce panic attacks among patients who experience panic disorders (e.g., Martinsen et al., 1989c; McDaniel, 1988; Pitts & McClure, 1967). However, if incorporated appropriately, exercise has been found in many studies to be an effective adjunct treatment with panic disorder and other anxiety-disorder patients (e.g., McDaniel, 1988). Some authors have demonstrated that aerobic exercise, relative to anaerobic, may not be necessary to obtain anxiety-reducing effects among anxiety-disordered patients (e.g., Martinsen, Hoffart, & Solberg, 1989a).

Unfortunately, the vast majority of studies in this area have used subjects who do not necessarily meet the *Diagnostic and Statistical Manual*, third edition (*DSMIII*) or third edition, revised (*DSMIII-R*) diagnostic criteria for an anxiety disorder. Most of the studies using anxiety-disordered patients tend to use case-study research designs (e.g., Driscoll, 1976; Muller & Armstrong, 1975; Orwin, 1974). Thus, although research is fairly consistent in supporting the notion that exercise will decrease state anxiety, especially immediately following an exercise workout, there have not yet been many studies examining clinical samples of anxiety-disordered patients using rigorous research methodologies.

## Psychoses Such as Schizophrenia

A handful of studies have examined the role of exercise on psychotic symptomatology (e.g., Clark, Wade, Massey, & Van Dyke, 1975; Dodson & Mullens, 1969; Kramer & Bauer, 1955; Lukoff, Wallace, Liberman, & Burke, 1986; Smith & Figetakis, 1970). Unfortunately, most of the studies in this area are case reports, anecdotes, or small group studies. Methodologically rigorous research has not yet adequately assessed how exercise may impact psychotic symptoms. The current research results suggest that exercise may assist these patients with mood and self-esteem factors much more than with thought disturbances associated with psychotic symptomatology. Therefore, exercise may be helpful to psychotic patients experiencing anxiety, depression, and/or low self-esteem rather than helping to reduce thought disorder per se.

## Alcoholism and Other Substance Abuse

A fairly small number of studies have examined the association between exercise and alcoholism or other substance abuse (e.g., Frankel & Murphy, 1974; Gary & Guthrie, 1972; Murphy, Bennett, Hagen, & Russell, 1972; Sinyor, Brown, Rostant, & Seraganian, 1982). Unfortunately, most of these studies, like those in the area of exercise and psychosis, depend on case studies and other uncontrolled research methodologies. Existing research suggests that exercise may help these patients with improved mood and self-concept. Some studies also claim that exercise may help these patients to achieve greater abstinence (Sinyor et al., 1982).

## Somatoform Disorders

Only a very small number of studies have examined the association between exercise and the treatment of conversion and somatoform disorders (Delargy, Peatfield, & Burt, 1986; Martinsen & Stangbelle, 1986). All of these studies support the notion that exercise may be beneficial in decreasing somatoform symptoms (i.e., hypochondriasis, somatization, and conversion reactions). However, these few studies are exploratory and lack adequate experimental designs.

## POSSIBLE MECHANISMS TO EXPLAIN THE CONNECTION BETWEEN EXERCISE AND MENTAL HEALTH

Exercise appears to be associated with modest gains in a variety of psychological variables. If exercise improves psychological functioning, then it is important to examine the possible mechanisms underlying this association. A number of biological and psychological mechanisms have been proposed to explain the connection between exercise and psychological health.

## Biological Mechanisms

Numerous biological hypotheses have been proposed to explain the connection between exercise and psychological health. One theory states that increases in body temperature due to exercise result in short-term tranquilizing effects (Von Euler & Soderberg, 1956, 1957). This theory is based on the notion that temperature changes in the brainstem result in decreased muscle-spindle activity and synchronized electrical activity in the cerebral cortex, causing a more relaxed state. A second theory posits that regular exercise facilitates stress adaptation because the increase in adrenal activity resulting from regular exercise increases steroid reserves, which are then available to counter stress (Hughes, 1984; Michael, 1957). A third theory proposes that reduction in resting muscle-activity potential following exercise causes tension release (deVries, 1968). A fourth theory suggests that exercise enhances the neurotransmission of norepinephrine, serotonin, and dopamine (Ransford, 1982), resulting in improved mood.

A popular biological theory states that psychological improvements resulting from exercise are due to the release of endogenous morphinelike chemicals (i.e., endorphins and enkephalins) synthesized in the pituitary gland (Farrell, 1981; Markoff, Ryan, & Young, 1982). Although a prevalent theory throughout the 1970s and early 1980s, the opiate hypothesis has recently been tempered by research suggesting that opiates may be associated with decreases in negative moods but not with increases in positive moods (Farrell, Gustafson, Morgan, Pert, 1982; Haier, Quaid, & Mills, 1981; Hughes, 1984).

Although biological factors may be related to the psychological improvements associated with exercise, they do not provide evidence compelling enough to explain adequately the relationship between exercise and psychological health. For example, the similar psychological gains achieved through either aerobic or anaerobic exercise (e.g., Doyne, Ossip-Klein, Bowman, Osborn, McDougall-Wilson, & Neimeyer, 1987), as well as the psychological gains associated with perceived fitness, relative to actual fitness (e.g., King et al., 1989), suggest that these biological theories cannot explain adequately the complex relationship between exercise and psychological functioning.

## Psychological Mechanisms

Many psychological theories have also been offered to explain improvements resulting from exercise. One theory suggests that improved physical fitness provides people with a sense of mastery, control, and self-efficacy (e.g., Bandura, 1977; Ismail & Trachtman, 1973). Another theory states that exercise is a form of meditation that triggers an altered and more relaxed state of consciousness (e.g., Buffone, 1980). A third theory proposes that exercise is a form of biofeedback, which teaches exercisers to regulate their own autonomic arousal (e.g., Hollandsworth, 1979). Another theory suggests that exercise provides distraction, diversion, or time-out from unpleasant cognitions, emotions, and behaviors (e.g., Long, 1983). A fifth theory states that because exercise results in the physical symptoms associated with anxiety and stress (e.g., sweating, hyperventilation, fatigue) without the subjective experience of emotional distress, repeated pairing of the symptoms in the absence of associated distress results in improved psychological functioning (Hughes, 1984). A sixth theory claims that the substantial social reinforcement afforded exercisers may also lead to improved psychological states (Hughes, 1984). A seventh theory suggests that exercise may act as a buffer, resulting in decreased strain caused by stressful life events (Kobasa, Maddi, & Puccetti, 1982). Finally, Schwartz, Davidson, and Coleman (1978) propose a systems model such that exercise competes with negative affects, such as anxiety and depression, in the somatic and cognitive systems.

Interestingly, until recently, investigators have not considered the possibility that many positive results may accrue because of psychological gains experienced from trying to get fit rather than, or at least in addition to, gains attributable to physical fitness per se. Yet the rapidity of the changes reported in most studies suggest that factors other than those stemming from increased fitness are likely to be responsible. The perception of fitness, rather than actual fitness, may be more closely associated with improvements in psychological functioning. King et al. (1989) found that perceived fitness was more closely associated with improvements in psychological variables among 120 middle-aged adults following a 6-month exercise program than were measures of actual fitness ($\dot{V}O_2$ max). Possibly, perceived fitness may improve psychological variables due to an enhancement of self-efficacy (Bandura, 1977; Ismail & Trachtman, 1973; Rodin & Plante, 1989). Perceived health and fitness may also result in an increase in behaviors that promote mental and physical health.

Although various biological and psychological theories have been offered to explain the connection between exercise and psychological health, no one theory or group of theories have been confirmed with sufficient scientific evidence. Furthermore, no integrated theoretical model has been either proposed or substantiated to explain cause-and-effect relationships between exercise and psychological health. This lack of clarity may well be due to methodological inadequacies that pervade the literature. The current lack of compelling data to support the array of largely untested theories calls for a sound and integrated theoretical and empirical approach to the problem.

## METHODOLOGICAL CONSIDERATIONS

Medhodological problems continue to plague this area of research. Although improved designs and procedures have been incorporated into a few notable studies published recently, the three types of studies that do not permit reasonable causal inferences (i.e., one-group posttest-only design, posttest-only design with nonequivalent groups, and one-group pretest–posttest design; Cook & Campbell, 1979) persist as the most prevalent research designs used currently.

Methodological flaws include threats to both internal and external validity. *Threats to internal validity* include nonrandom assignment into experimental and control conditions, the failure to use any control groups at all, examination of small numbers of subjects in relation to a large number of dependent variables, sole reliance on self-report information without examining the reliability of this information, and having numerous dropouts from the experimental condition relative to the control condition. *Threats to external validity* include the use of nonstandard measures of exercise, fitness, and/or psychological constructs, as well as the use of atypical exercise regimens.

Of further concern are the measures employed in these studies. The most frequently used measures include the Profile of Mood States (POMS; McNair, Lorr, & Droppleman, 1971) and the Spielberger State–Trait Anxiety Scale (Spielberger, Gorsuch, & Lushene, 1970). Other commonly used assessment devices include the Minnesota Multiphasic Personality Inventory (MMPI; Hathaway & McKinley, 1962), the Sixteen Personality Factors Questionnaire (16PF; Cattell, Eber, & Tatsuleo, 1970), the Jenkins Activity Rating (JAS; Jenkins, Rosenman, & Zyzanski, 1974), and the Beck Depression Inventory (BDI; Beck & Beamesderfer, 1974). Also, many studies employed unpublished author-developed measures without providing reliability and validity information on these assessment devices. Numerous studies used only one assessment device to examine the psychological construct of interest. Furthermore, high face validity in combination with important demand characteristics results in the need to be cautious in interpreting findings using these scales. More-sophisticated instruments, as well as the use of multimodal approaches, are needed to assess changes in psychological variables associated with physical activity. Examining perceived fitness and health, as well as subjects' attributions regarding the reasons for improvements in psychological functioning as a result of exercise activity, may also shed further light on the connection between exercise and psychological health.

## FUTURE DIRECTIONS

We recommend that a number of specific questions deserve to be highlighted in future research. These include psychological improvements that may be due to (1) exercise per se versus preexisting characteristics of exercisers, (2) the frequency and duration of exercise activity, and (3) the type of exercise.

## Exercise Activity and the Exerciser Role

Because most of the studies failed to randomly assign subjects into experimental and control conditions, it is difficult to determine whether exercise improves psychological functioning or whether exercisers, as a group, tend to be more psychologically fit than nonexercisers prior to embarking on an exercise program. Although a number of correlational studies have found that exercisers differ from nonexercisers on personality and other psychological variables (e.g., Hammer & Wilmore, 1973; Hartung & Farge, 1977), other studies report no psychological differences between these two populations (e.g., Goldfarb & Plante, 1984; Plante & Karpowitz, 1987). Therefore, the use of random assignment is strongly recommended in any future research in this area. Furthermore, research aimed at addressing the importance of engaging in exercise activity relative to the factors that motivate someone to become an exerciser would also assist in addressing the biological and psychological hypotheses concerning the relationship between exercise and psychological health. If being an exerciser were more closely associated with psychological improvements relative to exercise activity, intensity, or duration, then the evidence for some of the aforementioned psychological theories would be further substantiated.

## Exercise Duration and Frequency

Although research suggests that mood is sensitive to the short-term effects of exercise, it is currently unclear how long these effects last. It is impossible to determine either the minimal or the optimal frequency and duration of exercise necessary for achieving and maintaining significant psychological improvements.

The current research has not carefully addressed these important questions. While a few researchers have assessed changes in psychological states both during (e.g., Ewing & Scott, 1984) and immediately following (e.g., Berger & Owens, 1983, 1988) an exercise workout, the vast majority of studies wait until the end of an exercise program to obtain posttest psychological measures. Further confounding interpretation is the fact that these programs vary dramatically from a few weeks (e.g., Goldwater & Collins, 1985) to a few years (e.g., Tsai, Baun, & Bernacki, 1987). While some researchers have required subjects to participate in exercise activities three to five times per week (e.g., Jasnoski & Holmes, 1981), others have required only one workout per month (e.g., Tsai et al., 1987). While some investigators require 4 years of regular exercise participation (e.g., Tsai et al., 1987), others require only one exercise session (e.g., Ewing & Scott, 1984).

Future research should measure psychological functioning before, during, and immediately following exercise activity, as well as at various follow-up periods. Furthermore, future research should vary the frequency and duration of both exercise sessions and programs and should examine the differences, in order to establish a clearer understanding of the optimal amount of exercise necessary for maximum psychological benefit. Perhaps experimental conditions that include between 1 and 7 days per week of exercise activity could be considered. Varying the amount of time for each exercise period from very brief (5- to 10-minute) workouts to longer (45- to 60-minute) workouts should also be pursued. Finally, brief exercise programs (e.g., 6 weeks) versus longer programs (e.g., 18 months) should also be examined.

## Type of Exercise Activity

In addition, researchers must further explore and clarify the types of exercise that enhance psychological functioning. Although most research in this area studied some form of aerobic exercise (such as running, walking, biking, or swimming), many studies examined a combination of aerobic and anaerobic exercise, or anaerobic activity alone. Some researchers employed vigorous aerobic exercise protocols, while others define brief neck rolls and arm spins as exercise. Although most authors purport that aerobic exercise is the exercise of choice for enhancing psychological functioning, recent research has suggested that anaerobic exercise such as weight lifting may be just as effective in some cases (e.g., Doyne et al., 1987).

Furthermore, some researchers suggest that participation in nonexercise hobby activities may result in psychological improvements similar to those obtained through exercise (Blair, personal communication, December 1987; Plante & Karpowitz, 1987; Plante & Schwartz, 1990). Due to the social-reinforcement hypothesis of exercise benefits (Hughes, 1984), it is also important to assess the effects of individual versus group exercise participation. Therefore, future research should examine the type of exercise activity and its relation to psychological variables, using various hobby or other nonexercise activities as control groups. For example, examining the psychological effects of participation in hobby activities such as reading, music, art, board games, and gardening relative to similar amounts of time engaged in both aerobic and anaerobic activities may yield important information. The psychological benefits of exercising alone, as compared with exercising with a group, while keeping intensity, duration, and frequency constant should also be investigated.

## CONCLUSIONS

Current research suggests that although aerobic exercise is not the primary treatment of choice for major psychopathology such as major affective disorders, personality disorders, or psychoses, exercise can improve some of the symptoms associated with psychopathology. Exercise can improve mood, psychological well-being (especially immediately following exercise), and self-esteem, as well as decrease symptoms of depression and anxiety. In addition, exercise may improve some work-relevant behaviors. Exercise appears to have little effect on trait personality functioning, while the research concerning improvements in cognition (especially among nonelderly populations) is currently unclear. Exercise may help to prevent some forms of psychopathology by assisting people in managing some of the symptoms associated with psychopathology.

The most recent research suggests that the form of exercise may not have to be aerobic in order to obtain the desired therapeutic psychological effects. Thus, aerobic fitness may not be as important as once thought in improving many of the symptoms associated with psychopathology. Because the vast majority of studies in this area have significant methodological flaws, much more research should be done in order to better understand the association between exercise and mental health. In the meantime, because we clearly know that regular aerobic exercise can be very helpful regarding physical health, and many studies have suggested that exercise may be helpful for mental health, it appears reasonable to encourage people to participate in a regular exercise program.

## REFERENCES

Bandura, A. (1977). Self-efficacy: Toward a unifying theory of behavioral change. *Psychological Review, 84,* 191–215.

Beck, A. T., & Beamesderfer, A. (1974). Assessment of depression: The Depression Inventory. In P. Pichot (Ed.), *Psychological measurements in psychopharmacology* (pp. 1–10). Basel, Switzerland: Karger.

Berger, B. G., & Owens, D. R. (1983). Mood alteration with swimming. Swimmers really do "feel better." *Psychosomatic Medicine, 45,* 425–433.

Berger, B. G., & Owens, D. R. (1988). Stress reduction and mood enhancement in four exercise modes: Swimming, body conditioning, hatha yoga, and fencing. *Research Quarterly for exercise and Sport, 59,* 148–159.

Biddle, S. J. H., & Fox, K. R. F. (1989). Exercise and health psychology: Emerging relationships. *British Journal of Medical Psychology, 62,* 205–216.

Blumenthal, J. A., & Madden, D. J. (1988). Effects of aerobic exercise training, age, and physical fitness on memory-search performance. *Psychology and Aging, 3,* 280–285.

Blumenthal, J. A., Williams, S., Needels, T. L., & Wallace, A. G. (1982b). Psychological changes accompany aerobic exercise in healthy middle-aged adults. *Psychosomatic Medicine, 44,* 529–535.

Browman, C. P. (1981). Physical activity as a therapy for psychopathology: A reappraisal. *Journal of Sports Medicine, 21,* 192–197.

Buffone, G. W. (1980). Exercise as therapy: A closer look. *Journal of Counseling and Psychotherapy, 3*, 101–115.

Cattell, R. B., Eber, H. W., & Tatsuleo, M. M. (1970). *Handbook for the Sixteen Personality Factors Questionnaire (16PF) in clinical, educational, industrial, and research psychology.* Champaign, IL: Institute for Personality and Ability Testing.

Clark, B. A., Wade, M. G., Massey, B. H., & Van Dyke, R. (1975). Response of institutionalized geriatric mental patients to a twelve-week program of regular physical activity. *Journal of Gerontology, 30*, 565–573.

Clarkson-Smith, L., & Hartley, A. A. (1989). Relationships between physical exercise and cognitive abilities in older adults. *Psychology and Aging, 4*, 183–189.

Conroy, R. W., Smith, K., & Felthous, A. R. (1982). The value of exercise on a psychiatric hospital unit. *Hospital and Community Psychiatry, 33*, 641–645.

Cook, T. D., & Campbell, D. T. (1979). *Quasi-experimentation: Design and analysis issues for field settings.* Chicago, IL: Rand McNally College Publishing.

Delargy, M. A., Peatfield, R. C., & Burt, A. A. (1986). Successful rehabilitation in conversion paralysis. *British Medical Journal, 292*, 1730–1731.

deVries, H. A. (1968). Immediate and long term effects of exercise upon resting muscle action potential level. *Journal of Sports Medicine and Physical Fitness, 8*, 1–11.

Doan, R. E., & Scherman, A. (1987). The therapeutic effect of physical fitness on measures of personality: A literature review. *Journal of Counseling and Development, 66*, 28–36.

Dodson, L. C., & Mullens, W. R. (1969). Some effects of jogging on psychiatric hospital patients. *American Corrective Therapy Journal, 23*, 130–134.

Doyne, E. J., Ossip-Klein, D. J., Bowman, E. D., Osborn, K. M., McDougall-Wilson, I. B., & Neimeyer, R. A. (1987). Running versus weight lifting in the treatment of depression. *Journal of Consulting and Clinical Psychology, 55*, 748–754.

Driscoll, R. (1976). Anxiety reduction using physical exertion and positive images. *Psychological Research, 26*, 87–94.

Dustman, R. E., Ruhling, R. O., Russell, E. M., Shearer, D. E., Bonekat, W., Shigeoka, J. W., Wood, J. S., & Bradford, D. C. (1984). Aerobic exercise training and improved neuropsychological function of older individuals. *Neurobiology of Aging, 5*, 35–42.

Ewing, J. H., & Scott, D. G. (1984). Effects of aerobic exercise upon affect and cognition. *Perceptual and Motor Skills, 59*, 407–414.

Farrell, P. A. (1981). Exercise and endogenous opioids. *New England Journal of Medicine, 305*, 1591–1592.

Farrell, P. A., Gustafson, A. B., Morgan, W. P., & Pert, C. B. (1987). Enkephalins, catecholamines, and psychological mood alterations: Effects of prolonged exercise. *Medicine and Science in Sports and Exercise, 19*, 347–353.

Folkins, C. H., & Sime, W. E. (1981). Physical fitness and mental health. *American Psychologist, 36*, 373–389.

Frankel, A., & Murphy, J. (1974). Physical fitness and personality in alcoholism. *Quarterly Journal on Studies on Alcoholism, 35*, 1272–1278.

Gary, V., & Guthrie, D. (1972). The effects of jogging on physical fitness and self-concept in hospitalized alcoholics. *Quarterly Journal of Studies on Alcoholism, 33,* 1073–1078.

Goldfarb, L. A., & Plante, T. G. (1984). Fear of fat in runners: An examination of the connection between anorexia nervosa and distance running. *Psychological Reports, 55,* 296.

Goldwater, B. C., & Collins, M. L. (1985). Psychologic effects of cardiovascular conditioning: A controlled experiment. *Psychosomatic Medicine, 47,* 174–181.

Greist, J. H., Klein, M. H., Eischens, R. R., Gurman, A. S., & Morgan, W. P. (1979). *Comprehensive Psychiatry, 20,* 41–54.

Haier, R. J., Quaid, K., & Mills, J. S. C. (1981). Naloxone alters perception after jogging. *Psychiatry Research, 5,* 231–232.

Hale, R. E., & Travis, T. W. (1987). Exercise as a treatment option for anxiety and depressive disorders. *Military Medicine, 152,* 299–302.

Hammer, W. M., & Wilmore, J. H. (1973). An exploratory investigation in personality measures and physiological alterations during a 10-week jogging program. *Journal of Sports Medicine and Physical Fitness, 13,* 238–247.

Hartung, G. H., & Farge, E. J. (1977). Personality and physiological traits in middle-aged runners and joggers. *Journal of Gerontology, 32,* 541–548.

Hathaway, S. R., & McKinley, J. C. (1972). *MMPI manual.* New York: Psychological Corporation.

Hayden, R. M., & Allen, G. J. (1984). Relationship between aerobic exercise, anxiety, and depression: Convergent validation by knowledgeable informants. *Journal of Sports Medicine, 24,* 69–74.

Hollandsworth, J. G. (1979). Some thoughts on distance running as training in biofeedback. *Journal of Sport Behavior, 2,* 71–82.

Hughes, J. R. (1984). Psychological effects of habitual aerobic exercise: A critical review. *Preventive Medicine, 13,* 66–78.

Hughes, J. R., Casal, D. C., & Leon, A. S. (1986). Psychological effects of exercise: A randomized cross-over trail. *Journal of Psychosomatic Research, 30,* 355–360.

Ismail, A. H., & Trachtman, L. E. (1973). Jogging the imagination. *Psychology Today, 6,* 78–82.

Jasnoski, M. L., & Holmes, D. S. (1981). Influence of initial aerobic fitness, aerobic training and changes in aerobic fitness on personality functioning. *Journal of Psychosomatic Research, 25,* 553–556.

Jenkins, C. D., Rosenman, R. H., & Zyzanski, S. J. (1974). Prediction of clinical coronary heart disease by a test for the coronary-prone behavior pattern. *New England Journal of Medicine, 290,* 1271–1275.

Kavanagh, T., Shephard, R. J., Tuck, J. A., & Oureshi, S. (1977). Depression following myocardial infarction: The effect of distance running. *Annals of the New York Academy of Sciences, 301,* 1029–1038.

King, A. C., Taylor, C. B., Haskell, W. L., & DeBusk, R. F. (1989). Influence of regular aerobic exercise on psychological health: A randomized, controlled trial of healthy middle-aged adults. *Health Psychology, 8,* 305–324.

Klein, M. H., Greist, J. H., Gurman, A. S., Neimeyer, R. A., Lesser, D. P., Bushnell, N. J., & Smith, R. E. (1985). A comparative outcome study of group psychotherapy vs. exercise treatment for depression. *International Journal of Mental Health, 13,* 148–177.

Kobasa, S. C., Maddi, S. R., & Puccetti, M. C. (1982). Personality and exercise as buffers in the stress–illness relationship. *Journal of Behavioral Medicine, 5,* 391–404.

Kramer, R., & Bauer, R. (1955). Behavioral effects of hydrogymnastics. *Journal of the Association of Physical and Mental Rehabilitation, 9,* 10–12.

Ledwidge, B. (1980). Run for your mind: Aerobic exercise as a means of alleviating anxiety and depression. *Canadian Journal of Behavioral Science, 12,* 127.

Lichtman, S., & Poser, E. G. (1983). The effects of exercise on mood and cognitive functioning. *Journal of Psychosomatic Research, 27,* 43–52.

Lobitz, W. C., Brammell, H. L., Stoll, S., & Niccoli, A. (1983). Physical exercise and anxiety management training for cardiac stress management in a nonpatient population. *Journal of Cardiac Rehabilitation, 3,* 683–688.

Lobstein, D. D., Mosbacher, B. J., & Ismail, A. H. (1983). Depression as a powerful discriminator between physically active and sedentary middle-aged men. *Journal of Psychosomatic Research, 27,* 69–76.

Long, B. C. (1983). Aerobic conditioning and stress reduction: Participation or conditioning? *Human Movement Science, 2,* 171–186.

Lukoff, D., Wallace, C. J., Liberman, R. P., Burke, K. (1986). *Schizophrenia Bulletin, 12,* 274–282.

MacMahon, J. R. (1990). The psychological benefits of exercise and the treatment of delinquent adolescents. *Sports Medicine, 9,* 344–351.

Markoff, R. A., Ryan, P., & Young, T. (1982). Endorphins and mood changes in long-distance running. *Medicine and Science in Sports and Exercise, 14,* 11–15.

Martinsen, E. W. (1989). The role of aerobic exercise in the treatment of depression. *Stress Medicine, 3,* 93–100.

Martinsen, E. W., Hoffart, A., & Solberg, O. (1989a). Comparing aerobic and nonaerobic forms of exercise in the treatment of anxiety disorders: A randomized trial. *Stress Medicine, 5,* 115–120.

Martinsen, E. W., Hoffart, A., & Solberg, O. (1989b). Comparing aerobic and nonaerobic forms of exercise in the treatment of clinical depression: A randomized trial. *Comprehensive Psychiatry, 30,* 324–331.

Martinsen, E. W., Medhus, A., & Sandvik, L. (1985). Effects of aerobic exercise on depression: A controlled study. *British Medical Journal, 291,* 109.

Martinsen, E. W., & Stangbelle, J. K. (1986). Treatment of patients with chronic low back pain: Collaboration between physical medicine and psychiatry. *Tidsskr Nor Lageforen, 5,* 384–386.

Martinsen, E. W., Strand, J., Paulsson, G., & Kaggestad, J. (1989c). Physical fitness level in patients with anxiety and depressive disorders. *International Journal of Sports Medicine, 10,* 58–61.

McDaniel, W. W. (1988). Panic disorder and exercise. *American Journal of Psychiatry, 145,* 269.

McNair, D. M., Lorr, M., Droppleman, L. F. (1971). *Manual for the Profile of Moods States.* San Diego, CA: Educational and Industrial Testing Service.

Michael, E. D. (1957). Stress adaptation through exercise. *Research Quarterly, 28,* 50–54.

Mobily, K. (1982). Using physical activity and recreation to cope with stress and anxiety: A review. *American Correction Journal, 36*, 77–81.

Moses, J., Steptoe, A., Matthews, A., & Edwards, S. (1989). The effects of exercise training on mental well being in the normal population: A controlled trial. *Journal of Psychosomatic Research, 83*, 47–61.

Muller, B., & Armstrong, H. E. (1975). A further note on the "running treatment" for anxiety. *Psychotherapy: Theory, Research and Practice, 12*, 385–387.

Murphy, J. B., Bennett, R. N., Hagen, J. M., & Russell, M. W. (1972). Some suggestive data regarding the relationship of physical fitness to emotional difficulties. *Newsletter on Research in Psychology, 14*, 15–17.

North, T. C., McCullagh, P., & Tran, Z. V. (1990). Effect of exercise on depression. *Exercise and Sport Sciences Reviews, 18*, 379–415.

Oberman, A. (1984). Healthy exercise. *Western Journal of Medicine, 141*, 864–871.

Orwin, A. (1974). Treatment of a situational phobia: A case for running. *British Journal of Psychiatry, 125*, 95–98.

Parent, C. J., & Whall, A. L. (1984). Are physical activity, self-esteem, and depression related? *Journal of Gerontological Nursing, 10*, 8–10.

Pauly, J. T., Palmer, J. A., Wright, C. C., & Pfeiffer, G. J. (1982). The effect of a 14-week employee fitness program on selected physiological and psychological parameters. *Journal of Occupational Medicine, 24*, 457–463.

Perri, S., & Templer, D. I. (1985). The effects of an aerobic exercise program on psychological variables in older adults. *International Journal of Aging and Human Development, 20*, 167–172.

Phelps, J. R. (1987). Physical activity and health maintenance: Exactly what is known? *Western Journal of Medicine, 146*, 200–206.

Pitts, F. N., & McClure, J. N. (1967). Lactate metabolism and anxiety neurosis. *New England Journal of Medicine, 277*, 1329–1336.

Plante, T. G., & Karpowitz, D. (1987). The influence of aerobic exercise of physiological stress responsivity. *Psychophysiology, 24*, 670–677.

Plante, T. G., & Rodin, J. (1990). Physical fitness and enhanced psychological health. *Current Psychology: Research and Reviews, 9*, 1–22.

Plante, T. G., & Schwartz, G. E. (1990). Defensive and repressive coping styles: Self-presentation, leisure activities, and assessment. *Journal of Research in Personality 24*, 173–190.

Plummer, O. K., & Koh, Y. O. (1987). Effect of "aerobics" on self-concepts of college women. *Perceptual and Motor Skills, 65*, 271–275.

Raglin, J. S. (1990). Exercise and mental health: Beneficial and detrimental effects. *Sports Medicine, 9*, 323–329.

Ransford, C. P. (1982). A role for amines in the antidepressant effect of exercise: A review. *Medicine and Science in Sports and Exercise, 14*, 1–10.

Rippe, J. M., Ward, A., Porcari, J. P., Freedson, P. S. (1988). Walking for health and fitness. *Journal of the American Medical Association, 259*, 2720–2724.

Rodin, J., & Plante, T. G. (1989). The psychological effects of exercise. In R. S. Williams & A. Wallace (Eds.), *Biological effects of physical activity*. Champaign, IL: Human Kinetics.

Roskies, E., Seraganian, P., Oseasohn, R., Hanley, J. A., Collu, R., Martin, N., &

Smilga, C. (1986). The Montreal Type A intervention project: Major findings. *Health Psychology, 5,* 45–69.

Roth, D. L. (1989). Acute emotional and psychophysiological effects of aerobic exercise. *Psychophysiology, 26,* 593–602.

Sachs, M. L. (1982). Exercise and running: Effects on anxiety, depression, and psychology. *Humanistic Education and Development, 21,* 51–57.

Sachs, M. L., & Buffone, G. W. (1984). *Running as therapy.* Lincoln, NE: University of Nebraska Press.

Schwartz, G. E., Davidson, R. J., & Coleman, D. J. (1978). Patterning of cognitive and somatic processes in the self-regulation of anxiety: Effects of meditation versus exercise. *Psychosomatic Medicine, 40,* 321–328.

Simons, A. D., McGowan, C. R., Epstein, L. H., Kupfer, F. J., & Robertson, R. J. (1985). Exercise as a treatment for depression: An update. *Clinical Psychology Review, 5,* 553–568.

Sinyor, D., Brown, T., Rostant, L., & Seraganian, P. (1982). The role of a physical fitness program in the treatment of alcoholism. *Journal of the Study of Alcoholism, 43,* 380–386.

Sjoberg, H. (1980). Physical fitness and mental performance during and after work. *Ergonomics, 23,* 977–895.

Smith, W. C., & Figetakis, N. (1970). Some effects of isometric exercise on muscular strength, body-image perception and psychiatric symptomatology in chronic schizophrenics. *American Correction Therapy Journal, 214,* 100–104.

Sonstroem, R. J. (1984). Exercise and self-esteem. *Exercise and Sports Science Review, 12,* 123–155.

Sothmann, M. S., & Ismail, A. H. (1984). Relationship between urinary catecholamine metabolites, particularly MHPG, and selected personality and physical fitness characteristics in normal subjects. *Psychosomatic Medicine, 46,* 523–531.

Spielberger, C., Gorsuch, R., & Lushene, R. (1970). *Manual for the State–Trait Anxiety Inventory.* Palo Alto, CA: Consulting Psychologist Press.

Spirduso, W. W. (1980). Physical fitness, aging, and psychomotor speed: A review. *Journal of Gerontology, 35,* 850–865.

Steptoe, A., & Cox, S. (1988). Acute effects of aerobic exercise on mood. *Health Psychology, 7,* 329–340.

Stones, M. J., & Kozma, A. (1989). Age, exercise, and coding performance. *Psychology and Aging, 4,* 190–194.

Taylor, C. B., Sallis, J. F., & Needle, R. (1985). The relation of physical activity and exercise to mental health. *Public Health Reports, 100,* 195–202.

Tomporowski, P. D., & Ellis, N. R. (1986). Effects of exercise on cognitive processes: A review. *Psychological Bulletin, 99,* 338–346.

Tomporowski, P. D., Ellis, N. R., & Stevens, R. (1987). The immediate effects of strenuous exercise on free-recall memory. *Ergonomics, 30,* 121–129.

Tsai, S. P., Baun, W. B., & Bernacki, E. J. (1987). Relationship of employee turnover to exercise adherence in a corporate fitness program. *Journal of Occupational Medicine, 29,* 572–575.

Tucker, L. A. (1982). Effects of a weight-training program on the self-concepts of college males. *Perceptual and Motor Skills, 54,* 1055–1061.

Valliant, P. M., & Asu, M. E. (1985). Exercise and its effects on cognition and physiology in older adults. *Perceptual and Motor Skills, 63,* 955–961.

Von Euler, C., & Soderberg, U. (1956). The relation between gamma motor activity and electroencephalogram. *Experimentia, 12,* 278–279.

Von Euler, C., & Soderberg, U. (1957). The influence of hypothalamic thermoceptive structures on the electroencephalogram and gamma motor activity. *EEG and Clinical Neurophysiology, 9,* 391–408.

# PART IV

## OVERVIEW

# 14

## Current Status and Future Directions in the Field of Exercise Psychology

**PETER SERAGANIAN**

The aim of this concluding chapter is to provide an overview of some critical issues in the field of exercise psychology, as characterized in this volume. The research endeavor is scrutinized with respect not only to the present status but also to the directions in which the field is moving. The emergence of this edited book, in itself, indirectly reflects the increased attention given to issues at the interface of psychology and exercise. Psychologists, physiologists, and physical educators all have mapped out a common ground where it is recognized that some familiarity with each other's turf is a prerequisite for making headway on fundamental issues. A multidisciplinary band of researchers/practitioners now address themselves to fundamental issues that just a decade ago were largely unstudied. Accordingly, the contributors to this volume often moved somewhat afield of their own specialties in order to pool efforts in a collective, interdisciplinary undertaking. Such willingness to extend beyond conventional academic borders is confirmation of the growing maturation of the discipline.

In an effort aimed at the promotion of coherence across the chapters in this volume, a 2-day conference was held in Montreal, Canada, in December, 1990. At that time, 12 of the contributors or their proxies gave presentations based on chapter outlines and discussed their views with other contributors. Because the gathering cut across traditional disciplinary boundaries and brought together academics with widely disparate views of the field, many of the presentations were followed by brisk debate. In some instances, chapters subsequently underwent appreciable revision, to better incorporate points of view raised at that time. Conference presentations and the ensuing discussions also influenced the tone of this concluding chapter. Nevertheless, I retain ultimate responsibility for the views expressed herein.

Three principal issues are explored: (1) the status of measurement protocols in both the exercise and the psychological domains, (2) the role of experimental manipulation of aerobic fitness levels in laboratory and field studies, and (3) the merits of empirically driven versus theoretically driven inquiry. In all cases, both methodological and conceptual aspects of the issues are treated, in that the separation of such factors seemed artificial. Although it was tempting to foray into other areas, the pursuit of closure is better served by remaining focused on these three selected issues.

## MEASUREMENT PROTOCOLS

A feature that clearly differentiates the measurement of psychological, as opposed to exercise, variables is the degree of consensus associated with the quantification of fundamental processes. Oxygen uptake assessment is widely regarded as the "gold standard" by which to assess aerobic fitness level. One underlying factor that contributed to such consensus was the pioneering work conducted several decades ago by Archibald Hill. Hill (1927) first established a tenable methodology to accurately measure oxygen uptake during various degrees of physical exertion. Although the technology would be considered primitive by today's standards (i.e., collection of expired gas samples in cumbersome Douglas gas bags, followed by intricate off-line chemical analysis), the methodology revolutionized the discipline of exercise physiology. The awarding of the 1922 Nobel Prize in Physiology/Medicine to Hill justly recognized the significance of his contribution. For me, as a Canadian, an interesting reference point is that, in the following year, Frederick Banting was the recipient of the Nobel Prize for his discovery of insulin. The discipline of exercise physiology in general and the subspecialty dealing with the quantification of aerobic work capacity have been able systematically to build upon the firm foundation that Hill's research program provided. His clear, well-conceived research initiative coupled with an innovative methodology has supported decades of cumulative research. Although, as Boutcher's chapter (Chapter 3) indicates, the determinants of oxygen uptake are still being actively explored, the quantification of the construct does not seem contentious.

In marked contrast, in the psychological domain, no single research tradition dominates. The absence of a firm anchor is readily apparent. When delving into the realm of psychological well-being, what seems to characterize the literature is a bewildering variety of loosely formulated constructs that are often coupled to problematic measurement protocols. Without a strong unifying foundation such as that provided by Hill (1927) for exercise, the psychological domain seems relatively fragmented and idiosyncratic. Self-report questionnaires, profiles of mood states, behavioral response patterns, and autonomic reactivity are just a few of the quantification strategies employed to measure psychological constructs. Not only does the scaling of most measures have inherent problems, but also the relationships among the various indices can be murkier still. Although such a scenario in and of itself does not necessarily handicap psychological research, the absence of a unifying superstructure is noticeable.

Nevertheless, a certain degree of headway has been made. The review chapters by Salazar et al. (Chapter 5), and by Tuson and Sinyor (Chapter 4) provide an indication of promising, as well as suspect, psychological indices in the basic research area. In this vein, the identification of the merits and the pitfalls of both ends of the continuum of measurement protocols is vital, in order to help focus subsequent research initiatives on potentially productive avenues rather than on blind alleys. In the applied domain, Chapter 13, by Plante, clearly describes the assessment of psychopathology. The Gauvin and Brawley chapter (Chapter 6) describes an innovative social-psychological approach, which may provide a finer-grained perspective on subjective mood states. The Holmes chapter (Chapter 2) provides an interesting example of triangulating a psychological construct by systematically exploring different facets of the problem. Thus, despite the absence of a single dominant research tradition, several promising psychological assessment strategies hold promise for further clarifying the relationship between physical and psychological states.

## EXPERIMENTAL MANIPULATION

When assessing the impact of aerobic activities on psychological processes, traditional wisdom posits that the preferred research design involves experimental manipulation of aerobic activities. As outlined in

Chapter 8 by Jamieson and Flood, experimental studies, at the minimum, require the following: (a) a control condition that mimics in certain respects the aerobic activities received by experimental subjects, and (b) random assignment of individuals to experimental and control conditions. In a number of chapters (e.g., Chapter 13 by Plante, Chapter 8 by Jamieson & Flood, and Chapter 5 by Salazar et al.) an interesting contrast with regard to the findings from correlational versus experimental studies was noted. In correlational studies that permitted self-selection of activity patterns, an influence of aerobic activities on psychological factors was evident. However, in experimental studies that involved random assignment to treatment versus control conditions, the effects largely disappeared.

Such failures to replicate initial unsophisticated yet consistently observed correlational findings with more rigorous experimental research designs are not uncommon. Two examples from related fields are noteworthy. Impressive clinical case histories (e.g., Kavanaugh, 1976) attested to dramatic postmyocardial infarction recoveries associated with aerobic training. However, two ensuing large-scale randomized clinical trials (Palatsi, 1976; Shephard, 1980) carefully screened post-myocardial-infarction patients, who were then assigned at random to participate in structured aerobic exercise or control programs. With long-term follow-up, little difference in the incidence of reinfarction was seen across groups. Moreover, for some subgroups (e.g., older blue-collar workers) there was even a suggestion that participation in aerobic exercise might actually increase the likelihood of reinfarction. Thus, the contribution of aerobic exercise toward rehabilitation of heart-attack sufferers, which was manifested when patients self-selected whether to exercise, disappeared when patients were randomly assigned to experimental versus control conditions.

Moving even further afield to psychotherapy treatment evaluation, a related development can be discerned. Case histories and correlation studies first documented the efficacy of some psychotherapeutic regimes. More rigorous experimental research with random assignment of patients to treatment and control conditions has largely failed to replicate the promising changes seen in the less-well-controlled studies. This development is of such importance for both researchers and practitioners that a special issue of the *Journal of Consulting and Clinical Psychology* (1991, Vol. 59, No. 2) was recently devoted to the topic.

In this issue, Smith and Sechrest (1991) formulated an innovative approach to deal with the shrinking effect size typically associated with experimental manipulation of treatment conditions. First, they acknowledged the traditional argument. Because experimental manipulation of psychotherapeutic regimes fails to replicate findings seen with cruder designs, then it follows that a specific psychotherapy is, in and of itself, ineffective. Accordingly, the relationship seen in correlational studies reflects, in all likelihood, the influence of a confound that was eliminated with experimental manipulation.

Nevertheless, Smith and Sechrest (1991) outrightly reject this traditional argument. What they propose instead has been termed the "matching hypothesis": particular treatment x aptitude interactions are critical for an intervention to work. More specifically, when patients are allowed to self-select a psychotherapeutic regime, certain expectations and aptitudes regarding the intervention are argued to be at play. However, when patients are assigned at random to treatment versus control conditions, both matches and mismatches between what is expected and what is received are bound to occur. Such expectancies and attitudes are considered not merely as confounds, but rather as proactive forces that can dramatically modulate a treatment regime's efficacy.

Given such circumstances, the question then arises as to whether a design that includes experimental manipulation is optimal for the meaningful assessment of treatment effects (Institute of Medicine, 1989). The stringent requirements of experimental design in which patient expectancies or aptitudes are systematically counterbalanced across treatment conditions may actually attenuate a treatment program's true impact. To circumvent this roadblock, the proposal forwarded is that instead of asking, "Is a treatment effective?" we should inquire instead, "For whom might this treatment be indicated or contraindicated?" Existing designs involving experimental manipulation are not well suited to address this latter issue.

The literature exploring the linkage between physical activity and psychological states may be at a similar crossroads. Because many of the most interesting effects generated in correlational studies dissipate when more rigorous experimental manipulation is carried out, could a matching hypothesis also apply here? Perhaps some individuals are uniquely predisposed to exhibit psychological gains from participating in aerobic activities. For other individuals, aerobic exercise may have no effect on psychological states. For some, aerobic exercise might even detrimentally affect psychological states. If, for the sake of argument, one posits an equal number of individuals in each of these three categories, it becomes apparent that random assignment of individuals to exercise versus control programs is not an effective means of analyzing the problem. Instead, what would seem to be called for would be the search for biological and psychological factors that predispose a subset of the population uniquely to benefit from aerobic activities.

Some researchers might consider such a proposal as tantamount to scientific desecration. On a practical level, what is being proposed, however, is to let the question of interest rather than scientific convention drive choices as to research designs. If, for instance, only one third of the adult population as a whole stands to benefit psychologically from an aerobic-fitness program, greater efforts to precisely identify such a subset of the population seem necessary.

This issue may also have broader "applied," as opposed to "experimental," implications. Short of the political/military exigencies that bring on conscription into the armed forces and the ensuing physical training regime, most people self-select whether to regularly engage in physical activities. If such self-selection indeed influences the degree of psychological gains that are encountered, indiscriminate promotion of physical activity in the population as a whole becomes somewhat suspect. Given that the Canadian federal government has a program (Participation) that has, as a primary goal, promotion of a physically active life-style (see Chapter 10 by Brawley & Rodgers), the foregoing concerns might contraindicate the utilization of broadly based media campaigns for such ends. Coercive promotional techniques certainly do not seem appropriate.

One final issue related to the matching hypothesis stems from the fact that the bulk of the evaluative research that spawned this formulation was done with adults. When transposing the matching hypothesis to the influence of physical activity on psychological states, the issue could have distinct implications across different phases of the life span. For instance, one could hypothesize that in adulthood, there is a constriction in the subset of the population that stands to benefit psychologically from physical activity. In contrast, during earlier developmental stages and for the elderly, there could be a greater proportion of the population that stand to benefit psychologically from participation in physical activities. Such potential age-dependent relationships could markedly influence the degree to which one targets some subsets of the population for promotional efforts.

## EMPIRICAL VERSUS THEORETICAL INQUIRY

Another theme repeated in the chapters (e.g., Chapter 1 by Rejeski & Thompson, Chapter 7 by Péronnet & Szabo) is the difficulty of working at the exercise-psychology interface in the absence of a tenable theoretical model to guide and systematize the research undertaking. Despite the various conceptual models that have been entertained (see Chapter 9 by Fillingim & Blumenthal, Chapter 11 by Horn & Claytor), no one position has emerged to capture the interest of a critical mass of researchers. Moreover, there do not appear to be any prominent candidates waiting in the wings to burst forth on the scene.

What is less clear is whether the absence of a single dominant theoretical model has handicapped the study of the influence of physical activity on psychological processes. Some historical disputes in the psychological literature may shed some light on this topic. B. F. Skinner (1950), in his classic review article "Are Theories of Learning Necessary?" argued forcefully for the adequacy of conducting empirically based research without a structured theoretical framework. For instance, one does not have to be constrained by the constructs of a particular theoretical model but rather can explore a wider range of manipulations that influence control over dependent variables of interest.

I suspect that, given the current state of development of the field of exercise psychology, we continue to need both phenomenologically based empirical research as well as theory-driven conceptual formulations. To focus unduly on the search for a comprehensive theory might stifle the exploratory analysis of discrete phenomenon. Phenomenologically based inquiry directed at the characteristics and the limits of interrelationships between physical and psychological states might best foster the development of a critical mass of knowledge that could then better support theory emergence.

A final example from the psychological literature may make this point clearer. Long's chapter (Chapter 12), exploring the cognitive aspects of exercise, is representative of the substantial and growing impact of a cognitive—as opposed to a behavioral—outlook in contemporary psychological inquiry. The roots of the cognitive school trace back to the turn of the century, to the early German Gestalt psychologists, Wertheimer and Kohler. In the now-classic monograph entitled *Productive Thinking*, Wertheimer (1945) set himself the task of formulating a psychological model for creative thought processes such as insight and creativity. He had no systematic theoretical model to guide his inquiry. Instead, he gathered bits of information from highly disparate sources, which eventually started to fit together into a meaningful pattern. For example, in a chapter of his monograph, Wertheimer describes in intriguing detail many hours of interviews with Einstein, reviewing, decisive step by decisive step, the thinking Einstein had done in formulating the theory of relativity. From the content of these loosely structured interviews and other innovative observational techniques, Wertheimer gradually amassed sufficient data to formulate some of the fundamental tenets of Gestalt theory. A principal factor in productive thinking is to grasp the overall structure or configuration of the situation. Such thinking can relate specific problems at hand to the totality of the situation as a whole. Rather than a focus on the analysis of parts, the focus is on the part–whole relationships. The whole is greater than the sum of its parts. Thus, a theoretical model that has had far-reaching impact on contemporary psychology essentially emerged from disparate empirical observations. Perhaps the field of exercise psychology should not unduly despair at the absence of a unifying theory. Our research programs are still emerging. The continued empirical pursuit of meaningful relationships between physical and psychological processes may provide fertile grounds for theory germination.

## SUMMARY

This concluding chapter has provided a somewhat idiosyncratic view of some of the issues in the field of exercise psychology. There clearly are problems to surmount. Nevertheless, the wherewithal and the will to systematically confront these problems seem to be gathering momentum. The scope and caliber of the individual chapters in this volume reflect concerted interdisciplinary initiatives regarding issues of fundamental import. It is hoped that this volume will help the process along.

## REFERENCES

Hill, A. H. (1927). *Muscular movement in man*. London: McGraw-Hill.

Institute of Medicine (1989). *Prevention and treatment of alcohol problems*. Washington DC: National Academy Press.

Kavanaugh, T. (1976). *Heart attack? Counter attack!* Toronto, Canada: Van Nostrand.

Palatsi, K. (1976). Feasibility of physical training after myocardial infarction and its effect on return to work, morbidity, and mortality. *Acta Medica Scandinavica, 599*(Suppl.), 1–84.

Shephard, R. J. (1980). Recurrence of myocardial infarction: Observation of patients participating in the Ontario Multicentre Exercise-Heart trial. *European Journal of Cardiology, 11*, 147–157.

Skinner, B. F. (1950). Are theories of learning necessary? *Psychological Review, 57*, 193–216.

Smith, B., & Sechrest, L. (1991). Treatment of aptitude x treatment interactions. *Journal of Consulting and Clinical Psychology, 59*(2), 232–244.

Wertheimer, M. (1945). *Productive thinking*. New York: Harper & Row.

# Author Index

# Subject Index